Ecological Task Analysis and Movement

Walter E. Davis, PhD

Kent State University

Kent, Ohio

Geoffrey D. Broadhead, PhD

Kent State University

Kent, Ohio

Editors

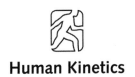

Human Kinetics

Library of Congress Cataloging-in-Publication Data

Ecological task analysis and movement / Walter E. Davis, Geoffrey D. Broadhead, editors.

p. ; cm.

Includes bibliographical references and index.

ISBN-13: 978-0-7360-5185-9 (hard cover)

ISBN-10: 0-7360-5185-6 (hard cover)

1. People with disabilities--Rehabilitation. 2. Task analysis. 3. Motor ability. I. Davis, W. E. (Walter E.) II. Broadhead, Geoffrey D., 1937-

[DNLM: 1. Motor Activity. 2. Task Performance and Analysis. 3. Disabled Persons--education. 4. Ecosystem. 5. Teaching--methods. WE 103 E193 2007]

RM930.8.E26 2007

362.4--dc22

2006027705

ISBN-10: 0-7360-5185-6

ISBN-13: 978-0-7360-5185-9

Copyright © 2007 by Walter E. Davis and Geoffrey D. Broadhead

Acquisitions Editor: Judy Patterson Wright, PhD; **Developmental Editor:** Christine M. Drews; **Managing Editor:** Maureen Eckstein; **Assistant Editor:** Heather M. Tanner; **Copyeditor:** Joyce Sexton; **Proofreader:** Pamela Johnson; **Indexer:** Betty Frizzéll; **Permission Manager:** Dalene Reeder; **Graphic Designer:** Fred Starbird; **Graphic Artist:** Kathleen Boudreau-Fuoss; **Photo Manager:** Laura Fitch; **Cover Designer:** Keith Blomberg; **Photographer (cover):** Neil Bernstein; **Photographer (interior):** © Human Kinetics unless otherwise noted; **Art Manager:** Kelly Hendren; **Illustrator:** Keri Evans; **Printer:** Edwards Brothers

Printed in the United States of America   10   9   8   7   6   5   4   3   2   1

Human Kinetics

Web site: www.HumanKinetics.com

United States: Human Kinetics
P.O. Box 5076
Champaign, IL 61825-5076
800-747-4457
e-mail: humank@hkusa.com

Canada: Human Kinetics
475 Devonshire Road Unit 100
Windsor, ON N8Y 2L5
800-465-7301 (in Canada only)
e-mail: orders@hkcanada.com

Europe: Human Kinetics
107 Bradford Road, Stanningley
Leeds LS28 6AT, United Kingdom
+44 (0) 113 255 5665
e-mail: hk@hkeurope.com

Australia: Human Kinetics
57A Price Avenue, Lower Mitcham
South Australia 5062
08 8372 0999
e-mail: liaw@hkaustralia.com

New Zealand: Human Kinetics
Division of Sports Distributors NZ Ltd.
P.O. Box 300 226 Albany,
North Shore City, Auckland
0064 9 448 1207
e-mail: info@humankinetics.co.nz

Ecological
Task Analysis
and Movement

Allen W. Burton
1954–2001

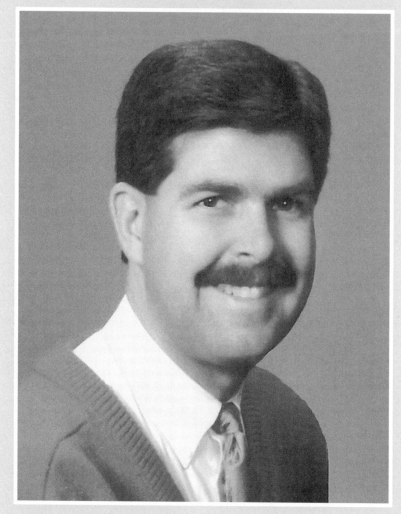

On the morning of September 11, 2001, my family and I were driving to the funeral of Allen Burton, who had died a few days earlier. I was quietly thinking about my eulogy for Allen and how deeply saddened I was at the passing of my good friend and colleague. My contemplation was shattered when my cell phone rang; it was my daughter in Texas calling to ask if I was listening to the radio. I said we were not, and she said, "You'd better turn it on." At the time we were about a mile and a half from the church where the funeral was being held, and we began listening to the news bulletins coming in about what was one of the most tragic days in American history, comparable only to perhaps Pearl Harbor. The funeral service proceeded with those attending not fully appreciating the impact of that day. It was only after the funeral that we began to realize what had transpired and its impact. In one sense, Allen's demise and our farewell to him occurring on September 11, 2001, might be seen as a tragic parallel between the personal loss that we, his many friends and colleagues, had suffered, and the national sense of loss and tragedy that we all endured on that day. Had these two events not coincided, Allen's loss would still have been premature. For Allen's friends, September 11 represents a double tragedy. Our personal loss was marked on a day of a national tragedy.

To paraphrase an old saying, "You can take the boy out of California, but you can't take California out of the boy!" I had known about Allen when he was an undergraduate student at UCLA. I was on sabbatical at UCLA in the spring of 1980, and Allen was completing his degree in kinesiology. Our paths did not cross until I arrived at Minnesota in 1986. Allen was a postdoctoral fellow working with Herb Pick at the Institute for Child Development. As fate would have it, as the incoming director of the School of Kinesiology, I knew we had a faculty vacancy for which Allen was a perfect fit. Allen began his career at Minnesota in the fall of 1986, and from that time onward we all began to appreciate Allen both as a colleague and as a truly remarkable man. Allen was deeply spiritual and had a strong and enduring set of principles that were clearly part of his Christian faith. I can think of no person who lived out the values of his faith more than Allen. He was a very supportive colleague; he was a great teacher, an outstanding mentor, and an insightful thinker. While his faith was part of his daily life, he was always respectful of others' views; and as he once remarked to me with a mischievous glint in his eye, "You know, Mike, folks at my church might be surprised about my politics."

The individuals who have contributed to this book all share a personal and a professional relationship with Allen and his ideas on skill development, especially as it relates to children. And as such, it is a fitting tribute to the enthusiasm he had for life and his work. My earlier remark about not being able to "take California out of the boy" is made in the context of observing Allen on a daily basis. Allen would travel around campus on his skateboard, in baggy shorts, well into the fall, which those of you who live south of Minnesota will recall often ends in late September. Allen was a true Californian, the real deal. He still enjoyed the music of California—the Beach Boys—and he brought all of this joy not only to his relationships but to his classes and his students in a way that blended a lot of life with a strong work ethic, fulfilling obligations, and always a positive perspective regardless of the many frustrations and challenges that academe seems to generate. The field at large may never fully appreciate the legacy of Allen, simply because it was ended in midcareer. This book provides a suitable memorial to a colleague and friend who continues to be missed. This book celebrates an individual whose warmth and ability touched us all.

Michael G. Wade

Allen Burton was not just an admired and respected colleague; he was a friend to many of us contributing to this book. He was indeed a careful and dedicated scholar who was excited by discoveries. He combined innovative research with a devotion to his subjects. Like many of us, he loved to share his newly acquired insights, but his sharing was one of exuberance. His positive outlook was contagious.

I first met Allen when we both applied for the adapted physical education position at the University of Minnesota. We immediately struck up a friendship, finding that our commonalities went far beyond the job application. They included a love of science, a dedication to the populations we both studied and served, and a love of sports, especially basketball. In those early years we'd make a point of working in pickup games between presentations at academic conferences. Those were the days of Larry Bird and Magic Johnson, and because I was a Celtics fan and Allen was naturally a Lakers fan, this made for another enjoyable connection through friendly competition.

Although I was very interested in going to Minnesota to be in a department headed by Michael Wade, I knew at the time that Allen was a better fit. I understood the choice and felt that it was a real privilege for me to continue our friendship as well as a professional relationship. With Allen having studied under Herb Pick and my graduating from the University of Connecticut, an appreciation for ecological psychology was another common bond. So when I went to Allen with my ideas about what was to develop into our 1991 paper on Ecological Task Analysis, it was the beginning of a delightful and meaningful collaboration. Our work together was highlighted in producing the *Human Movement Studies* paper on intrinsic measures, for which we did an exchange of writing and commenting. In the end neither of us could remember for sure who had written which part.

Allen and I did not talk much about religion, though it was obvious to me that he was devoted. Having grown up with a religious background, I appreciated that part of Allen. I attended a liberal arts college sponsored by our church, and there I asked some serious "why" questions about life. The answers I received from my religion came up short. Eventually, I turned to science to pursue my interests in finding truth. Once again, serious "why" questions arose, and again the answers came up short. I have since turned to metaphysics and to a newer paradigm in which science and spirituality are confluent. It is unfortunate in this much lesser sense that Allen has left, for herein lies another bond. I know that he is pleased with the direction toward which our ETA model is heading, because spirituality is yet another quality that Allen exemplified.

It is a real honor and privilege for me that this book is dedicated to Allen W. Burton. It is a testament to Allen that so many people eagerly offered to make a contribution.

Walter E. Davis

CONTENTS

Chapter 7   **Enhancing Responsible Student Decision Making in Physical Activity** **141**

Linda M. Carson, EdD • Sean M. Bulger, EdD
J. Scott Townsend, EdD

Chapter 8   **Ecological Task Analysis in Games Teaching: Tactical Games Model** **161**

Steve Mitchell, PhD • Judy Oslin, PhD

Chapter 9   **Systematic Ecological Modification Approach to Skill Acquisition in Adapted Physical Activity** **179**

Yeshayahu Hutzler, PhD

A.E. Wall, PhD • Greg Reid, PhD • William J. Harvey, PhD

Walter E. Davis, PhD • Geoffrey D. Broadhead, PhD

CONTRIBUTORS

Geoffrey D. Broadhead, PhD
  Kent State University, Ohio

Sean M. Bulger, EdD
  West Virginia University

Linda M. Carson, EdD
  West Virginia University

Walter E. Davis, PhD
  Kent State University, Ohio

Nancy Getchell, PhD
  University of Delaware

Donna L. Goodwin, PhD
  University of Alberta, Edmonton

Henriëtte Groeneveld, PhD
  H. G. Consulting, Edmonton, Alberta

William J. Harvey, PhD
  McGill University, Montreal, Quebec

Yeshayahu Hutzler, PhD
  Zinman College at the Wingate Institute
  Israel Sport Center for the Disabled

Kimberlee Jordan, PhD
  University of Colorado, Boulder

Lynn Kidman, PhD
  Christchurch College of Education, New Zealand

Steve Mitchell, PhD
  Kent State University, Ohio

Gerald Mullally, MSc
  Accenture, Dublin, Ireland

Mary Mullally, DipPhysio
  Paediatric Physiotherapy Clinic, Templemore, Ireland

Karl M. Newell, PhD
  The Pennsylvania State University

Judy Oslin, PhD
  Kent State University, Ohio

Greg Reid, PhD
  McGill University, Montreal, Quebec

Sarita Sanghvi, MPT
  Orthopedic and Sports Medicine Center, Annapolis, Maryland

Dan Southard, PhD
  Texas Christian University

Joyce Strand, PhD
  University of Minnesota, Duluth

Jane Taylor, PhD
  Lakehead University, Thunder Bay, Ontario

J. Scott Townsend, EdD
  Appalachian State University, North Carolina

Richard E.A. Van Emmerik, PhD
  University of Massachusetts

Adri Vermeer, PhD
  Utrecht University, The Netherlands

A.E. Wall, PhD
  McGill University, Montreal, Quebec

Jill Whitall, PhD
  University of Maryland, Baltimore

PROLOGUE

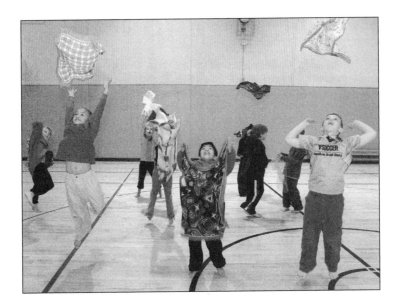

The book describes and advances an approach to understanding human movement originally developed by Allen Burton and Walter Davis (Burton and Davis 1992, 1996; Davis and Burton 1991) as the Ecological Task Analysis (ETA) model. The ETA includes a global theoretical model designed to provide insight into the dynamics of movement behavior through examination of the interacting constraints of performer, environment, and task. It also includes an applied model for movement skill assessment and instruction grounded in the theoretical model.

Theoretical Background and Tenets

The basic tenets of the original ETA theoretical model are as follows.

- The movement solution is separate from the task, allowing for any variation in movement from a modal pattern to be not a problem to be corrected (as in traditional task analysis), but a window into the dynamics of the person-action system.
- Actions are relations, not parts, and thus tasks should be categorized by function and intention, rather than mechanism or names.

- Invariant features of a task and variations within a task may be defined in terms of essential and nonessential variables (task dimensions), respectively. Thus the goal of a task remains constant across instructional variations of the task.
- Direct links should be established between the constraints of the task goal, the performer, and environment through the use of performer-scaled or other intrinsic dimensions.

The intent was to develop an applied model firmly grounded in the theories and research that were emerging as a challenge to the machine model embodied in information processing, behaviorism, and the medical model. Indeed, in the decade since the inception of ETA, all these supporting theories have had a revolutionizing impact on several major fields including biology, psychology, and evolution, as well as human movement science. Forming the backbone of the seminal paper by Burton and Davis is Karl Newell's (1986) triangle of constraints model (see also Keogh and Sugden 1985) suggesting that human movement is dynamically constrained (both limited and enabled) by three essential elements: task, context, and performer. Other important theoretical influences in the development of ETA include the broad-based approach of Peter Kugler and Michael Turvey (1987), which brought together several important philosophical assumptions, theoretical perspectives, and research tools to bear on the understanding of rhythmic movement, including Gibson's theory of affordance; Bernstein's physical and neurophysiological approach; dynamic systems, general systems, and chaos theory; and biological systems as open self-organizing systems. Also important to the development of the ETA approach was Ed Reed's (1982) theory of action, which stressed the functional classification of action systems, the use of functionally relevant variables in task manipulation, and a rejection of the central–peripheral dichotomy in motor control.

James Gibson's (1979) ecological psychology, which brought to the fore the context conditioning of perception and action and had a revolutionizing impact on all of psychology, is influential in all of the work just cited and is reflected in all the chapters here. Thus, the term ecological is applied to task analysis.

Research Support

Allen Burton's own research innovations help substantiate the claim that the principles embodied in ETA theory are equally suited for research as for instruction. Davis and Van Emmerik (1995b) identified five general strategies for conducting empirical work within the ETA framework:

- *Choosing affordances.* From the perspective *of the participants,* how do they perceive their environment with regard to what it offers for action?
- *Detecting higher-order variables.* Both the physical and social environments are structured through energy distributions and through abstract rules and regularized practices. These structures are higher-order variables that may be described generally or given a more precise mathematical description.
- *Measuring affordances.* This is also referred to as "the perception-action coupling" paradigm. Intrinsic measures are used to identify the critical point, which corresponds to phase transitions in behavior (e.g., at what body-scaled height does a participant go over rather than under a barrier?), and the optimal point, which corresponds to stable, successful, preferred regions of minimum energy expenditures during goal-oriented behavior (e.g., at what body-scaled height does the participant successfully negotiate the barrier to achieve the goal of "go as fast as you can"?).
- *Changes in movement coordination.* This is an investigation of the relationship between limbs (e.g., during bimanual movements) in terms of phase transitions and phase relations.
- *Stability and variability.* What is the functional role of these elements in the formation of movement patterns?

ETA Applied Model

Davis and Burton developed the ETA applied model from the broad-based theoretical support just described, from discussions at many venues, and from Davis' (Davis and Klingler 2004) several years of coordinating an on-campus hands-on teaching laboratory. The model includes four fundamental procedures or steps, which are applied to assessment, instruction, and research alike, making the approach unique in human movement theory and practice.

The first step in the applied model requires structuring the physical and social environment to clearly specify the task goal. This recognizes the goal directedness of human action and the significance of its context conditioning.

The second step is the heart of the ETA applied approach and requires that the students, participants, and subjects be given choices regarding how to solve the movement problem as specified by the structured environment and task goal. This participant-centered, participant-empowering approach stands in stark contrast to the teacher-directed approaches that dominate the current education system. Thus, choice as conceived in ETA is clearly more than an important strategy to facilitate movement learning; it also infuses the learning and experimenting processes with the importance of developing self-determination in all persons. Self-determination is the overarching goal for developing both movement competence and competence as members of a democratic community.

The third step requires the instructor to manipulate relevant task variables, making the task easier (for success) or more difficult (for challenge) in order to elicit further responses from the participants. This is a direct tie-in to dynamic systems theory advocating the scaling of control parameters.

The fourth step is to provide further instructions as the teacher or researcher deems necessary and appropriate. This step includes intrinsically measuring and comparing qualitative and quantitative movement forms and outcomes. This last step recognizes the expertise of the instructor and researcher without taking away the agency of the performers. This step makes ETA the open-ended model that is necessary in the ever-changing context of the dynamical learning process.

The ETA applied model is not a cookbook. Rather it is based upon principles and concepts that apply in different settings and with all populations (shown most clearly in part II of this book) and requires competent critically thinking practitioners. It is believed to be more efficacious than the categorical approach in special education and adapted physical activity, the teacher-directed approach in physical education, and the prescriptive approach in the therapies, all of which still dominate today.

Utility of This Book

The chapters in this book provide meaningful and usable methods and strategies for implementation in both research and instruction. We believe that this collection of papers will, in and of itself, encourage more individuals to understand and inquire about, discuss and debate, borrow from and fully utilize, and critique and further develop the ETA model.

We do not see the model as static, devoid of weaknesses or misconceptions and beyond improvement. Rather we see it as a model and approach connected to several other related models and approaches—and one full of potential for influencing how people think about action. Thus, knowledge of the contents of *Ecological Task Analysis Perspectives on Movement* can become a powerful tool for those who observe, study, instruct (in the broadest sense), or participate in physical activity in a variety of settings.

This book is the first concerted effort to bring the work of other scientists together to further develop, expand, and promote the ETA model. One impetus behind the ETA model has been a need to connect the distinct but related forms of scientific inquiry: philosophy, theory, research, and practice. Thus, the book is organized into two parts: part I, "Strengthening the Foundation of Ecological Task Analysis," and part II, "Enhancing Instruction Using Ecological Task Analysis." An introduction to each part highlights the connections between the parts and the chapters. Readers should note that the references from all the chapters are compiled into one list, with bracketed numbers following each entry indicating which chapter or chapters that particular source is cited in. It is our hope that this book encourages students and researchers to study, challenge, and further develop the ETA model.

Strengthening the Foundation of Ecological Task Analysis

Geoffrey D. Broadhead, PhD

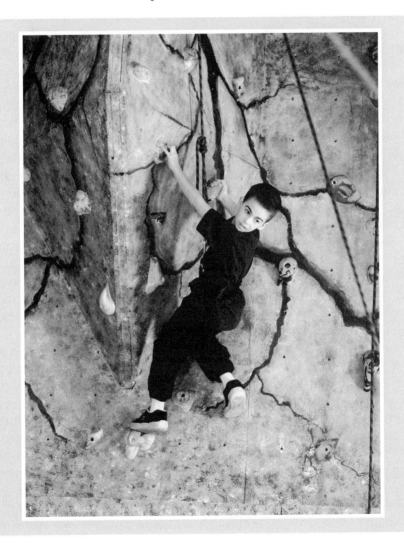

Part I includes chapters that remind us of the foundations of the Ecological Task Analysis (ETA) model and investigate the theoretical details of the model. These chapters trace some of the theoretical advances that have taken place since the inception of the model in 1991 and broaden the vision of ETA.

The first chapter, by Newell and Jordan, "Task Constraints and Movement Organization: A Common Language," is an update of the original tenets of the movement constraints theory (Newell 1986), which is noted to be one of the bases of the ETA model.

The authors retrace the development of the constraints model, citing research that has interpreted it and emphasizing the importance of what they call an overarching self-organization metaphor for learning and control. In discussing task constraints, Newell and Jordan counsel researchers to ensure that the task is rich enough to engender the full range of movement dynamics while avoiding overconstraining the situation.

Van Emmerik (chapter 2) examines how variability in movement influences coordination and disability. Although some researchers propose that improved levels of skilled motor performance are accompanied by decreases in performance variability, Van Emmerik cites literature suggesting that it is actually decreased variability that is associated with performance decline or decrement.

To Van Emmerik, the presence of variability brings performance benefits to conditions associated with competence in motor skill and maintenance of healthy body systems, and is attributed to research into nonlinear dynamical and complex systems. Thus, he emphasizes the essential nature of performance variability to ETA and to the scaling of performer attributes.

In chapter 3, Davis and Strand explore the concept of choice as a central feature of the ETA applied model. They suggest that there are at least seven levels or perspectives from which choice may be viewed. They also discuss acts or situations that eliminate choices, noting that persons with limited intellect, emotional instability, or physical or sensory disabilities have been unnecessarily limited in their opportunities for choice. They cite research demonstrating that increased productivity accompanies increased choices and that this is true for all populations investigated. Through an extensive review of these seven aspects of choice, Davis and Strand present ETA as a window through which to broaden our vision of movement.

Chapter 4 demonstrates the efficacy of testing the principles of the ETA model through sound research studies. Whitall, Sanghvi, and Getchell (chapter 4) examine the perceptual-action judgments of children with learning disabilities (LD) following the applied research process described by Burton and Davis (1996). They used a stepping-over task with elementary-aged children with and without LD. The choice of subjects is very important because of the large number of school-aged children who are given the LD label. Thus the research question has considerable practical application. Whitall and colleagues make the point that a well-documented characteristic of children with LD is lack of competence in motor skills. The research question was whether such children differed from typically developing children in the way they made decisions in a perception-action task.

Subjects were asked to state whether they could step over a bar at a self-perceived height and later asked to demonstrate actual competence. Because decision time for correct performance was longer for children with LD, it follows from a pedagogical standpoint that such children should be given a little more time in order to perform optimally.

Southard (chapter 5) follows the tenets of dynamical systems theory to examine velocity as a control parameter leading to a change of movement pattern in the overarm throw. One link to the ETA model for this study is via the element of self-discovery. By providing choice of task velocity, Southard sought to discover not only whether the movement pattern would change but also whether changing the scale would result in increased velocity of throw. Results of the study showed that for these subjects, movement patterns changed without instruction and were guided by an order parameter identified by Southard as the open kinetic link principle, which allows the upper limb to conserve angular momentum during a throwing motion. These findings are discussed in relation to ETA principles.

We think the chapters in part I help to extend our understanding of what the ETA model is, as well as indicating efficacy and adaptability. They help provide the theoretical and research bases for the applied chapters in part II.

Task Constraints and Movement Organization: A Common Language

Karl M. Newell, PhD, and Kimberlee Jordan, PhD

Action goals and task demands have a long history in general learning theory (e.g., Tolman 1932), but they are constructs that have had an uneven place in theories of motor learning and control. The traditional theorizing about development, learning, and motor performance has often given emphasis to the role of goals and the relative influence of the environment and the organism (or performer) in organizing behavior. There has, however, been less importance placed on directly linking task constraints with environmental and organismic constraints so as to understand the role of task goals in organizing the coordination and control of movement in action. In this chapter we approach this issue directly and further develop the theorizing for the role of task constraints in the coordination and control of action (Newell 1986), a viewpoint that has relevance to motor performance and the change of behavior that reflects motor learning and development.

The constructs of tasks and actions have been used and emphasized differently in the various subdomains of psychology and in other movement-related disciplines such as physiology and engineering. This chapter outlines a basis from which to consider these constructs in a coherent fashion and to place the role of task constraints in a unified framework for action along with the influence of both the organism and environment. The notion of tasks was developed in the traditions of experimental psychology and the emerging field of human learning and performance (cf. Fleishman and Quaintance 1984). The construct of action has a much longer history and broader position in the study of behavior, including the influences of philosophy (Mischel 1969) and development (Juarrero 1999).

In this chapter we outline a framework for how the study of movement provides a context in which to integrate the traditional notions of actions and tasks. A key element of this approach is having a common framework and language from which to describe both the goals of tasks and the properties of movement within the context of action. Traditionally goals and movements have been described in different languages, often from different theoretical perspectives—a feature that has made it difficult to bring these constructs together into a common theory of motor learning and control. For example, the early work in motor learning driven by the traditions of experimental psychology emphasized task goals and downplayed the analysis of the movement properties (cf. Schmidt and Lee 1999). In contrast, biomechanics and the physiology of motor control emphasized movement description through kinematics and kinetics but without often recognizing the significant influence of task constraints (Nigg and Herzog 1994). Today, the more interdisciplinary field of motor control is integrating task constraints and movement properties more vigorously and rigorously than heretofore, although there is still considerable progress to be made in this regard.

This chapter also provides an update and additional perspectives with respect to the constraints on action framework of Newell (1986). Since the publication of that paper there have been several elaborations that implicitly or explicitly build on aspects of the original theoretical framework (e.g., Burton and Davis 1992, 1996), together with experimental investigations that were guided by the constraints perspective (Cesari and Newell 1999; Newell et al. 1989a). The Ecological Task Analysis (ETA) model of Burton and Davis places emphasis on the process of changing the relevant dimensions of a functional task to gain insights into the dynamics of the behavior of the performer and to provide the instructor clues for developing instructional strategies. In the long run it is hoped that the ideas expressed on tasks and movement will move us closer to a theory of tasks for the movement domain (Greene 1972), and in a fashion that is more firmly grounded in motor control than the early work in this area from experimental psychology (Fleishman and Quaintance 1984).

Role of Constraints on Action

We now consider the role of task constraints in action from several perspectives. The first section recaptures the role of the ecological approach to perception and action in introducing this theme. The second section provides an outline of the categories of constraint to action.

Ecological Approach to Perception and Action

The introduction of the coordinative structure theory by Kugler, Kelso, and Turvey (1980, 1982) provided a sharp contrast to the then-prevailing prescriptive theories of the motor program (Keele 1968) and schema (Schmidt 1975). Indeed, the central construct of self-organization in the coordinative structure view reflected what Kuhn (1996) would describe as a paradigm change from the prevailing notion of the motor program. The coordinative structure theory was part of the emerging and broader ecological approach to perception and action (Gibson 1979; Kugler and Turvey 1987; Michaels and Carello 1981).

One can understand the importance of constraints in the ecological approach to perception and action by considering Kugler and colleagues' statement that "the order in biological and physiological processes is primarily owing to dynamics and that the constraints that arise, both anatomical and functional, serve only to channel and guide dynamics; it is not that actions are caused by constraints it is, rather, that some actions are excluded by them" (1980, p. 9). This kind of thinking about emergent processes and properties, which had been originally promoted in the physical sciences, helped lead to a paradigm shift in the motor behavior domain whereby the order and structure of movement in action emerge from constraints that eliminate certain configurations of self-organizing optimality of the biological system, rather than the specification from the prescriptive symbolic knowledge structure of programs.

The introduction of self-organization as the overarching metaphor for motor learning and control held many far-reaching implications, a number of which have been outlined or investigated in the subsequent 25 years or so (Kelso 1995; Kugler and Turvey 1987; Turvey 1990). Furthermore, as even a cursory review of the experimental journals would reveal, a prodigious amount of quality experimental work has developed under the ecological approach to perception and action and under the related, though in many ways distinct, dynamical systems approach. Indeed, there are many scholars who would see these approaches as currently the most influential theoretical force in the behavioral study of human motor learning and control.

Nonetheless, it could be argued that the emerging experimental work in this area has often little to do directly with the construct of self-organization. This leaves self-organization as an overarching or guiding metaphor rather than a construct that is being examined theoretically and empirically in a rigorous program of scholarship. It is as if we are in a period of normal science (Kuhn 1996), in which the primary focus of scholars is just to get on with investigating the experimental aspects of the prevailing theoretical work without questioning or challenging the metaphor of the framework. The same normal-science state of affairs is largely the case for the cognitive approach to human movement and action (cf. Newell 2004).

This brief digression to metaphor is important in the context of this chapter because the notion of constraints is intimately linked to the construct of self-organization. In other words, empirical examinations of the self-organization metaphor will be in part addressed by manipulation of constraints and an examination of the consequences on the qualitative and quantitative properties of movement. As Kugler and colleagues (1980) originally noted, the study of constraints is also another way of considering the degrees of freedom problem (Bernstein 1967). The number of papers that have pursued this line of inquiry within the ecological approach to perception and action has been relatively few, as scholars have emphasized other aspects of the agenda, including movement coordination and perceptual variables such as time to contact (Haken, Kelso, and Bunz 1985; Lee 1980). The net result is that the overarching metaphor of self-organization has not been challenged or developed to any significant degree since its introduction to the movement field. It is now either generally accepted and sometimes used as a guiding metaphor by those working within the ecological approach to perception and action or ignored and unaccepted, as in much of the cognitive-action domain.

One area of research that has progressively used the self-organization construct as a guide to the manipulation of constraints is motor development (Smith and Thelen 1993; Thelen and Smith 1994). In the study of motor development we are increasingly seeing how even small changes in the initial conditions to action, by manipulations of the infant, environment, and task, lead to either the early emergence of the fundamental movement patterns or the generation of new patterns of coordination that heretofore have not been observed. The recent demonstration of the leg and foot instrumental behavior by young infants in the study of Angulo-Kinzler, Ulrich, and Thelen (2002) is a novel and interesting example of this work, with profound implications for the theory of motor development, and more generally motor control.

The success of the infant and motor development work on constraints is based in part on not having the participant overconstrained in an experimental protocol so that only two degrees of joint space freedom are the measured movement properties, a limiting feature of the hammer swinging (Kugler and Turvey 1987) and finger wiggling (Kelso 1995) tasks. Important theoretical and empirical work has arisen from or because of these protocols, but clearly these movement conditions are limiting to the full expression and study of the dynamics of self-organization in the movement domain. The ecological approach to perception and action emphasized the significance of Bernstein's (1967) degrees of freedom problem (Saltzman 1979; Turvey, Shaw, and Mace 1978), but then followed the overconstraining traditions of experimental psychology in task selection for empirical studies of motor control. The challenge is to find tasks that are rich enough to engender the full range of movement dynamics, as well as the problems of many degrees of freedom and system degeneracy (Tononi, Sporns, and Edelman 1999), while at the same time being sufficiently manageable in terms of measurement and modeling. In the practice of experimentation, this collective of experimental conditions is a tall order to realize but is a direction we need to move further toward if the constructs of constraints and self-organization are to be investigated beyond contemporary experimental work with any sense of adequacy.

Categories of Constraints on Action

Constraints are interpreted as boundary conditions that, in the case of action, limit the configurations of the system. There are constraints at all levels of analysis of the system, including biochemical, morphological, neurological, and behavioral. These boundary conditions at each level of analysis may be spatial, temporal, or, usually, spatial and temporal. In the case of the ecological approach to perception and action it is important to note that the action system (or, often just the system) is defined over the organism, environment, and task. System is not referring to the biological system, as it is in many other theoretical perspectives of the life sciences.

Most constraints to action are changing over time to varying degrees and thus are what Kugler and colleagues (1980) described as relatively time independent or dependent. The rate of change of their influence leads to a wide range of time scales from very slow (considered to be almost no change) up to more rapid and obviously apparent change over time. This continuum of the rate or time scale of change provides the basis for considering biological constraints as either structural (relatively time independent) or functional (relatively time dependent). For example, anatomy is generally interpreted as a structural constraint because the rate of change of the body form is considered nonexistent within the context of a given action and relatively slow even when viewed in the big picture of the life span of the individual. In contrast, heart rate, for example, can change over time on the order of seconds within a given action so as to provide a rapidly changing functional constraint on movement organization and performance.

A standard approach to the constraints of development has been to view the three major time scales of influence on the emergence of movement forms as the very slow time scale of evolution, the more rapid time scale of ontogenetic development, and the much more rapid time scales of biological processes (e.g., Mittenthal and Baskin 1992; Waddington 1957). This traditional categorization, however, has tended to ignore or play down the role of task constraints and the relatively short time-scale influence of intention on the changes in the landscape dynamics supporting action (Newell, Liu, and Mayer-Kress 2003). However, there are many ways to consider or organize the constraints to action, and Eckhardt (2000) has provided a comprehensive framework outlining environmental influences and population response over time.

Figure 1.1 provides a schematic of the constraints on action framework originally outlined by Newell (1986). The central proposal was that the categories of environment, organism, and task provide a complete though general basis on which to consider the constraints to action. The distinctive contribution was to place task constraints in a cohesive framework with those of the organism and environment, so that the interaction of these sources of boundary conditions provides the confluence of constraints to action. This framework has been highlighted and elaborated

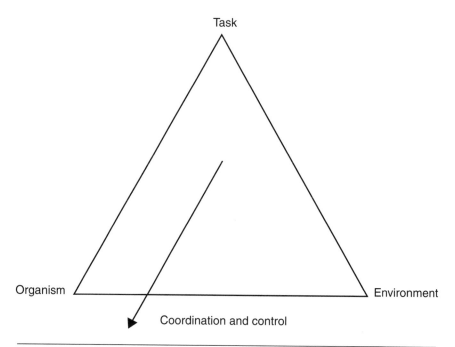

Figure 1.1 Schematic of the constraints on coordination.

Adapted, by permission, from K.M. Newell, 1986, Constraints on the development of co-ordination. In *Motor development in children: Aspects of coordination and control,* edited by M.G. Wade and H.T.A. Whiting (Heidelberg, Germany: Springer-Verlag GmbH), 348. With kind permission from Springer Science and Business Media.

in several more recent papers (Burton and Davis 1992, 1996; Davis and Burton 1991; Shumway-Cook and Woollacott 2001).

Organismic Constraints

The operational distinction between organismic and environmental constraints is generally considered to be straightforward. Organismic constraints are those of the biological system as defined at each level of analysis, such as chemical, neural, and morphological. In the area of human movement, the organism is the performer, or the individual performing the task. The most obvious and commonly measured constraints to human action are at the behavioral level, as in the physical properties of height, weight, and shape of the individual, together with the properties of the effectors (e.g., strength and flexibility) that are available for action. In Newell 1986, several candidate examples of organismic constraints to action were discussed (see also Thelen 1986), but since then there have been limited advances in understanding the short- or long-term changes in the more relevant micro-level constraints to movement in action and the impact of such properties on the movement domain.

One exception to this has been the significant work documenting the adaptive plasticity of the central nervous system and the cortical sensorimotor brain areas (e.g., Merzenich and Jenkins 1993). This experimental work has shown that the traditional textbook account of the homunculus-like representational map is much too static an image of both brain structure and function. The experimental findings also show clearly that practice and experience can change the neural constraints to action, in addition to adaptation and learning leading to the individual's being better able to take advantage of them in system organization. This mutual influence on and from constraints through the engagement of movement in action contributes to the adaptive nature of system change.

It would seem that the not too distant future also holds the potential and promise of the experimental manipulation of genes as a vehicle for enhancing movement behavior. The concept of gene therapy has already been implemented as an experimental medical intervention in movement disorders such as Parkinson's disease. Gene manipulation for the enhancement of human functions, such as sport performance, is also now viewed as a realistic possibility in the near term (Marcus 2004).

Environmental Constraints

The environmental constraints are those physical properties that are external to the organism. Both the organism and the environment can be analyzed at many of the same levels of analysis as already outlined for the action system. Most research in motor learning and control is conducted within the confines of a laboratory setting where the ambient environmental properties of altitude, temperature, wind, and so on are viewed as "normal" (within standard ambient range) and "controlled" so as not to influence performance. These ambient conditions are in effect viewed as "neutral" and are the norm in both theoretical and experimental movement research, although it is obvious that even small departures from this "typical" environment can and do influence movement in action. Moreover, it should be recognized that the "controlled" conditions of the laboratory are providing a particular confluence of constraints to action. The laboratory is not a vacuum, and even if it were, a vacuum holds its own set of constraints. At the other end of the continuum is the strong manipulation of environmental constraints on human movement as in, for example, the gravity-free environment of space or the medium of water.

In Newell 1986, the distinction was made between environmental constraints to action that are general or ambient and those that are task specific. It is much cleaner in a definitional sense not to force this distinction, and it is more coherent to consider environmental constraints as all those physical boundary conditions external to the organism. This amendment has been the only modification to the original constraints on coordination outline of Newell (1986; see also Davis and Burton 1991).

Task Constraints

The task constraints are reflected in two categories. These are (a) the goal of the task and (b) the rules specifying or constraining the movement dynamics to realize a goal. Within this framework, most actions in everyday life are constrained only by the goal of the task. This goal can have more than one dimension, for example, space and time; or the goal of the task could reflect several component goals, as in dual task performance.

However, in music, sport, and some other movement contexts there are often also rules specifying or constraining (or both specifying and constraining) the movement properties so as to impose additional performance constraints beyond those of the action goal. For example, certain sports, such as swimming, have boundary conditions on the pattern of limb movement that can take place while one is attempting to swim a certain distance in a minimum time or a time less than an opponent. Newell (1986) provided an extensive discussion of the influences of goals and rules with many examples of the role of task constraints in action.

Task constraints may be determined externally to the individual or by the participant him- or herself. These constraints may be explicit, as when they are written in the rules of games and sports, for example; or they may be implicit as in a child's play behavior. Thus, task constraints can impose a physical boundary to movement in action that can be measured in space, time, or both, but they can also reflect "imaginary" boundary conditions that are more difficult although not necessarily impossible to measure in the same language.

The idea of task constraints can be elaborated to consider the role of a teacher, coach, or therapist as that of a change agent who is imposing additional constraints in the learning or relearning context (Newell 1991, 1996; Newell and Valvano 1998). These additional constraints can take the form of changing the goals of subtasks in learning or the environmental conditions of practice. One advantage of this extension of the original constraint framework is that it also allows the role of interventions to be considered in the same language as the other subdomains of movement in action. Thus, augmented information, for example, can be viewed as a control parameter in a dynamical systems framework to motor control. The challenge for the change agent is to find the most effective and relevant control parameter(s) to induce task-adaptive change in the organization of movement output.

Finally, it should be noted that the view has been advanced that the construct of task constraints as expressed in Newell (1986) holds a different ontological status than that of organismic and environmental constraints as originally expressed by Kugler and colleagues (1980). In this view, the triangle of constraints framework is not uniformly coherent in a theoretical sense with the principles of the ecological approach to perception and action. The construct of task constraints can be viewed as more compatible with the theorizing of cognitive symbolic approaches to action. Nevertheless, the notion of task constraints has been embraced experimentally within the ecological approach to perception and action. Clearly there is some theoretical work still to be done on this important issue.

Confluence of Constraints

A central and significant element of the constraint triangle in figure 1.1 is that the coordination and control of movement in action are emergent from the confluence of the boundary conditions represented in the categories of organismic, environmental, and task constrains. In this view, all constraints are contributing to the channeling of the system dynamics, though clearly some boundary conditions play a more important role than others in motor learning and performance. An emerging view is that these constraints at multiple levels of the system have multiple time scales of influence. Unfortunately, we have not progressed much on the time scales of constraints that have either developmental or life span influence and those that regulate behavior in the short term.

The triangle notion of constraints (Newell 1986) has been redrawn as a circle, presumably to "round out" literally the distinctive categorizations reflected in the triangle schematic (Burton and Davis 1992, 1996). The categories of organism, environment, and task have also been sub-categorized to varying degrees, thus creating a hierarchy of constraints to action. These developments have not changed the original formulations of the constraints on action framework and may have helped its interpretation and promotion.

Mapping Movement to Task Constraints

As outlined earlier, the traditional disciplinary approaches in motor learning and control have tended to keep the description of action goals and task constraints distinct from observations of the movement properties, that is, not in the same dimension or language. But if the idea of task constraints as the complement of degrees of freedom in action (Kugler et al. 1980) is to receive any principled examination, we will need to have the description of the task constraints in the same language as is used to describe the movement. Theoretical developments in the movement domain in recent years have approached this theoretical and operational problem directly.

McGinnis and Newell (1982) proposed the application of topological dynamics to the representation of movement and task criteria. "Topological" is used here in the sense of properties of geometric configurations of movement that are invariant under transformation by continuous mappings. The approach is sometimes referred to more generally as qualitative dynamics. The framework is based on classical mechanics and the representation of a particle or system of particles in space (e.g., Rosenberg 1977).

This topological approach allows one to represent and analyze any generalized dynamical system, be it mechanical, electrical, hydraulic, or other. The orientation is based on the assumption that a particle, in this case some point of the human body or an extension of it, can occupy only one position in space at any given instant of time. This concept of impenetrability implies that no two points of the body can occupy the same point in space at the same time. The position or motion of a system of particles may be represented within some boundaries or living space. There are several frames of reference, for example Cartesian 3D space or relative motion space, in which this motion could be described.

The topological framework could also accommodate force as a control variable, as in the analysis of isometric actions or any number of physiologically controlled parameters.

McGinnis and Newell (1982) outlined several control space frames of reference that could be used to analyze movement and represent task constraints. These included configuration space, event space, state space, and state-time space (see figure 1.2). These frames of reference have different kinematic properties to define the dimensions of description, and the choice for use in experimental analysis is question and task specific. For example, configuration space represents the movement in spatial coordinates without direct consideration of time, and this may be sufficient and appropriate in certain circumstances. Event space plots the position of the system point in question over time, a common

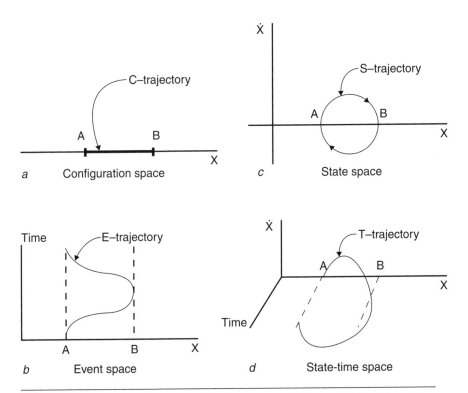

Figure 1.2   Trajectories of a pen-positioning movement shown in *(a)* configuration space, *(b)* event space, *(c)* state space, and *(d)* state-time space. The movement was constrained in one dimension in configuration space.

Reprinted from *Human Movement Science,* Vol. 1, No. 4, P.M. McGinnis and K.M. Newell, "Topological dynamics: A framework for describing movement and its constraints," pgs. 289-305, Copyright 1982, with permission from Elsevier.

representation in biomechanics. Indeed, the control space framework approach to the description of movement in different control spaces is standard in biomechanics given its origins in engineering and physics.

The movement representations shown in the different control spaces of figure 1.2 are of the same discrete movement. This illustration clearly shows that different properties of the movement are emphasized in each frame of reference. The qualitative property of the movement trajectory is also distinct in each control space. Each space or frame of reference has its uses to uniquely reveal properties of the movement depending on the research question. For example, the roles of movement time or velocity are not revealed in configuration space, as many movements could have the same configuration but different dynamics. This can be highlighted by a consideration of the movement properties in the control space that best reveal the unique qualitative properties of the movement.

The more interesting use of this analysis approach, given the thrust of this chapter, is the linking of the task constraints to those of the movement properties in this topological framework. Thus, the goal and the constraints on movement can be represented in space or time (or both) within this framework in the same way that the movement properties are. This allows a comparison of the imposed task constraints in the same language that is being used to describe the movement. Furthermore, there may be physical constraints in the environment that act to preclude the realization of certain positions in space, and these too can be represented in the same framework. Figure 1.3 presents an illustration of the representation in the same language of both the movement and the task constraints imposed by the physical properties of objects in the action context.

Of course, many internal physiological or morphological constraints are not known a priori, and the analysis of performance in this framework may help identify these heretofore hidden constraints. One might consider the representation of movement in this framework as standard biomechanics so that the major contribution of the approach is the simultaneous representation or identification of either task or other constraints. The tendency in biomechanics, however, has been to emphasize the quantitative aspects of movement rather than the qualitative properties.

It follows that this framework also provides a principled basis from which to consider the application of augmented information in motor skill learning (Newell and McGinnis 1985). Here augmented information can be viewed as a constraint that channels the movement dynamics in learning. The challenge has been to select the appropriate information

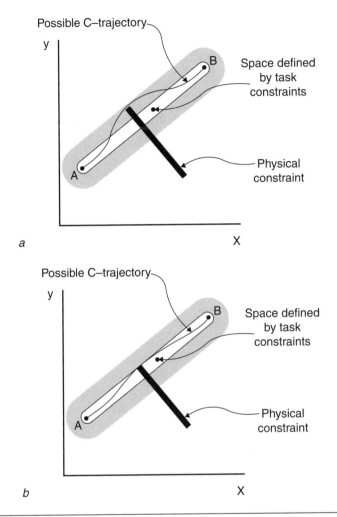

Figure 1.3   An example *(a)* of a physical constraint that prevents any acceptable C-trajectories defined by the task constraints and *(b)* of a physical constraint that reduces the space of acceptable configurations defined by the task constraints.

Reprinted from *Human Movement Science,* Vol. 1, No. 4, P.M. McGinnis and K.M. Newell, "Topological dynamics: A framework for describing movement and its constraints," pgs. 289-305, Copyright 1982, with permission from Elsevier.

that brings about effective and efficient change in the movement (Newell 1991, 1996).

The topological dynamics approach allows one to examine the qualitative and quantitative features of movement and task constraints. There has, however, been very little consideration of the qualitative properties of movement. One reason is that there are few theoretical perspectives that motivate such an orientation to movement analysis, given that most focus on quantitative properties of movement. Secondly, there is the difficulty of assessing a qualitative form from a movement trajectory. Sparrow and colleagues (1987) created an approach to measure the qualitative aspects of movement (see also Whiting and Zernicke 1982), but these are isolated efforts in this area. The net result is that the topological aspects of movement have actually rarely been assessed operationally.

The qualitative properties of movement can also be considered from the perspective of nonlinear dynamics (Abraham and Shaw 1982). This approach gives emphasis to the qualitative properties of the time-evolutionary properties of the dynamics of the system output. It is based on the idea that motion in dissipative dynamical systems tends to settle to some long-term recurrent behavior or stable attracting solutions. Here dynamics does not refer to the classic engineering categories of kinematics and kinetics but rather the qualitative or dynamical topologies of the time-dependent system output.

This approach gives emphasis to the categorical types of attractors and their qualitative dynamics. The most basic attractor forms are those of the point attractor, periodic or limit-cycle attractor, and chaotic attractor (Thompson and Stewart 1986). The use of dynamical systems theory and analysis techniques has become a central approach within the ecological approach to perception and action and movement science more generally. Indeed, there are now many analyses of the dimension of the attractor that is organizing the qualitative and quantitative properties of movement output.

It was from this dynamical systems framework that Saltzman and Kelso (1987) proposed a task dynamic approach to the consideration of skilled actions. This approach to the analysis of movement and tasks has four levels: task space, body space, task network, and articulator network. A key element of the task dynamic approach is the mapping of the qualitative distinctions among task properties to the corresponding qualitative properties of the movement dynamics. Thus, as an example, the task constraint of posture might be viewed as the production of point attractor behavior where the goal is that of no movement. The expectation, therefore, is that the qualitative properties of the postural system will map to the qualitative properties of the task. This strategy of mapping the qualitative properties of the movement to those of the task can be generalized to all tasks.

However, the mapping of the dynamical degrees of freedom to the dimension of the task constraints is not necessarily a one-to-one relation.

That is, the qualitative properties of the movement output do not have to match those of the task constraints so as to realize the task demand. The properties of the system dynamics can be qualitatively different from those of the task goal. Furthermore, because most task criteria tend to have few dimensions, this has helped support the postulation that the number of dynamical degrees of freedom controlled is reduced as a function of practice. However, the dimension of the control system can increase or decrease with practice, according to the constraints on action, particularly the influence of task constraints (Newell and Vaillancourt 2001).

These important issues—the mapping of movement output to task constraints and the direction of change in the dimension of the output—were both addressed by Newell and colleagues (2003) experimentally in an isometric force control study. The task constraint of a constant isometric force output has a dimension of zero. Thus, as described earlier, the task demand can be considered to be that of a point attractor. In contrast, a sinusoidal-like isometric output has a dimension of 1, as in a limit-cycle or periodic attractor. Experiments have shown, however, that subjects reduce error in the constant-level force task by increasing the dimension of the force output. Thus, there is not even an approximate mapping of the dimension (qualitative properties) of the force output with that of the task demand. Indeed, the minimization of error in the constant force target is approached only through the introduction of more dimensions of control into the motor output; and these dimensions are typically those with shorter time scales, as these tend to have smaller force amplitudes, thus leading to reduced force error in the output. In contrast, the sinusoidal task with a dimension of 1 is essentially mapped by the dimension of the subject's output with some additional variability.

This contrasting pattern of findings as a function of task demand shows (1) that there is not necessarily a direct mapping between the dimension of the motor output to that of the task constraint and (2) that the direction of change through practice in the dimension of control is dependent on the task constraints. Vaillancourt and Newell (2002, 2003) have also proposed that this more adaptive potential bidirectional change in the dimension of output leads to a different interpretation of the "loss of complexity" hypothesis with aging (Lipsitz and Goldberger 1992), in that older adults can have either increased or reduced dimension compared to young adults depending on the task demands. Overall, these findings provide further evidence of the strong and sometimes counterintuitive role of task constraints in the organization of motor output.

Actions, Tasks, and Theories of Motor Learning and Control

In this section we briefly consider two related themes. First we examine the relation between actions and tasks. In the second theme the focus is on tasks and theories.

Actions and Tasks

Movement is a necessary but not sufficient condition for action. Similarly, tasks are an integral feature of actions, but they are not the same construct. In general, action is the more inclusive term for considering human movement in the context of behavior. Actions are usually identified, in part, by the goal(s) to which they are directed (e.g., pick up the teapot) or by specification of certain criteria that the individual performer complies with in what he or she does (e.g., walking, hopping). This feature of action is what tasks are about and reflects what is referred to here as the task constraints.

The concept of action is a slippery term in philosophy and psychology (Mischel 1969). Nevertheless, many definitions of action incorporate most if not all of the following features: (a) an intention to realize a particular goal (read task constraints), (b) selection among appropriate means for achievement of the act, and (c) sustained direction of behavior during deployment of the means (Bruner 1973, p. 2). This definition points up the importance of being aware that there can be a distinction between viewing the task constraints from the perspective of the individual and independent of the individual as defined by, for example, an experimenter.

In most experimental situations the assumption is that the individual's perception of the task constraints is the same as that defined externally by the experimenter. This assumption is not always justified, particularly early in stages of learning a task or with particular subpopulations, such as young children. Nevertheless, for purposes of our exposition here about task constraints, we assume that there is a mapping between the externally defined goal(s) and those intended by the participant.

Finally, it is worthwhile to reemphasize that a variety of potential movements may be generated to complete any single act (the long-standing idea of motor equivalence), and that a variety of movements may be identified as being as a particular act. However, movement itself is not sufficient to define an action or determine if there was an intended goal. For example, if an individual leaned against a door to rest and the door suddenly opened due to a faulty catch, we could not describe this as the act of opening the door on the part of the performer, even if the kinematics and end product of the movement were identical to those produced in the everyday act of opening the door. Thus, movement in action is intentionally generated to realize a particular set of task constraints.

Tasks and Theories

There has been a strong trend in contemporary motor learning and control to limit theorizing to a particular category of tasks or, in even more restrictive circumstances, to a single task (e.g., Adams 1971). This is in sharp contrast to the all-encompassing theories of behavior of the early 20th century as, for example, with behaviorism. The narrowing of the boundaries of tasks for study seems a natural and almost essential requirement for engagement in the study of human motor learning and control. This approach follows nicely the standard scientific maxim of not going beyond one's data; but the flip side of this approach is that generalization is often lost, or not even considered, in both experimental and theoretical orientations. This has led to the position that most theories, models, and hypotheses about motor learning and control are task specific (Newell 1989).

There are different theories and models for (a) slow movements and fast movements; (b) movements constrained by a single biomechanical degree of freedom and those involving multiple degrees of freedom—although usually only two; (c) movements that are repetitive or oscillatory in nature and those that are discrete and settle on a single space point; (d) movements that are terminated by the individual performer and those that are terminated by contact with the environment; (e) the initiation of movements as opposed to their subsequent control during execution; (f) isometric tasks and those that involve movement in body or limb position; (g) simple movements as opposed to complex movements; and (h) phylogenetic movements as opposed to ontogenetic activities. This fractioning of the study of task influence has been magnified by the parallel constraining of theorizing to particular subpopulation groups so that, for example, the study of motor learning has been predicated on a very different set of tasks from the traditions of motor development (Newell and Van Emmerik 1990). Of course, we can add to this the disciplinary specialization in distinct levels of analysis, and it is not surprising that the scientific outcome is that of task and theory specificity.

One of the original attractions of the ecological approach to perception and action was that it seemed to offer theoretical perspectives that held the promise to cut across the many task boundaries that have been created. And, in the last 20 years or so there has been more generalization of theory across a range of what were formerly considered distinct task categories. For example, Schöner has developed a dynamical systems approach that holds principles for both discrete and rhythmical movement tasks (Schöner 1989, 1990) and that can be extended to the initiation of movement phenomena (Erlhagen and Schöner 2002). Indeed, the dynamical systems approach to movement in action seems to offer principled ways to consider the development of a general theory of motor learning and control that is also not confined to the performance of young-adult students.

These criticisms of the traditions of task and theory specificity should not be taken to mean that progress was not made with this approach, but rather to make the point that it does hold limitations. We would begin with the Occam's razor perspective, that the goal of our science is a unified theory of motor learning and control that generalizes across tasks and task categories. In other words, we do not expect that at the end of the day it will be necessary to have a distinct theory for walking and running, walking and standing, and even walking and grasping. This is a large claim, and one that we are probably not in a position to justify, beyond a philosophical stance. Nevertheless, it is a principled position to have as a theoretical backdrop, even if the ongoing work requires some halfway steps, so to speak, by being task oriented.

The approach of task and theory specificity has fostered the development of ideas that are clearly wrong (even without the benefit of experimentation) when considered in a broader context. We believe that it is this kind of experimental agenda that should be minimized if not avoided. In other words, there should naturally be some consideration in theorizing of the generalization of the ideas to action broadly defined. And finally, a practical outcome of the constraints on action framework is the recognition that the task always brings some constraints to action and thus will inevitably influence in some way the variables under study. Thus, gone should be the days when a task is just pulled out of the experimenter's bag or off of the laboratory shelf in order to run a study, as in much of the social psychology of physical activity research. As much consideration needs to be given to the potential influence of task constraints as to properties of the environment or the individual in the study of movement in action.

KEY POINTS

- The confluence of task, organismic, and environmental constraints channel the movement dynamics.
- Action goals and task demands play an important role in channeling the qualitative and quantitative properties of movement dynamics.
- The boundary conditions of task constraints can be described in the same language as that used to describe movement.
- The intervention of instructors can be described in the same language of constraints and movement.

Summary

In summary, the increasing focus on the role of task constraints to action has facilitated a growing appreciation of the more general influences of the task in our theorizing about motor learning and control. To paraphrase, it is increasingly recognized that a task is not a task is not a task. Each task brings its own set of constraints that meld to form the confluence of constraints to movement in action (Newell 1986). This realization of the influential role of task constraints not only influences descriptions of movement in action, but also provides boundary conditions to theorizing about motor control.

The ETA model of Burton and Davis is clearly a development from and is compatible with the constraints perspective to motor learning and development outlined in Newell 1986. The ETA model places emphasis on the process of changing the relevant dimensions of a functional task to gain insights into the dynamics of the behavior of the performer, as well as to provide the instructor clues for developing instructional strategies. Ecological Task Analysis seems to be a very useful perspective for the dual consideration of learning and teaching in physical activity.

Functional Role of Variability in Movement Coordination and Disability

Richard E.A. Van Emmerik, PhD

Current research emerging from nonlinear dynamics and chaos theory has challenged traditional perspectives that associated high variability with performance decrements and pathology. These new insights in biological function provided by dynamical systems approaches are finding their way into clinical applications, such as the diagnosis and treatment of heart disease, neurological disorders, schizophrenia, sleep disorders, and many more (Glass 2001; Glass and Mackey 1988). In the human movement domain, the Ecological Task Analysis model by Burton and Davis (Davis and Burton 1991) signifies the primary effort to implement dynamical systems perspectives into clinical practice, learning, and rehabilitation. The ETA model was designed to provide insight into the dynamics of movement behavior from the perspective that the emergence of human movement is dynamically constrained by three essential elements, namely the performer, context or environment, and the task (Newell 1986).

The basic tenets of the ETA model are that

1. variation is essential, not a problem to be corrected;
2. actions are defined in terms of relations, not parts;
3. the goal of a task remains constant across instructional variation of the task, defining the essential and nonessential variables; and
4. performer-scaled or intrinsic dimensions should be used to classify and assess performance.

These four basic tenets of the ETA model are critical for developing proper diagnosis and intervention strategies for older people and those who have physical and mental disabilities.

Coordination in human movement involves the integration of multiple degrees of freedom into coherent functional units. This integration is important not only within levels of analysis (e.g., motor unit, muscle, joint) but also between different levels or subsystems, as in the coordination of locomotion and respiration (McDermott, Van Emmerik, and Hamill 2003). In research on human and animal movement, it is widely accepted that there is redundancy: Our action systems enable different solutions to a particular task. Bernstein (1967) defined coordination as overcoming excessive degrees of freedom, thereby turning joints, segments, muscles, and motor units into controllable systems. Especially in the early phases of acquiring new movement repertoires, elimination or freezing is considered a strategy to allow controllability of the redundant degrees of freedom in the action system (Bernstein 1967; Vereijken et al. 1992). Later in learning, degrees of freedom are released and optimized. More current views are moving away from defining coordination as overcoming excessive or redundant degrees of freedom and argue that all degrees of freedom contribute to the task, offering both stability and flexibility (e.g., Latash, Scholz, and Schöner 2002). In a similar approach proposed by Riccio (1993), the interaction between subsystems (such as the postural and manual) is critical for successful task performance.

Whether the multiple degrees of freedom underlying human movement are considered redundant or not, it is without question that the presence of these different elements is a major source of variability in human movement. Variability has traditionally been considered detrimental, and researchers have often avoided or eliminated variability as a source of error in their data. In the assessment of coordination changes due to aging and disease, the presence of variability is still regarded as one of the most powerful indicators of performance decrement.

A substantial and growing body of literature in the biological and physical sciences stresses the beneficial and adaptive aspects of variability in system function. These developments are in remarkable contrast to previous perspectives in which decreased variability was universally associated with increased competence, skill, and health. Instead, the path to frailty or disease cannot be identified solely by increased variability in fundamental variables reflecting biological function (Lipsitz 2002). More and more, research based on nonlinear dynamical and complex systems approaches is beginning to explore the role of variability in pattern formation. In this endeavor, critical elements are the assessment of the nature of variability, the dynamics under which systems change from regular to irregular behavior (or vice versa), and the role of variability in pattern change.

This chapter presents an overview of this emerging line of research and makes a strong case for the functional role of variability in movement coordination. It is shown that reductions in variability may be associated with performance decrement, frailty due to aging, and disability. Tools and methodologies that have emerged from dynamical systems perspectives and the ETA model are discussed in the context of coordination during postural control and locomotion. The following sections focus primarily on the implication of these emerging concepts for understanding stability and transitions in movement coordination, and in particular how aging and disease affect persistent and transitory aspects of human motor behavior.

After an overview of key issues regarding the role of variability in motor control, the chapter presents theoretical and empirical evidence that variability can play a functional role in maintaining pattern stability and in movement transitions. This is followed by an overview of current research on the role of variability in aging and disease. Implications of these dynamical systems concepts of stability and change for further research and practice are discussed.

Current Perspectives on Variability and Stability in Coordination

Research based on nonlinear dynamics and complex systems approaches is changing our perspectives regarding the role of variability in movement coordination. This section presents an overview of the different aspects of variability and the implementation of the functional aspects of variability in movement coordination and perception research.

Sources of Variability

Biological systems exhibit variation in performance that is visible both within and between measurements. This variation can be fundamentally of two different forms, namely noise due to measurement error and variation due to inherent dynamics of the system (Kantz and Schreiber 1997). The first source of variability, measurement noise, is independent of and additive to the dynamics of interest. Equipment noise, electrical interference, and movement artifacts are examples of sources contributing to this measurement noise. Traditional filtering techniques in biomechanics and motor control focus on separating measurement noise from the original signal.

A second source of biological variation is dynamical variability, which arises from within the system to be studied. In this case no clear separation can be obtained between the "original" signal and variability. This form of variability emerges from underlying nonlinearities and is important for pattern formation, sensation, and perception in biology (Glass 2001; Schöner and Kelso 1988a).

In most research in motor control and biomechanics, variability has been treated primarily as emerging from measurement noise. More specifically, in motor learning and development, increased movement skill has been associated with decreased variability. Similarly, increased variability is often used to identify the detrimental aspects associated with aging and disease. Current developments in nonlinear dynamics and complex systems perspectives are now emphasizing the functional aspects of variability intrinsic to nonlinear systems (Glass 2001). There is growing awareness that aging and disease can be associated with a loss of complexity and variability (Lipsitz 2002; Vaillancourt and Newell 2002; Van Emmerik and Van Wegen 2002). The degree of complexity is typically associated with the number of system elements and their functional interactions. Research supporting this change in perspective on the role of variability has emerged in a wide range of different domains, such as in the function of the heart, brain, and locomotor system in health and disease (Glass 2001; Lipsitz 2002).

Variability in Movement Coordination and Perception

According to Turvey and Carello (1996), fundamental principles of movement coordination are revealed most elegantly through the study and modeling of rhythmic movements. A major impetus for the development of such models was provided through the work of the physiologist Von Holst (1939/1973). Modeling approaches at the level of synergies, inspired by the work of Von Holst (1939/1973) and Bernstein (1996), have focused on the level of observables without making assumptions about the internal details of the component oscillators. Specifically, phase relations between oscillators are the variables through which basic principles of coordination can be discovered. Proponents of both the synergetics (e.g., Haken, Kelso, and Bunz 1985; Kelso 1995) and the natural-physical approaches to movement coordination (Kugler and Turvey 1987; Turvey and Carello 1996) have advocated this approach. In the synergetics approach, a distinction is made between collective or *order parameters* and *control parameters.* Order parameters identify the macroscopic aspects of the system and specify the collective behavior of the components involved. The stability and transition dynamics of a synergy can be revealed by the systematic manipulation of a control parameter. Such control parameters can be used to reveal regions of stability and instability in coordination and also establish the role of variability in pattern change.

The importance of control parameters is clearly emphasized in Glass and Mackey's (1988) dynamical diseases approach. In dynamical diseases, loss or reduction of function emerges when regular spatiotemporal processes break down and are replaced by some abnormal dynamic. The nature of these normal and abnormal biological rhythms is typically examined on the basis of nonlinear mathematical models, in which control parameters are essential in inducing a pattern change (Glass 2001; Glass and Mackey 1988; Winfree 1980, 1987). In the dynamical diseases approach, three types of qualitative change in oscillatory behavior can emerge, namely (1) the appearance of regular oscillations in a biological control system that normally does not show oscillatory behavior; (2) the appearance of new periodicities in a process that is already periodic; and (3) the disappearance of rhythmic processes.

In movement coordination, increased variability in the coordination dynamics has been observed before a transition to a new pattern. This has been shown in work on bimanual coordination (Kelso 1995; Schöner and Kelso 1988a) in which subjects were asked to oscillate both index fingers in an anti-phase mode while gradually increasing movement frequency. Movement frequency was used as a control parameter in these experiments, whereas the relative phasing between the hands was the order parameter. At a critical frequency, an abrupt change to an in-phase pattern was observed (see figure 2.1). These transition patterns are characterized by increased fluctuations (higher variability) in the relative phasing of the two limbs. In locomotion, increased fluctuations have been observed in segmental coordination in the transition from walking to running (Diedrich and Warren 1995). Reduced variability in the coordination dynamics during locomotion has been associated with an inability to switch gait patterns in Parkinson's disease (Van Emmerik et al. 1999) and lower extremity injury (Hamill et al. 1999; Heiderscheit, Hamill, and Van Emmerik 2002).

In research on sensory detection, Collins, Imhoff, and Grigg (1996) have shown that when a given input noise is added to very weak local indentations to the tip of the finger, detection of touch is significantly enhanced over that with a stimulus with no superimposed noise. These results suggest that noise can provide information and could play a critical role in exploration (Riccio 1993). More recently, Priplata and colleagues (2002) and Gravelle and colleagues (2002) have shown that added noise to the feet or lower extremity can enhance balance control in older and younger individuals. These results suggest that randomly vibrating shoe inserts may compensate for sensory loss or elevated perceptual thresholds due to aging and disease. Added noise could also be used in the design

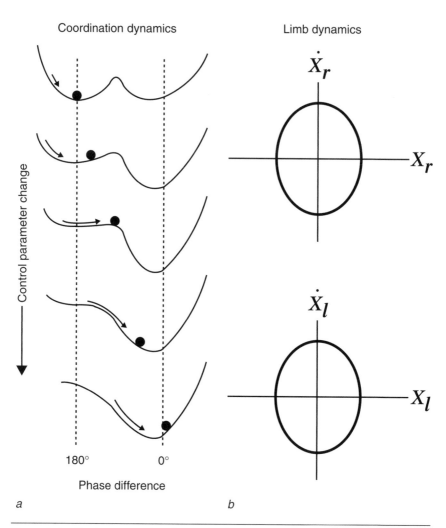

Figure 2.1 Control parameter change leading to a transition in pattern dynamics from anti-phase to in-phase coupling in bimanual finger coordination. *(a)* Coordination dynamics of the relative phase are expressed in the form of point attractors. Zero degrees relative phase represents in-phase coordination, while anti-phase coordination is indicated by a relative phase of 180°. *(b)* Individual limb oscillations can be expressed in the form of limit-cycle oscillations. x_l and x_r represent left and right limb oscillation amplitude; overdots indicate velocity.

of haptic interfaces and virtual environments and may aid in detection of stability boundaries during postural control.

Vaillancourt and Newell (2002) have recently proposed that the beneficial aspects of variability may be task dependent. In more discrete output tasks, such as tracking a required level of isometric force with the index finger, increasing force variability enhances performance. In contrast, in more rhythmic tracking tasks, decreasing the level of force variability may enhance performance (Newell et al. 2003). But it is also possible that the functionality of variability may change with different types of variables, such as movement outcome (a pattern drawn in handwriting) versus performance variables (underlying joint, segmental, and muscular coordination; see Latash, Scholz, and Schöner 2002). Collectively, these results show that different task, organismic, and environmental constraints could have a significant impact on the role of variability in human performance.

One of the conclusions to be drawn from this brief review is that the association of health and disease with either low or high levels of variability might not provide sufficient insights into the role of variability in movement control. The significance of variability for movement coordination and control will emerge more clearly when deeper insight is established regarding (1) the role of variability in maintaining stable movement and postural patterns, (2) the role of variability in pattern change, and (3) the nature or structure of variability and its role in stability and adaptability of human motor performance. The following sections address these three aspects of variability in more detail.

Role of Variability in Maintaining Stable Movement Performance

Much of the research on the control of locomotion and posture has focused on variability as a negative aspect, often used to identify pathology and performance decrement. In addition, increased variability has often been assumed to identify less stable patterns. The next sections offer a different perspective that emphasizes the functional role of variability in the control of posture and locomotion.

Gait Variability and Stability: Are They the Same?

A common assumption in gait studies is that increased variability in traditional gait parameters (such as stride length and stride frequency) is associated with instability and increased risk for falling during locomotion (e.g., Gabel and Nayak 1984). Although increased variability in the spatiotemporal patterns of footfalls might indeed be indicative of risk of falling, this association leaves open the question of how falling and overall gait instability are related to dynamics of segmental coordination in the upper and lower body. As indicated earlier, in multiple degrees of freedom systems, variability in performance is an inevitable and necessary condition for optimality and adaptability. Variability patterns in traditional gait parameters, therefore, might not reflect variability patterns in segmental coordination of upper body and lower extremity segments (Heiderscheit 2000; Van Emmerik et al. 1999).

Another challenge to unequivocally linking degree of stride variability to risk of falling is based on recent findings that the structure of variability might reveal significant differences between gait patterns of healthy and disabled individuals. Hausdorff and colleagues (1996) have developed variability analyses based on fractal techniques, and have suggested that adaptability in gait is linked to changes in variability patterns of stride intervals.

Finally, current developments in stability analyses based on nonlinear dynamical techniques (Dingwell et al. 2001) have questioned the link between gait variability and stability measures. Dingwell and colleagues found no association between upper and lower body stability measures and variability in stride parameters. The stability analyses used by Dingwell and colleagues were based on methods developed by Rosenstein, Collins, and De Luca (1993) in which the degree of convergence and divergence of these patterns are assessed (see also Hurmuzlu, Basdogan, and Stoianovici 1996). These authors assessed local dynamic stability of trunk translational and rotational motions. Although global stability measures accommodate finite perturbations (as might occur during a slip or fall), local stability measures capture very small ongoing perturbations to locomotion. The stride-to-stride fluctuations that occur during locomotion are thought to reflect the presence of these local perturbations. The relation between variability and stability in the trunk, however, needs further examination, especially under more challenging postural conditions.

Segmental Coordination, Variability, and Gait Stability

Humans have the ability to choose movement patterns that minimize metabolic energy expenditure, a process that has been referred to as self-optimization (Holt et al. 1995; Sparrow and Newell 1998). Stride frequency has been identified as a parameter that is chosen to minimize metabolic cost for a given locomotor speed. Holt and colleagues (1995) had subjects walk on a level treadmill at their preferred stride frequency and at frequencies above and below preferred. The legs were modeled as a pair of periodically forced harmonic oscillators. This model predicted that, at resonance, a minimum forcing would be necessary to maintain the oscillatory pattern. Subjects chose preferred stride frequencies that were the same as predicted by the model at resonance. A U-shaped oxygen consumption curve was also reported in response to the varying stride frequencies, with the minimum at the preferred stride frequency. These findings have been reproduced during running as well (Hamill, Derrick, and Holt 1995). Walking at the preferred frequencies resulted not only in minimal metabolic cost but also in maximal stability of the head and joints. These findings suggest a complementary relationship between physiological and stability constraints at the preferred frequency of locomotion (Holt et al. 1995). It is now well established in movement research that preferred modes of coordination (defined in terms of frequency and phase relationships between components) arise because of stability constraints (Kelso 1995; Kugler and Turvey 1987).

Another significant finding from the Holt and colleagues (1995) study was that spectral power of the preferred frequency increased systematically from distal segments (e.g., ankle) to proximal segments (head). The authors interpreted these differences in spectral power as systematic shifts in stability of segments from distal to proximal. These shifts would allow flexibility to adapt to perturbations and maintain a stable visual platform at the head (Holt et al. 1995; Pozzo, Berthoz, and Lefort 1990).

In comparison to the extensive gait literature on lower extremity function, relatively little is known about the contribution of the upper body to locomotor stability. Saunders, Inman, and Eberhart (1953) identified pelvic and trunk motion as essential determinants of bipedal gait, and coordination between the trunk and pelvis has been demonstrated to be an important aspect of postural stability during locomotion (McGibbon and Krebs 2002; Murray, Kory, and Clarkson 1964; Van Emmerik and Wagenaar 1996b). In human walking, the coordination between pelvis and trunk in the transverse plane changes in young healthy subjects from being close to in-phase at low speeds to out-of-phase patterns at higher speeds. This increased counterrotation is necessary to reduce the overall momentum of the trunk and maintain gait stability at higher walking speeds (see figure 2.2).

Stability and Variability in the Control of Upright Stance

A substantial body of research on postural control assesses postural stability on the basis of the excursion of the foot center of pressure. The center of pressure represents the point of application of the reactive forces at the support surface. Most studies report larger degrees of excursion and

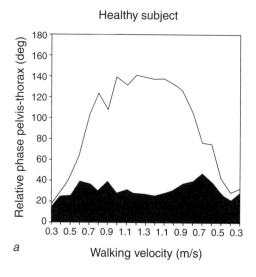

Healthy subject

a Walking velocity (m/s)

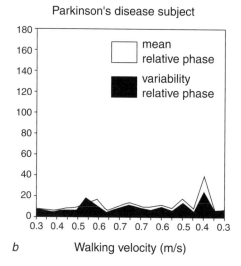

Parkinson's disease subject

mean
relative phase

variability
relative phase

b Walking velocity (m/s)

Figure 2.2   Examples of coordination changes in the relative phase between pelvic and thoracic rotations under systematic manipulation of walking speed. *(a)* Healthy subject. *(b)* Parkinson's disease subject. The patient with Parkinson's disease shows lack of adaptation in the coupling of the trunk with changes in movement velocity. This inability to change pattern is accompanied by a marked reduction in variability of relative phase.

greater variability of the center of pressure in older subjects as compared to younger subjects. This higher variability of center of pressure patterns is then often used as a measure of postural stability (e.g., Maki, Holliday, and Topper 1994). However, this assumed relation between increased center of pressure variation and loss of stability does not take into account (1) the fact that movement of the center of pressure corrects or controls for movement of the body center of mass (Winter 1995), (2) the structure or dynamics of these postural center of pressure patterns (Newell et al. 1993), or (3) the fact that upright posture is almost never an isolated task but integrated or "nested" within other task goals (such as opening doors or picking up an object).

An example of different time scales and variability patterns of the centers of pressure and mass and their role in postural control is illustrated in figure 2.3. The center of pressure (COP) patterns in figure 2.3 exhibit higher frequency characteristics than the center of mass (COM). The higher frequencies in the COP are a necessary aspect to control or correct the COM position (Winter 1995). It is said that the center of pressure

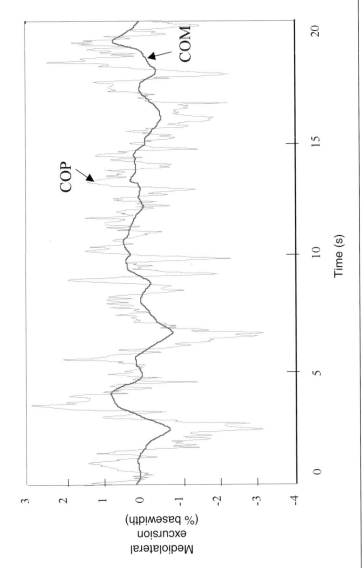

Figure 2.3 Mediolateral center of pressure (COP: thin line) and center of mass (COM: thick line) trajectories during quiet stance in a healthy subject. The mediolateral excursion is expressed as a percentage of the lateral distance between the feet.

"corrals" the center of mass. These higher frequency aspects in the COP, however, not only reflect compensatory activity, but also could result from exploratory activity that may contribute to postural stability.

Recent nonlinear analysis techniques emphasize the assessment of pattern dynamics in state space (Kantz and Schreiber 1997; Strogatz 1994). The state space represents the essential state variables that define a system. Proper reconstruction of this state space enables an accurate description and assessment of system complexity, stability, and change. Preferred regions in this state space onto which the dynamics settle are called "attractors." In figure 2.4, different types of state space patterns are drawn. In random patterns there is no preferred region of the center of pressure in state space, and the number of state space variables is infinite and lacking in attracting properties. An example of such an apparently random pattern is presented in figure 2.4a, where the axes could represent the anterior-posterior and mediolateral dimensions of the center of

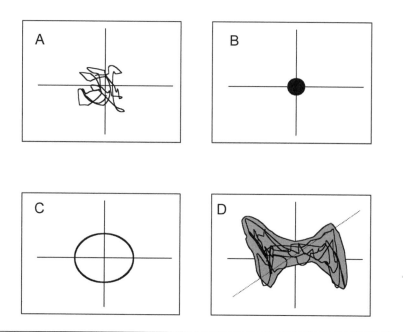

Figure 2.4   Different types of attractors in state space. *(a)* Random pattern without attracting properties. *(b)* Fixed-point attractor: The center of pressure pattern converges onto a fixed point in the postural state space, formed by the anterior-posterior and mediolateral components of the center of pressure. *(c)* Limit-cycle attractor. The postural dynamic converges to a stable cycle in state space. *(d)* Chaotic attractor in higher-dimensional state space. The dimensionality of the state space and attractor increases from point to limit-cycle to chaotic attractor.

pressure. Attraction to a single point in state space is called fixed-point attraction (figure 2.4*b*). Regions in state space that are attracting can also be in the form of a cycle or limit-cycle attractor. In this case, postural states are being attracted toward a cyclic pattern with minimally two state space dimensions (figure 2.4*c*). This type of dynamic shows resistance to perturbations but is less flexible and adaptable when a change in postural state is needed. In higher-dimensional state spaces (three and up), quasi-periodic and chaotic attractors can emerge (figure 2.4*d*). The chaotic attractor shows both stable attraction to a region in state space and variability. These dual features are now associated with the higher pattern complexity that is reflective of healthy and expert systems. As an example, increased heart rate variability is considered an important indicator of healthy heart function, reflecting a degree of complexity in organization in which disruptions can be compensated for and changes in rhythm occur more easily (Glass 2001; Lipsitz 2002).

The control and maintenance of upright posture are, in most natural activities, nested within other task goals of the organism. Upright stance is a fundamental prerequisite in, for example, opening doors, picking up objects, and observing different aspects of the environment. Increased sway can arise from exploratory activity, which may or may not be destabilizing (Riccio 1993; Van Wegen, Van Emmerik, and Riccio 2002). In order for exploratory behavior not to interfere with the required movement pattern, variability due to exploratory dynamics occurs at smaller time scales (lower amplitude and higher frequency) than the actual movements (Riccio 1993). However, in most postural control research, higher-frequency components have traditionally been eliminated as unwanted sources of noise.

Adaptive Control and the Perception of Stability Boundaries

A critical element in the proposal that variability plays a role in facilitating adaptive postural control is that it allows for the exploration of the limits of current states and boundaries between different postural configurations. In the control of quasi-static upright stance, the center of mass needs to remain within the base of support formed by the boundaries of the feet. This base of support forms the limit for which a change in postural state (e.g., a step, a fall, a reach to hold on to a supporting object) is not required and perturbations can be reversed. Current research on postural control increasingly focuses on the role of these boundaries in the maintenance of upright balance (Slobounov et al. 1998; Van Wegen, Van Emmerik, and Riccio 2002). Changes in control with respect to these boundaries may also be playing a role in loss of stability due to aging and Parkinson's disease (Van Wegen et al. 2001; Van Wegen, Van Emmerik, and Riccio 2002).

A central requirement for the robust and adaptive control of human movement is the ability to perceive the range of effectiveness of a variety of action systems. Action systems can be operationalized within the same musculoskeletal segments, as can be seen, for example, in ankle and hip compensatory strategies (Horak, Henry, and Shumway-Cook 1997). However, these action systems could also involve overlapping or nested segments, as in the interaction of postural and manual control. Detection of effectiveness of stability boundaries implies observability of one's own postural state relative to these boundaries. Riccio and colleagues have developed an approach that emphasizes the functional role of variability in the detection of these stability boundaries (Riccio 1993; Riccio and Stoffregen 1988; Van Wegen, Van Emmerik, and Riccio 2002). Exploratory behavior is critical and provides persistent excitation of adaptive perception-action systems. A central element in this approach is that the most important and elementary aspects of the animal–environment interaction are the affordances of postural behavior (Riccio 1993). These affordances refer to the consequences that certain body configurations have for the pickup of information and achievement of task goals. An essential element of postural control is therefore the maintenance of orientation and stability of motor and sensory systems (such as the head and upper body) over variations in the organism, environment, and task. Movement variability in the form of exploratory dynamics provides robustness in the postural system and the freedom to adopt orientations that are not optimal with respect to particular task-relevant criteria (e.g., stability; Riccio and Stoffregen 1988).

The ability to perceive the spatiotemporal proximity to a stability boundary has been proposed as an important determinant for postural stability (Riccio 1993). In visual perception, time-to-contact information can be obtained through retinal changes due to optic flow. Time to contact is the time that remains before an approaching object "hits" the observer or before a surface is contacted, and reflects position and velocity information. An object that is threatening to hit you (such as an approaching ball) would be characterized by a symmetrical outflow of the optic pattern from the center of the ball, signaling the closing in of the ball to the target. Lee and colleagues have shown that organisms use time-to-contact information from this optic flow to guide the timing of purposeful actions and to maintain postural stability (Lee and Reddish 1981; Lishman and Lee 1973).

The time-to-contact approach has recently been extended to sensory and perceptual aspects of posture other than the visual system (Haddad et al. 2006; Slobounov et al. 1998; Van Wegen et al. 2001; Van Wegen, Van Emmerik, and Riccio 2002). The time to the stability boundary in upright stance can be obtained from distance and velocity of the center of pressure with respect to the base of support provided by both feet. An example of a time series of the temporal margin to the anterior stability boundary is shown in figure 2.5.

The spatiotemporal margin of the center of gravity or center of pressure with respect to these stability boundaries might be a key variable for

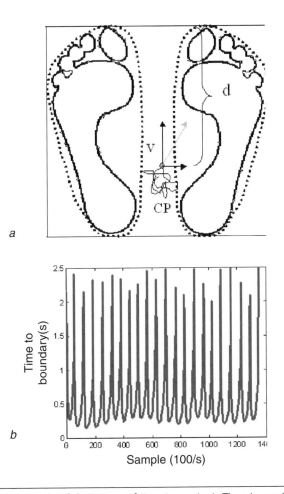

Figure 2.5 *(a)* Schematic of derivation of time to contact. Time to contact is obtained by the ratio of the distance, d, to the boundary and the instantaneous velocity, V, for every data point. *(b)* A time series of assembled temporal margins to the anterior-posterior stability boundary (see Van Wegen, Van Emmerik, and Riccio 2002 for a more detailed description). CP = foot center of pressure.

upright postural control. Techniques developed by Schöner and colleagues could reveal the importance (i.e., whether this is an essential or nonessential variable) of this time-to-contact variable for postural control (e.g., Latash, Scholz, and Schöner 2002). Research along these lines should elucidate whether these boundaries are in fact perceivable, and if variation in task dimensions (e.g., reaching distance or platform perturbations) leaves aspects of boundary-relevant dynamics (such as minimum time-to-contact threshold) relatively invariant. Support for the invariance of boundary-relevant measures comes from observations that time-to-contact measures do not appear to be less than 200 to 300 milliseconds (Riccio 1993).

In sum, postural control strategies that allow and optimize on exploratory behavior are anticipated to benefit the detection of these stability boundaries. Adaptability in postural control might therefore emerge from the ability to control behavior with respect to these stability boundaries.

Nested Systems: Interaction Between Postural and Manual Control

Performance on many manual tasks is dependent on body configuration as well as movement. Postural adjustments are essential in tasks involving, for example, looking at or looking around objects or people, reaching, and touching (Gibson 1966; Riccio 1993). Body movements (i.e., variations in posture) influence the precision of visual and prehensile tasks. In other words, configuration and stability have consequences for the ease or difficulty of seeing or manipulating objects (Riccio and Stoffregen 1988; Riccio 1993). Visual or manual performance, therefore, should not only be evaluated in isolation; it may also serve as an evaluation function for body configuration. As such, body configuration may be perceived and controlled with respect to performance on suprapostural tasks. These suprapostural tasks can change optimal regions in postural configuration space. Riccio (1993) described techniques to assess the effects of body configuration on performance in suprapostural tasks, such as during interval production. In this experiment subjects performed a manual task under different postural configurations (see figure 2.6). The manual control task in this study required that subjects tap at a constant rate and with constant force on an electronic keyboard. The results revealed a strong quadratic relation between postural configuration and variability of force. The manifold is shaped like a saddle, with the inflection point close to erect stance, showing distinct increases and decreases in variability in force production with different body postures (see figure 2.6).

Very few attempts have been made to analyze postural control and stability during manual tasks. In a recent study, Whittlesey (2003)

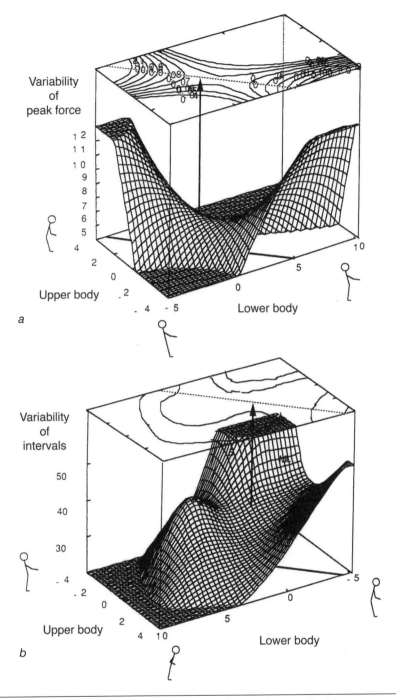

Figure 2.6 Effects of postural orientation (in degrees from vertical for upper and lower body) on *(a)* variability in peak force and *(b)* intervals between consecutive taps during a finger tapping task during upright standing. The response surfaces are derived from quadratic regression. Bold arrows represent erect stance.

Reprinted, by permission, from G.E. Riccio, 1993, Information in movement variability. About the qualitative dynamics of posture and orientation. In *Variability and Motor Control*, edited by K.M. Newell and D.M. Corcos (Champaign, IL: Human Kinetics), 347.

explored the forces, body accelerations, moments, and alignment of forces during a series of nested postural and manual tasks. A central element in this study was the calculation of moments of manual forces about the feet. Another important measure that was developed was that of whole-body center of pressure. This body center of pressure was used as an analogue to the foot center of pressure usually calculated in quiet upright stance research. In postural-manual control, the body center of pressure represents the balancing point of the body. Another critical element in the work by Whittlesey (2003) is the formal assessment of the necessity to lean in the direction of the force required through manual action. Therefore, body lean and associated changes in variation in center of pressure movement (e.g., variability) are critical elements under the dual task constraints of manual performance and the maintenance of a stable postural configuration (see also Van Wegen, Van Emmerik, and Riccio 2002). In other words, during nested tasks such as in postural and manual control, the foot position, stepping strategies, and variation in degree of body lean become essential performance variables. These variables, however, are typically constrained or controlled for in much of the research on postural control (such as a fixed foot position). Most research on postural control regards adaptations of ankle and hip strategies as primary, with a stepping strategy as a "last resort." The work by Whittlesey (2003) clearly challenges this view, demonstrating that stepping is an important strategy and that during manual exertion, foot placement and body orientation or lean are critically important and effective in maintaining balance. In the ecological assessment of postural control, ankle and hip strategies, considered the preeminent strategies in much of the work on upright postural control, might be used only to fine-tune other, more common postural strategies.

Role of Variability in Pattern Change

The research presented in the previous section clearly established the functional role of variability in maintaining stable coordinative patterns under different sets of postural and movement constraints. This section presents research that provides evidence for the functional role of variability in movement pattern change.

Variability and Change in Bimanual Coordination

Over the past two decades, between-limb coordination has been studied extensively on the basis of the Haken, Kelso, and Bunz (HKB) model

(Haken et al. 1985). The HKB model has made fundamental contributions to our understanding of stability and change in pattern formation in human movement. A key element of the synergetic theory of self-organization is that nonequilibrium phase transitions are characterized by instabilities (Kelso 1995). Essential aspects of these instabilities are (1) a strong enhancement of fluctuations *(critical fluctuations)* and (2) a large increase in the time it takes to recover from a disturbance and return to steady state *(critical slowing down)*.

Critical fluctuations in complex systems arise due to influences of elements at a more microscopic level compared to the level of interest. These microscopic influences, together with environmental fluctuations, "pull" the system away from its current attractor state. Fluctuations in relative phase characterize the transition point from anti-phase to in-phase finger movements (Kelso, Scholz, and Schöner 1986). Similar fluctuations have been observed in the transition between walking and running (Diedrich and Warren 1995) and upper body phase couplings in the human walking mode (Van Emmerik and Wagenaar 1996b; Wagenaar and Van Emmerik 2000).

Critical slowing down around the transition point is best shown by the changes and deformations in the potential landscape around the anti-phase attractor in figure 2.1. As the control parameter reaches its critical point, the potential well becomes more and more shallow, and a disturbance away from the fixed point will result in a slow relaxation back to the potential minimum (i.e., the relaxation time will be longer compared to that in the situation at lower frequencies when the potential well is steep; Scholz, Kelso, and Schöner 1987).

Variability and Coordination Change in Gait Patterns

Humans and animals move about in their environment through a variety of distinct locomotor patterns or gaits. Quadrupedal gaits are often distinguished on the basis of changes in interlimb coordination or footfall patterns (as in the walk, trot, and gallop in horses). In humans, different gait modes (e.g., walk, run) are typically distinguished on the basis of the presence or absence of a bipedal flight phase. This criterion, however, does not provide sufficient insights into the different coordination patterns that may emerge in bipedal locomotion (Van Emmerik, Wagenaar, and Van Wegen 1998).

Physiological and mechanical factors, such as metabolic energy usage and mechanical loading of the limbs and torso, have been proposed as "triggers" for changes in these gait patterns (Hutchinson et al. 2003).

Alternatively, the role of stability in gait transitions has been assessed on the basis of coordination dynamics within and between limb segments (e.g., Diedrich and Warren 1995; Schöner, Jiang, and Kelso 1990; Wagenaar and Van Emmerik 2000). This research is based on a dynamical and complex systems framework and has yielded new insights into the mechanisms of coordination change, the emergence of stable gait modes, and the role of variability in pattern change. Through use of this approach, increased variability in segmental coordination in the lower extremities has been observed before a transition from walking to running (Diedrich and Warren 1995). Observations of increased variability at certain walking speeds in the coordination dynamics of the upper body have resulted in the suggestion that there are at least two qualitatively different patterns within the human walking gait (Van Emmerik and Wagenaar 1996b; Van Emmerik, Wagenaar, and Van Wegen 1998; Wagenaar and Van Emmerik 2000). These coordinative modes are characterized by different relative phase patterns (see figure 2.2) as well as different frequency ratios between arm and leg oscillations.

Assessing the Nature of Variability

As indicated in the introduction to this chapter, the association of health and disease with either low or high levels of variability might not be productive in an assessment of the role of variability in movement control. More recent work from the perspective of nonlinear dynamics and complex systems approaches has made inroads in examining more closely the temporal structure and nature of variability in stride intervals during locomotion (e.g., Hausdorff et al. 1996) and in the control of upright stance (e.g., Collins and De Luca 1995). In addition, Newell, Liu, and Mayer-Kress (2001) have provided a theoretical foundation for the role of variation at different temporal scales in learning and development.

Time Scales and Variability in Postural Control

Different approaches have emerged to investigate changes in the pattern of variability across time. Collins and colleagues have developed spatiotemporal analyses to assess postural center of pressure patterns (Collins and De Luca 1995; Collins et al. 1995). This analysis technique can reveal the time scales over which particular postural strategies show "persistence" (continue with current strategy) or "antipersistence" (reverse or change strategy). Changes in these time scales have been observed in older adults and patients with Parkinson's disease when compared to younger healthy individuals, suggesting a more lenient postural strategy with aging and disease (Collins et al. 1995; Mitchell et al. 1995). From this perspective, loss of stability might not be associated with center of pressure excursion or variability per se, but with changes in temporal windows over which postural strategies change.

The different time scales underlying postural control have also been divided into the temporal aspects that reflect control and modification of actuators (relatively long) and those that reflect observability and information gain (relatively short) (Riccio 1993). From this perspective, short-duration, high-frequency temporal aspects not only are reflective of corrective actions, as has been shown in the research by Collins and colleagues, but also can be a sign of exploratory behavior with the goal of changing ongoing (lower frequency) control of actuators.

Time Scales and Variability in Rhythmic Movement

Recent developments in research on locomotion based on nonlinear dynamical techniques have emphasized the importance of the temporal structure in variability. Rather than focusing on degree of variability, techniques such as detrended fluctuation analysis (DFA) seek self-similarity in patterns (Hausdorff et al. 1996, 1997). The DFA analysis demonstrates that variability in stride intervals is not simply attributable to uncorrelated random fluctuations in the form of white noise. In contrast, the stride interval fluctuations exhibited long-range power law correlations. These long-range correlations are signatures of fractal processes in which fluctuations at one (shorter) time scale are statistically similar to fluctuations at another (longer) time scale. In Gaussian distributions, population mean and variance converge to finite values when the number of observations is increased. In contrast, in fractal processes (such as coastlines, branchings in lung alveoli), population mean and variance are meaningless. The mean and variance of these fractals depend on the resolution of the measuring device used. Scaling functions emerge in which changes in fluctuations under different resolutions of measurement can be assessed. The fractal nature of stride interval fluctuations indicates positive correlations in the duration of subsequent steps at time scales ranging from milliseconds to seconds to hours. The DFA analysis quantifies the nature of these fluctuations that can range from random to highly correlated. Correlated fluctuations have been found to be indicative of healthy and optimal system function. Detrended fluctuation analysis is a modified random walk analysis, in which self-similar scaling can be observed if the fluctuations at different observation windows scale as a power law with the window size.

Scaling exponents for white noise are expected to be found at $\alpha = 0.5$. For $0.5 < \alpha < 1$, there are long-range fractal correlations. An $\alpha < 0.5$ indicates antipersistent correlations.

Current Perspectives on the Role of Variability in Disability

Recent research on the control of posture and locomotion has begun to provide evidence against the traditional association between postural instability and the greater variability observed in some performance variables in people with disabilities. The following sections provide an overview of recent findings from this dynamical systems research.

Postural Stability and Variability

Postural instability is regarded as one of the major symptoms of individuals with Parkinson's disease. Research on postural control has shown increases as well as decreases in the variability of the center of pressure in these patients (see Van Wegen et al. 2001 for an overview). Although differences in study methodology and patient population could partially contribute to these different findings, it is also possible that the variability of the foot center of pressure may be necessary but not sufficient for assessing postural stability problems in patients with Parkinson's disease. Instead, postural control measures that reflect the relationship between the organism and task-relevant stability boundaries may be a necessary addition to postural stability research in aging and disease.

Several studies have examined the time to contact of the center of pressure to the stability boundary (Slobounov et al. 1998; Van Wegen et al. 2001; Van Wegen, Van Emmerik, and Riccio 2002). This research revealed a reduction in time to stability boundaries in older adults as compared to younger adults, indicating that these measures could be useful for the study of populations that suffer from postural instability. In the studies by Van Wegen and colleagues (2001, 2002), older subjects did not show the increase in variability in center of pressure usually observed in older populations (figure 2.7a). These older subjects did, however, show reductions in mediolateral temporal margins (see figure 2.7b). Patients showed further reductions in lateral stability margins compared to healthy older adults (see figure 2.7b).

These results suggest that variability measures of the center of pressure alone might not be sufficient to reveal changes in the postural system

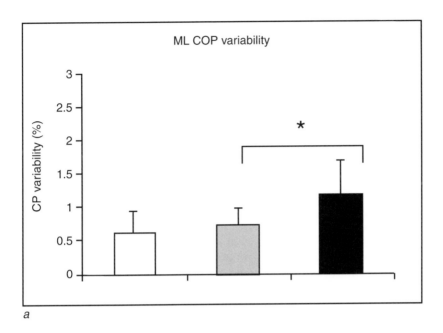

a

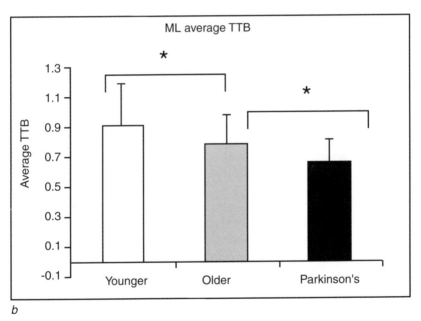

b

Figure 2.7 Changes in mediolateral foot center of pressure (CP) in healthy young and older age groups as well as in individuals with Parkinson's disease. *(a)* Variability of CP; *(b)* average minimum time to contact(s) to stability boundary (TTB). Error bars reflect both between-subject variation and within-subject variation due to averaging a variety of lean conditions. Asterisk indicates statistically significant difference at *p* = .05.

Data from Van Wegen et al. 2001, 2002.

that may lead to a loss of balance. This suggestion emerges from the observation that the older individuals clearly show changes in boundary-relevant measures that are not revealed by traditional center of pressure variability variables. In addition, the postural instability observed in many patients with Parkinson's disease could be related to reduced time to the lateral stability boundaries and not merely be the result of an increase in mediolateral sway variability.

Reduced Variability in Locomotion

Reduced variability in the coordination between lower extremity segments has been found in individuals with various pathologies. Jeng and colleagues (1996) found reduced variability in coordination between lower extremity joints in the affected limb during walking in children with spastic hemiplegic cerebral palsy. Using relative phase analysis, Hamill and colleagues (1999) observed reduced variability in intralimb couplings of the lower extremity during running in individuals with orthopedic injuries. The authors suggested that the reduction in variability might emerge from the selection of a few available movement patterns. Using vector coding techniques to assess variability in lower extremity angle–angle coordination patterns, Heiderscheit and colleagues (2002) did not observe reduced variability in individuals with patellofemoral pain when analyses were performed across the entire stride cycle. However, individuals with orthopedic injury showed reductions in variability in thigh-leg rotation around heel strike. Collectively, these data on lower extremity coordination demonstrate that pathological gait can be characterized by decreases in variability in the coordination between segments.

Van Emmerik and colleagues (1999) found changes in variability of the relative phase between the trunk and pelvis in the transverse plane in patients with Parkinson's disease during walking at a variety of speeds. This variability reflects the within-subject variation from stride to stride. Patients had significantly reduced levels of relative phase variability compared to age-matched healthy control subjects. An example of such a reduction in relative phase variability, and the related inability to change coordination patterns in the upper body, is presented in figure 2.2b. These observations of reduced variability are in direct contrast to the common assumption in gait studies that increased variability in traditional gait parameters (such as stride length and stride frequency) is associated with instability during locomotion. Instead, decreased variability can be interpreted as signifying a more rigid, less adaptive coupling between upper and lower body segments. This more rigid coupling, in turn, can be a contributing factor to transition problems in movement coordination often observed in these patients.

These changes in coupling between upper body segments might also play an important role in the recovery from perturbations to the gait pattern. Particularly relevant is how shock transmission is attenuated by coordination in the upper body and to what degree this attenuation is affected by locomotor speed and cadence. These issues have mainly been addressed in locomotion in healthy young persons (e.g., Hamill, Derrick, and Holt 1995). It is unknown at present whether and how these shock absorption mechanisms change with age and in individuals with disabilities.

The research discussed so far has identified reduction in variability with disability. Recently, Hausdorff and colleagues have also shown that the structure of variability changes with disease. Hausdorff and colleagues (1997) observed reductions in the scaling exponent α with aging and neurological disease (e.g., Huntington's disease). This reduction in scaling exponent indicates a more random pattern in stride interval fluctuation with aging and disease. These changes in the structure of variability are not necessarily related to the magnitude of the fluctuations, as no differences in stride interval variability were observed between groups. The results of these studies clearly demonstrate the importance of assessing the structure of variability in gait variables.

Implications for Further Research and Clinical Practice

This section presents implications for the further development and implementation of ETA principles in disability research in conjunction with summarizing the critical developments in dynamical and complex systems perspectives. The summary focuses in particular on aspects of variability, coordination, the identification of relevant variables that characterize performance, and the use of performer-scaled or intrinsic variables.

The different perspectives on the role of variability in movement performance are steadily making an impact on assessment of movement disorders. Lack of variability is increasingly regarded as a signature of pathology, injury, and aging (Hamill et al. 1999; Van Emmerik and Van Wegen 2002). Further development of nonlinear dynamical analysis techniques such as those presented in this overview will help in assessing the structure of variability and its role in learning, development, and disease.

Assessments of perceptual-motor performance are increasingly focused on relational (i.e., coordinative) aspects rather than performance statistics of individual elements. Biomechanical studies of lower extremity function are recognizing coordinative measures in the form of relative phase more and more as essential levels of system assessment (Hamill et al. 1999; Peters et al. 2003).

Many approaches in motor control continue to associate invariance in observable parameters as signatures of "internal" system control. The assumption is not only of a close one-to-one mapping between these internal control parameters and biomechanical observables, but also of reduced variance in a variable as indicative of control. Control variables should no longer be rigidly associated with invariance (e.g., Scholz and Schöner 1999). Instead, differential stability of variables may separate primary from secondary control variables in the central nervous system. The relative importance of different task variables in the control aspects of the task is evaluated by the degree of variability in joint configurations. Although the idea of assessing performance aspects by separating essential and nonessential variables was proposed a long time ago (Gelfand and Tsetlin 1971), Schöner and colleagues have recently developed methods to empirically distinguish these essential from nonessential variables (Scholz and Schöner 1999; Latash, Scholz, and Schöner 2002).

Recent developments have begun to incorporate stability boundaries and time-to-contact measures to these boundaries in the assessment of postural control. These measures no longer emphasize absolute body sway as a critical measure of disturbances of postural control, but instead emphasize postural variables with respect to subject-relevant boundaries or thresholds that may or may not elicit a change in postural strategy. In addition, recent research has begun to focus more on the interaction of postural and manual control (Whittlesey 2003). Although from the current research on posture and balance it is suggested that variability is important in the detection of stability boundaries, more direct evidence of the functionality of variability and its role in exploratory behavior is needed. However, the research clearly shows the importance of stability boundaries in the assessment of postural instability due to aging and disease. For the treatment of balance-impaired populations such as older adults and patients with Parkinson's disease, this notion can have a large impact: Instead of focusing on the reduction of postural variability, treatment could be aimed at increasing adaptability by stimulation of exploratory behavior with respect to stability limits.

KEY POINTS

- Variability may be beneficial rather than detrimental to system function and performance.
- In research studies, variability should not necessarily be eliminated or viewed as a source of error in data.
- Movement control variables should no longer be rigidly associated with invariance.
- Intervention strategies should not focus on reducing postural variability but on exploiting variability for the purpose of improving perception, exploration, and adaptability.
- Measures that reflect subject-related or intrinsic postural stability boundaries are performer-scaled and may offer new insights in changes in static and dynamic stability with aging and disability.

Summary

New insights into the role of variability in pattern formation have emerged with developments in nonlinear dynamics, chaos theory, and complex systems approaches. These developments have begun to challenge the long-held notion that increased variability is a sign of frailty due to aging or pathology, or that increasing skill level in perceptual-motor performance is universally associated with decreased variability. Dynamical systems approaches to movement coordination and control have emerged out of these nonlinear approaches and have yielded new perspectives and tools to assess stability and change in human movement. This chapter provided an overview of research on postural control and locomotion in which these tools from dynamical systems have been applied. This work so far has shown the importance of variability in gait transitions, has provided evidence that reduced variability and complexity are associated with frailty and pathology, and has demonstrated the role of variability in exploration and detection of stability boundaries in postural control. The ongoing research on the control of posture and locomotion will add to our understanding of basic control mechanisms as well as contribute to the clinical realm in the form of diagnosis and treatment. These current developments will strengthen the clinical application of the ETA model in all of its four basic tenets, in that new methods have been developed to assess (1) the functional role of variability for adaptation and exploration, (2) relational aspects of movement through new relative phase techniques

(McDermott, Van Emmerik, and Hamill 2003; Peters et al. 2003), (3) the nature of the control variables underlying coordinated performance, and (4) ecologically relevant behavioral measures that are performer scaled and represent the organism–environment–task interaction.

Conceptualizing Choice as Central to the ETA Applied Model: Broadening the Vision

Walter E. Davis, PhD, and Joyce Strand, PhD

> I never realized how many decisions I have had in my lifetime and how few of them I have made myself.
>
> *—Participant in decision-making seminar*

> To be imprisoned in one's own body is dreadful. To be confined to an institution for the profoundly retarded does not crush you in the same way. It just removes all hope.
>
> *—Crossley and McDonald,* Annie's Coming Out, *1980*

People make choices on a daily basis, many of which significantly affect their education, work, marriage, and family, and yet many of these choices are taken for granted. Indeed, much of behavior is "routinized," as sociologist Anthony Giddens describes it, and as such, unmotivated. Nevertheless, people often like to make decisions and to have choices, which are motivating in and of themselves. But "choices" are also often "made for us." To paraphrase Karl Marx, we make our own history but not under circumstances of our own choosing. We are all born into roles and resources that we do not select for ourselves. When we think about how we "choose" our profession, for example, we know there are many influential factors. Culture and beliefs are particularly important, especially our beliefs about nature and human nature (i.e., our world view). Also, one can be in the right (or wrong) place at the right (or wrong) time.

We thank Alan Costall, University of Portsmouth, for his review and comments.

A choice may be considered as an opportunity to make an unco-erced selection from two or more alternative events, consequences, or responses. But for Piaget, being an independent decision maker is not a right, but a capacity; and this is elaborated on in the theories of Giddens (agency), Mithaug (equal opportunity), and Deci (self-determination) as discussed later.

All this suggests that understanding choice is not as straightforward as it might seem at first, and that choosing is *not* something we should take for granted. Indeed, we argue that the idea of choice is extremely complicated and has far-reaching ramifications. What we intend to show is that "choice" is central to understanding human behavior and necessary for democracy. Thus, choice has tremendous implica-tions for educational practice. We consider several aspects of choice and show some of the many connections of choice to broader issues. We also discuss how choices are taken away from people. We offer that choice is not simply an individual act but is limited by, and contributes to, many social structures and social systems. People do not live in iso-lation but are connected to others spatially (globally) and temporally (historically).

What adds to the importance of this chapter is that choice, and indeed motivation in general, have not been given deserved attention in the textbooks and journals for adapted physical education. Motivation is perhaps the single greatest concern of those who work with students with disabilities. Two major funding efforts in special education have attempted to give people with disabilities more choices and enable them to become more self-determined (Wehmeyer 1998). It is important to know what choices we make for ourselves and when, and what choices are made for us and how, by whom, and by what.

Several ideas regarding choice are found in the literature dating back to antiquity. But two extreme notions we want to dismiss at the outset: Jean-Paul Sartre's idea of complete free will ("man makes himself") and Pierre Simon de Laplace's idea of absolute determinism. Clearly both the provision and the elimination of choices come about in many ways as people relate to their physical and social environments (e.g., Gove 1994). However, it is the deliberate elimination of some people's choices by others (though sometimes with good intention) that is of major concern here. The elimination of choices occurs particularly for those people believed incapable of making good decisions for themselves, which in today's society includes children, certain ethnic groups, females, persons who are elderly, and especially those with severe mental dis-abilities. "Persons with severe handicaps are probably one of the most vulnerable groups of persons at risk for having their choices limited by others and for experiencing learned helplessness" (Guess, Benson, and Siegel-Causey 1985, p. 83).

Special education professionals have studied the phenomena of choice and learned helplessness for several decades. However, neither issue has been given much consideration in adapted physical education, with at least one exception: Choice is an important feature in the Ecological Task Analysis model. In this chapter, we first conceptualize choice at several levels in an attempt to help fill the discussion void on choice and motivation in the adapted physical activity literature. In doing so, we attempt to show how choice can be viewed in many ways and is thus connected to many issues that are broader than the learning of movement skills. By connecting to these broader issues we hope to elevate the importance, indeed the necessity, of choice. We continue to broaden the vision in the second section when we discuss eliminating choice under the headings of structures of domination and the legacy of behaviorism. In the final section we provide ideas for creating opportunities for student choices within ETA.

Conceptualization of Choice

Choice is inherent in the second step of the ETA applied model (figure 3.1). Choice is not merely selecting among alternatives, having preferences, or making decisions but in fact does entail all of these and more. Here we conceptualize choice as seven different aspects of a more fundamental phenomenon. We discuss choice (a) at a systems level, (b) as a constraint, (c) as movement skills, (d) as having agency or power in

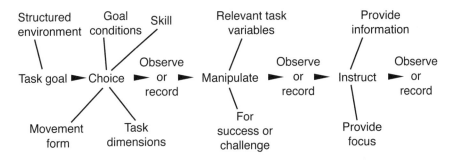

Figure 3.1   Ecological Task Analysis applied model: ETA model for assessment and instruction of movement tasks.

Reprinted, by permission, from W.E. Davis and A.W. Burton, 1991, "Ecological task analysis: translating movement theory into practice," *Adapted Physical Activity Quarterly* 8(2): 154-177.

a social context, (e) as decision making, (f) as intrinsic motivation, and (g) as self-realization or freedom in the highest sense. Clearly these seven aspects are both related to and distinct from one another. In addition, each choice situation entails a no-choice situation, and so each must also be conceptualized within a dialectical logic (Bhaskar 1993).

Choice at a Systems Level

Three types of systems have been described within systems theory: (a) open, (b) closed, and (c) isolated. We explain these here for heuristic purposes. An open system exchanges both matter and energy and can evolve. A closed system exchanges energy but not matter and does not evolve. An isolated system exchanges neither energy nor matter, and its movement is completely determined by the external energy gradients (e.g., gravity, inertia). Inanimate objects are isolated systems whose activity is determined by Newtonian laws. For example, the external force applied to the ball and the surface on which it travels determine a billiard ball's trajectory and that of any objects in its path. The behavior of isolated systems is completely governed by high-level energy or force fields.

In contrast, open systems, including the universe itself and all living systems, have on-board potential energy, which means that they are not tied to the external energy gradients (Kugler and Turvey 1987). Thus, for example, humans not only initiate their own movement; unlike a billiard ball, they can generally choose to avoid collisions with objects in their paths.

Closed systems include machines supplied with energy that, in some ways, appear to behave as humans. A prime example is a digital computer, which is distinguished from all other machines by two essential features: (a) its ability to store and execute programs that carry out conditional branching (that is, programs that are controlled by their own results to an arbitrary level of complexity) and (b) its ability to manipulate any kind of symbolic information at all, including numbers, characters, and images. "These features allow the same computer to 'be' many different machines: a calculator, a word processor, a control system, or a communication device" (Edwards 1996, pp. 27-28). Computers (and clocks) do not do physical work; rather they organize other machines or people that do the physical work. Such complexity gives computers the appearance of being humanlike, and they are indeed prominent as a model for humans in fields like cognitive psychology.

We believe, however, that machines of any sort are inappropriate models for humans because they differ from living systems in some very important ways. One reason a computer is not like a human is that the energy that is necessary for computers to work is not on board; it must be supplied to the computer. Thus, computers do not make choices in the same sense that humans do because they are not self-initiating or self-organizing; they have not evolved in the manner of humans, nor do they have the same kind of internal complexity. Some machines do have sensing devices but they do not have affective systems, which also distinguishes them from living systems.

Also, recent chaos theory suggests that living systems exhibit autopoiesis but machines do not (e.g., Capra 1998; Lovelock 2000). Thus every living organism "couples structurally" to its environment; it responds to environmental influences with structural changes, which will in turn alter its future behavior. Living systems are learning systems because they have continual structural changes in response to their environment—they continually adapt, learn, and develop. "Because of its structural coupling, we call the behavior of an animal intelligent but would not apply that term to the behavior of a rock. Thus the new systems view sees living nature as intelligent without the need to assume any over all design or purpose" (Capra 1998, p. 44).

Humans, as well as other living organisms with perceptual systems, are sensitive to the structured ambient energy, which provides information in the specificational sense (Gibson 1979). This perceptual information as low-level energy is coupled with the high-level energy of the motor system and allows for an exploration of one's environment, a discovery of the affordances, and an attempt to realize these affordances. All living systems are considered to exhibit exploratory behavior, but to varying degrees. There are wide variations between species and between individuals within species, but all have exploratory capacity. Living systems also utilize environmental affordances to create new affordances (Reed 1996). Thus, at a most fundamental level we understand why living systems can "make choices" and also understand that this naturally evolving exploratory behavior can be encouraged or discouraged.

Exploratory behavior is related very closely with affect or emotions (Epstein 1994). The world affords activities and events that have both negative and positive consequences. The appraisal of this information is through the perceptual systems but also involves both emotions (an affective system) and cognition. According to Gibson's (1979) theory of information pickup, there are two kinds of information always available: "one about the environment and another about the self" (p. 239). This relational information is provided simultaneously.

Awareness, as Gibson (1979) stated, is of "something in the environment or something in the observer or both at once. Perceiving is a psychosomatic act, not of the mind or body but of a living observer" (pp. 239-240). Perceiving is not restricted to the senses but is an activity of an observer as an irreducible unit, which must include affect. Hobson (1993) suggests that "understanding oneself and others as persons is constituted by mutual interpersonal transactions in which feelings play a pivotal role" (p. 227). A person has first contact with self and with his or her caregivers as not-self through the affective system (Hobson 1990; Zajonc 1980). Thus, affect is fundamental to how people relate to and value one another and their surroundings (Koehn 1998; Noddings 1984). Emotions, of course, have physiological and anatomical support, which are currently not viewed as sensory; but the functional outcome of their activity is informational in the Gibsonian sense. In fact, Davis and Van Emmerik (1995a) suggested that affect be conceptualized as a higher-order perceptual system. Therefore, it follows that affect is very much associated with both motivation and morality.

Choice as Constraint

The choices we have are limited. An important and useful, but abstract, concept for understanding the provisions and restrictions on choices is that of constraints. Kugler and Turvey (1987) define a constraint as simultaneously a limitation and an enablement (see also Bhaskar 1989). In this definition we recognize the dialectical logic.

Constraints are associated with degrees of freedom formally understood from this formula:

$$Df = ND - C,$$

where N is the number of elements in the system, D is the dimensionality of the system, and C is the number of equations of constraint (Fitch and Turvey 1977). Here we explore many of the numerous types of constraints. Some constraints are rather permanent or enduring and others only temporary. Constraints that are relatively long in comparison to the phenomena of interest may be termed *structural.* They more or less permanently freeze out some of the degrees of freedom. Constraints that are relatively short in comparison to the phenomena of interest may be termed *functional:* They effectively select one trajectory from among the virtual trajectories that a system might exhibit. Social as well as physical constraints are either functional or structural. A constraint does not, however, cause behavior; rather it limits or enables behavior. Physical and social laws guide behavior but do not determine it (Warren 1988).

Physical constraints consist of all physical objects, surfaces of support, and the physical laws, such as gravity, that govern their relationships. Thus, one could not choose to run 300 miles per hour because such speed exceeds the physical limitations of a human living on the earth. Social constraints consist of social structures, social institutions, and social systems. We believe that the most advanced understanding of social structures is found in Giddens 1984.

Giddens (1993) stresses the dual nature of social structures: They condition social action, but at the same time structures are reproduced or transformed by those very actions. Giddens' theory of duality of structures and agency in the social world is consistent with Gibson's (1979) theory of perception and action in the physical world. Social constraints are perhaps the least understood but are extremely important in understanding choice and its implications for practice.

There are also "psychological" constraints, which limit and enable people's behavior through their own feelings, beliefs, and desires. Beliefs, as Bhaskar (1989) explains, are causes. Beliefs and desires arise out of one's experiences in the physical and social worlds. Thus, for one to make a choice and act upon it, one must not only have the opportunity and capacity to act, but also the desire to do so. Desire (goals), opportunity (context), and capacity (attributes) are elements of the ETA theoretical model.

Choice as Possessing Skills

Consider the following question regarding the relationship of movement skill acquisition and choice. Can you choose *not* to dunk a basketball? Only if you can in fact dunk a basketball can you answer affirmatively. If you cannot dunk a basketball, then the choice is made for you. Dunking a basketball requires a certain amount of skill, but most of all it requires the capacity to hold a basketball in the hands and to jump high enough to put the ball above the rim of the basket and then slam it through. Of course it is possible to both reduce the size of the ball and lower the height of the basket, allowing those who could not, under normal circumstances, dunk a basketball to now make a decision to dunk or not to dunk.

This example illustrates several important points. Primarily, we emphasize the fact that the more movement skills one possesses the more choices one has, which illustrates the value of skill acquisition in physical education for all individuals. Skill development is brought about as limits on the degrees of freedom are provided on the one hand, and the degrees of freedom are increased or released on the other. It is believed that young children "freeze" some of their degrees of freedom in order to provide for postural stability and greater limb control, which then enable them to accomplish a movement task (e.g., Vereijken et al. 1992). Thus, some choices, in terms of mechanical variables, must be eliminated. Generally speaking, fewer degrees of freedom means an easier control problem. However, the ease of control must also be considered in the context of the task requirements. Some tasks require more degrees of freedom than others. In general, the more degrees of freedom, the more numerous are the tasks that can be achieved. Thus, there is a trade-off between control and maximizing the number of degrees of freedom (see Van Emmerik, this volume).

We examine this trade-off in more detail. Biological systems such as humans are constituted by numerous elements that function at different levels of time and space (e.g., neural nets, muscles, limbs). From the perspective of ETA, coordination is defined as the process that establishes the relationship among the various elements (Newell 1985). Absolute coordination means that two or more elements are in perfect synchronization (Turvey 1992). Coordination can thus occur at the level of neural units or at the level of limbs (Kelso 1995). Coordination also involves relations between the elements at different levels. Neural activity must be coordinated with limb activity. Control is the process by which, theoretically speaking, values are assigned to the coordinated elements and thus determine their speed or force of movement (Newell 1985). Skill is the degree to which the values assigned to the coordination variables are optimal for achieving the task goal. Absolute coordination is generally not desirable in a task involving a large number of degrees of freedom because there must also be flexibility in the system (Beek and Turvey 1992). In other words, one must be able to adjust to changes in the context, in the effector system, or in the task goal.

Overall, a biological system should increase the absolute number of elements and thus increase the total degrees of freedom while also increasing the number of possible temporary constraints, which then allows for accomplishing a maximum number of tasks in efficient ways. Therefore, a balance between degrees of freedom and degrees of control is necessary.

Consider the degrees of freedom and control as they relate to the task goal and the environmental conditions. Through change in the conditions of the surface, the dimensions of the objects (such as a basketball), or the goal conditions, new opportunities (choices) are made available to students as we describe in more detail at the end of the chapter. We believe these arguments we make for physical skills can be made for cognitive, social, and affective skills.

Choice as Having Agency or Power

People do have agency, even though it is constrained by both goals and context (Giddens 1984). The term *agency* is used in the sociology literature to mean acting in the world so as to make a difference, to alter the events. To be redundant: Human behavior is guided but not determined by social and physical laws; people can and do make choices, but to actualize them, they must have power, an opportunity, and a disposition to act.

Giddens (1984) described power as the "utilization of resources." In this chapter, we stress the importance of power as enablement and power as domination. For one to act in such a way as to make a difference in the world, that is, to affect an outcome, one must have power, which comes from both authoritative and allocative resources. Allocative resources are material resources, which include (a) material features of the environment (raw materials, material power sources), (b) means of material production and reproduction (instruments of production, technology), and (c) produced goods (artifacts created by the interaction of a and b). Authoritative resources are all nonmaterial resources, which include (a) organization of social time-space (temporal-spatial constitution of paths and regions), (b) production and reproduction of the body (organization and relation of human beings in mutual association), and (c) organization of life chances (constitution of chances of self-development and self-expression) (see Giddens 1984). Any social or biological system existing across time and space necessarily involves a combination of these two types of resources.

People with more resources have more and different choices than people with fewer resources. For example, people who have the necessary skills and access to technology can use them to benefit themselves and others or utilize them to dominate others. Since power is needed to enable, as well as to limit people, we should not seek to eliminate power as such, but to reduce it as domination. An important insight of Jacques Ellul (1967) is that often technology (*technique* is his term), in turn, does come to control even those with much power. "Neither nations nor individuals are free from the domination of means which instrumental reason has produced" (Benello 1981, p. 102). For example, people's lives are sometimes very dramatically changed when their computer breaks down even for a short period of time, and built-in obsolescence "forces" people to continually purchase newer and "better" technology.

Choice as Decision Making

First, we make a distinction between choices, preferences, and opportunities. Preferences are defined along a continuum of acceptance-rejection.

One can have both preferences and choices. Choosing an alternative does not mean that the choice is a preference. For example, a student may be given a choice between playing softball or basketball but in fact prefer neither. When the alternatives are limited, one may still choose but not be able to select one's preference.

Decision making is the highest level of choice and, as Bouffard and Wall (1991; Wall, Reid, and Harvey, this volume) point out, requires knowledge. One decides on the basis of "knowing" or having experience with at least some of the alternatives. The special education literature examines choice as a behavior to be learned (Newton, Horner, and Lund 1991; Reichle, Sigafoos, and Piche 1989). That is, choice entails knowledge and experiences, which are to be gained. Specific strategies to teach choice through self-determination, self-advocacy, self-efficacy, independence, and empowerment are numerous. Integral to these strategies is increasing the capacity to make decisions and to be aware of the consequences resulting from those decisions.

However, hidden factors can affect an individual's capacity to make a choice that indeed is a preference. One example of a hidden factor is the influence of response bias. From the research literature, three response biases are discerned. For example, individuals with limited verbal expressive language learn simple responses of "yes" or "no" and use them for all questions. An individual's preference may be inhibited by "automatically" replying "yes" no matter the content of the question (Seligman 1975). A response bias also occurs when an individual provides the information he or she perceives is desired by the person asking or soliciting information. As another example, lack of experience limits an individual's ability to make a choice because only a few of the alternatives offered may be familiar.

Although many factors prevent a choice of one's true preference, all individuals, even those with severe disabilities, have the capacity to make such choices. Providing opportunities for *all* individuals to choose their preferences and to realize the consequences (both intended and unintended) of those choices is critical to the teaching-learning process. Unfortunately, this contrasts with many of the recommendations made in traditional education.

Choice as decision making goes beyond simply being given one's preferences. Decisions can be rank ordered to a certain extent in terms of importance. Importance relates to both the individual and the social groups to which the individual belongs, from small to global. From a global perspective the most important decisions made in society concern the production and distribution of resources and the control over the means and use of violence (Giddens 1984). State sovereignty requires being able to independently make these decisions. And the extent to which the majority of people belonging to a given state are involved in making these most important decisions determines the degree of democracy of that state. As it stands today, only a few people who have a great deal of power—allocative and authoritative, as already discussed—make most of these decisions in nearly all nation-states, including the United States. As Marx noted, those who control the allocative power control the authoritative power.

Therefore, if democracy is to be established and preserved, it is necessary for all citizens to know how these decisions are made and by whom. In turn, for instructors and scientists, it is essential to know who makes the decisions about resources in the schools and the universities, which are important institutions in nation-states, and how the decisions are made. The relevance of these arguments to persons in adapted physical education can be seen in the literature on social control, academic freedom, and learning (e.g., Barrow 1990; Chorover 1979; Edwards 1996; Schrecker 1986; Simpson 1994); but these issues are only briefly considered here.

Choice as Intrinsic Motivation

The concept of intrinsic motivation developed from the recognition that persons and other animals with perceptual systems explore their environment in an active and curious manner, and that they also seek to have some control over that environment (White 1959). Deci and colleagues (1991) define intrinsically motivated behavior simply as behaviors that are "engaged in for their own sake—for the pleasure and satisfaction derived from their performance" (p. 328). Extrinsically motivated behaviors are those that occur primarily for purposes external to the act itself. Taking this further, Ryan, Connell, and Deci (1985) distinguish between external, introjected, and identified regulation of behavior. *External regulation* refers to behaviors for which the locus of initiation is external to the person as in the case of rewards, contingencies, avoidance of punishment, and compliance with existing rules. In contrast, *introjected regulation* involves internalized rules or demands that people set for themselves and that then pressure them to behave accordingly. Schafer (1968) notes that *internalization* is a proactive process through which people transform regulation by external contingencies into regulation by internal processes. When internalized rules are buttressed with threatened sanctions or promised rewards, they are not considered part of the integrated self and thus are not self-determined (Deci and Ryan 1991; see also Ikuenobe 1998). *Identified regulation* of behavior occurs when one engages in an activity for the values of the activity itself. We believe that this adheres to the highest ethical standard as explained by Arnold (1997).

Having choices and making decisions are central to Deci's (1980) theory of self-determination. "Simply stated, motivation, performance, and development will be maximized within social contexts that provide people the opportunity to satisfy their basic psychological needs for competence, relatedness, and autonomy" (Deci and Ryan 1985, pp. 327-328). These ideas have been given considerable empirical support. Research suggests that when people are given choices, performance, self-confidence, and self-satisfaction increase. "Problem behaviors" are also shown to decrease (e.g., Dyer, Dunlap, and Winterling 1990). Even though society highly values expressions of free choice, not all people are socialized to make choices or even decisions (see Gatto 1992). Very often the choices people could or should make for themselves are made for them by others. The social and physical environments also "make decisions" for people, as the example of choosing not to dunk a basketball illustrates.

An individual's participation level, progress, and overall performance can be affected by the number of choices available. All persons, but some more than others, are context conditioned. Motivation for action comes from the immediate social and physical surroundings. Active, vibrant surroundings energize people into action; but on occasion, for some people, the opposite can be true as well. Choice can affect motivation, and the motivation level can also affect performance. "Intrinsic motivation is based in the innate, organismic needs for competence and self-determination" (Deci and Ryan 1985, p. 32). Also, feeling competent in an activity seems to help one reach optimal performance levels.

Reaching achievable but challenging goals also increases intrinsic motivation. "The intrinsic needs for competence and self-determination motivate an ongoing process of seeking and attempting to conquer optimal challenges" (Deci and Ryan 1985, p. 32). Most people pursue activities that are suited to their competencies and that offer challenge, yet allow for some success. When people find optimal challenges, they persistently work to conquer them. The need for competence and self-determination keeps people involved in ongoing cycles of seeking and conquering optimal challenges.

Choice as Self-Determination and Freedom

Piaget (1970) noted that choice is not the right to make a decision but the capacity. As already discussed, freedom as a capacity requires agency. Thus, rationality and knowledge are necessary for freedom, but as Bhaskar (1980) notes, they are not sufficient. "For to be free is (i) to know, (ii) to possess the opportunity and (iii) to be disposed to act in (or towards) one's real interests. . . . It is salutary to remember that there is a logical gap between 'knowing' and 'doing,' which can only be bridged by 'wanting in suitable circumstances'" (Bhaskar 1980, p. 16). We note that the three items listed by Bhaskar correspond to the three elements of the ETA model.

Mithaug's (1996) equal opportunity theory is consistent with these ideas, resolves the discrepancy between the *right* and the *experience* of self-determination, and justifies social redress on behalf of individuals less well situated due to circumstances beyond their control. Equal opportunity theory claims that (a) all persons have the right to self-determination; (b) psychological and social conditions of freedom cause some individuals and groups to experience unfair advantages in determining their future; (c) declines in self-determination prospects for the less fortunate are due (in part) to social forces beyond their control; and (d) as a consequence of these declines, there is a collective obligation to improve prospects for self-determination among less well-situated groups (Mithaug 1996, p. 2).

People are not born with the same roles, resources, and other circumstances, nor do they generally choose the label or conditions of their ethnicity or their disability. Even so, this does not completely resolve individuals of their responsibility for changing, if necessary, their own conditions as we shall discuss further. Rather it is a recognition that both individual attributes and social context are determining factors in life chances. Unavoidably, resources become distributed unequally to a certain extent. It is also the case, however, that certain individuals and groups have been *unnecessarily* restricted from resources and opportunities required for expressing themselves and for making decisions, which in turn limits the possibility for improving their capacity to make decisions. In contrast, other individuals or members of certain groups are given more opportunities for expressing themselves and making decisions for themselves, disproportionately to, and sometimes at the expense of, others.

Furthermore, some people are given, unnecessarily and without justification, the opportunity to make decisions for others—decisions that others should make for themselves. Under such a social arrangement, systems of privilege are created for some and "nautonomy" created for others. Nautonomy is defined by Mithaug (1996) as the asymmetrical production and distribution of life chances that limits and erodes the possibilities of political participation. When power generates nautonomic outcomes, participation is involuntarily restricted or artificially limited.

Because of nautonomy, whether necessary or unnecessary and intended or unintended, there should be social means of redressing imbalances. Democratic processes provide one just means. The details of how this is to be accomplished are not discussed here. The point we want to underscore is that it takes power (capacity), as already defined, opportunity, and motivation to have self-determination and freedom, which are composed of having choices.

The power to make decisions gives one the freedom to act. But all actions result in both intended and unintended consequences. Thus, freedom is necessarily connected to responsibility as we discuss further on. Davis and Chandler (1998) defined freedom as maximizing the degrees of freedom for each individual of the collective and thus for the collective as a whole. Freedom therefore is making decisions. Decision making is social as well as individual; a person's decisions are constrained by the decisions other people make. Naturally, conflicts will arise and compromises must be worked out. Democracy is a process of group decision making that maximizes the degrees of freedom of each individual and thus the collective.

Unfortunately, and contrary to popular beliefs, very few social systems today are truly democratic in the classical sense of equality and rule by the consent of the governed (see Gutmann and Thompson 1999; Wood 1995). For example, schools today teach democracy, but students mostly learn authoritarianism because the latter is practiced and the former is only read about. In institutions for individuals with disabilities, democracy is often neither practiced nor taught. Schools and institutions are authoritarian by design; and they use laws, rules, and beliefs to help achieve this domination-subordination goal. As an example, consider a student code of conduct from a local school assumed to be typical of many schools in the United States (see figure 3.2).

Figure 3.2
Example of a High School Code of Conduct

INSUBORDINATION OR DEFIANCE

A student shall not refuse to comply with reasonable requests, orders, and directions of teachers, substitute teachers, teacher aides, administrators, or other authorized personnel during any period of time when the student is properly under the authority of school personnel. Insubordination includes but is not limited to the following:

- Disobedience or disrespect toward any staff member
- Not serving assigned detentions
- Not following school rules or proper procedures
- Not following assigned schedule/being in unauthorized area
- Chronically tardy to school or class
- Repeated misbehavior after warning

At first glance, this policy may seem innocuous enough, but when it is examined closely and put in a historical and social context, a different picture emerges. If one is not insubordinate, then one must be subordinate: Subordinate can be defined as "belonging to a lower or inferior class or rank" or "subject to the authority or control of another."

Should citizens of a true democracy be subordinate? Is subordination what we really want to impose on our students? We would argue that subordination has no place in most theories of ethics or in an egalitarian democratic community. Egalitarianism connotes mutual respect between people even when power is imbalanced. Respect is demanded from but not necessarily given to students by instructors and administrators. Likewise, when instructors use the term *cooperate* to mean that they want students to obey, the word is corrupted. Cooperation means working together to achieve a mutual goal.

In a true democracy, laws, when deemed necessary, are made by consensus, not by authority. That means that all or nearly all people who are subject to the laws must agree on them. Schools that operate undemocratically are not very effective in teaching students democratic principles and practices. Democracy is more than a form of government; it is a process and a way of acting. It is also a way of thinking, a belief system, and part of a world view. It is well established that students learn most effectively by doing, by putting into practice and experiencing that which they read about. If students are involved in making the laws and rules of the school, they are much more likely to understand, appreciate, and follow them. Most important in this process of learning is the connection of actions to both the intended and unintended consequences. Making these connections is how responsibility is best acquired, not by simply obeying laws made by someone else. Of course, as we discuss later, values are superior to laws and whenever possible should be used instead. Award-winning educator John Gatto (1992) had this to say about education:

> I've come to believe that genius is an exceedingly common human quality, probably natural to most of us. . . . Bit by bit I began to

devise guerrilla exercises to allow the kids I taught—as many as I was able—the raw material people have always used to educate themselves: privacy, *choice,* freedom from surveillance, and as broad a range of situations and human associations as my limited power and resources could manage." (pp. xi-xii, our emphasis)

In the present chapter, we examine some of the ways in which choices are taken away, particularly from people with disabilities and those in other socially devalued groups. Thus, we further show how choice is connected to a broad range of important issues. We begin with some overarching constraints, which we can only briefly describe here.

How Choice Is Unnecessarily Eliminated

In the previous section we discussed several ways of conceptualizing choice, showing some of the manifestations. In this section we continue to show the broader implications of choice by describing two important means by which choices are directly, though perhaps unintentionally, eliminated: structures of domination and behaviorism and other forms of social control.

Structures of Domination

Social hierarchies are structures of domination. We conceptualize *domination* as one or more acts whereby an individual (or group) takes away, eliminates, or reduces another individual's (or group's) allocative and authoritative resources, effectively reducing the other's opportunities, choices, rights, and freedoms and enhancing his or her own resources, opportunities, privileges, and freedoms. *Structures of domination* are social hierarchical structures reproduced through regularized social practices, which constrain behaviors in such a way as to produce domination and subordination actions and relationships.

Structures of domination span the range from two individuals to relations between and within groups. Groups range from a small family to the largest nation-states and empires. Thus, structures of domination vary considerably in details but exhibit some essential commonalities. Structures of domination serve to privilege one individual (or a group) and to limit the choices of another individual (or group).

Structures of domination include persons acting alone or within an identity group—for example, a relationship between a husband and a wife resulting in the husband's dominating the wife, as is the general case today. It is important to note that the social evolution literature strongly suggests that for the first 90 thousand years or so, human societies were rather egalitarian. It has been only in the last 10 thousand years or so that male domination over females has become more prevalent (Eisler 1987). Structures of domination also exist when owners and managers of corporations (including universities) dominate the workers. Structures of domination exist between nation-states as well. For example, the United States dominates other nations belonging to the United Nations through use of a veto power not given to all members, by withholding payment of dues, or by other means of coercion based on its economic and military hegemony.

Although all hierarchical relationships are not necessarily structures of domination, all structures of domination are hierarchically organized social structures (Davis and Chandler 1998). In a hierarchy, B must accept A's decision because A has the authority to make the decision. In contrast, if A must secure B's wholly voluntary agreement, as in a heterarchical system (see Davis and Chandler 1998), the decision becomes collective (communal) or joint and is no longer an individual decision (see Thayer 1994, for details on this line of reasoning). Today social hierarchies are ubiquitous, but the most ominous (and destructive) ones are empires, especially the United States (e.g., Blum 1995; Cook 1962; Drinnon 1997; Jones 1972; Parenti 1995; Smith 2002; Stannard 1992; Watson 1997).

Over the past several thousand years, social relationships among groups have all too prominently included several forms of oppression and destruction ranging from genocides (90 million people in the 20th century alone), wars, mass murders, and slavery to ownership of one's labor by another. Much of this destruction has been carried out in the name of empire building in which a few enrich themselves at the expense of the majority (Williams 1980). There is no question that empires competing for the world's wealth have great impact on the daily lives of all individuals. In Parenti's (1995) words,

> Imperialism has been the most powerful force in world history over the last four or five centuries, carving up whole continents while oppressing indigenous peoples and obliterating entire civilizations. Yet, empire as it exists today is seldom accorded any serious attention by our academics, media commentators, and political leaders. When not ignored outright, the subject of imperialism has been sanitized. . . . (p. 1)

Although today's imperialism does not receive serious attention by most writers, it is very well documented (Blum 2000; Foster 2001; Hanson 1993; Johnson 2000, Semmel 1993).

It is important to understand the behavioral constraints of all these systems, because much of human behavior is routinized (Giddens 1984), and people more often guide their behavior using their "experiential self" (emotions and tacit knowledge) than their "rational self" (pure reason) (Epstein 1994). The essence of these understandings is captured well by Iris Marion Young (1992):

> In its new usage, oppression designates the disadvantage and injustice some people suffer not [necessarily] because a tyrannical power coerces them, but [often] because of the everyday practices of a well-intentioned liberal society. . . . Oppression in this sense is structural, rather than the result of a few people's choices or policies. Its causes are embedded in unquestioned norms, habits, and symbols, in the assumptions underlying institutional rules and the collective consequences of following those rules.

The relevance here is that all structures of domination unnecessarily eliminate choices for some people while giving undeserved privilege to others.

Legacy of Behaviorism and Other Forms of Social Control

The assumption of behaviorism is that living organisms are like machines; they have no internal complexity and no onboard potential energy. Instead, to the behaviorist, all living organisms are simply guided by the external energy gradients. Although behaviorism has been discredited as a theory to explain the complexities of human learning (e.g., Schwartz 1990), its principles for practice remain entrenched in education and are central to economic, political, and other institutions in the United States. One of the most important legacies of behaviorism is the use of rewards or punishment, or both, as the means of human motivation and thus their use by some to control others. This is illustrated in the following quotes from two of the most prominent proponents of behaviorism. John Watson (1930, p.11) stated, "The interest of the behaviorist in man's doings is more than the interest of the spectator—he wants to control man's reactions as physical scientists want to control and manipulate other natural phenomena." B.F. Skinner (1983) expressed similar ideas about the control of behavior.

What does it mean to control the behavior of another person? Simply put, it means you take away the person's choices. You force people to do what you want them to do by simply giving them something they want, removing an aversive condition, or putting them into an adverse situation or threatening to do so when they respond or do not respond the way you want. Why would a pigeon peck at a metal bar except that it provides something she wants? Why would the dolphin jump high and touch the suspended ball? Pecking and jumping are certainly within the repertoire of behavioral possibilities (choices) for these animals. The animals could certainly act otherwise, as some of the behaviorists' own experiments show. If there was food next to the bar or in the tank and the animals were hungry, they most likely would not peck the bar or jump to the suspended ball but would choose instead to simply eat the food.

How often do people act a certain way because others tell them they must or because the laws, rules, policies, or regularized practices established by others require them to do so in order for them to achieve another goal that they really desire? Yes, living organisms can and very often do allow themselves to be guided by the external energy fields. Behaviorism is intoxicating because it works! On the other hand, animals, including most people, can and do, on a daily basis, choose to act otherwise. Behaviorism unnecessarily and sometimes destructively reduces people to machines by eliminating choices. Thus, it is necessary to revisit this legacy in more detail, as an antimony of choice.

Rewards and Punishment

Punishment has a long history in human evolution, including its use in schools (e.g., Hyman 1990), and remains pervasive in U.S. society (over 2 million citizens are incarcerated). The negative impact of punishment is well documented, and many educators throughout history have opposed its use in schools. A popular belief is that rewards, on the other hand, result in only positive outcomes. However, Alfie Kohn (1993), with his book *Punished by Rewards,* has led the proponents of a different view. We first briefly discuss punishment and then deal more extensively with rewards as means of social control.

Punishment is crudely defined as delivering pain. It is an antinomy of choice because it is also intended to eliminate choices of those being punished. It is an effort to force people to conform to the desires of those responsible for enforcing laws or rules and is believed to serve as a redress for damages and pain caused by the offenders (e.g., Tam 1996). We do not suggest that people do not need to be held accountable to others and to society as a whole, but question whether punishment is the best way to accomplish this redress as a purported goal of authority. In our earlier discussion of accountability, punishment has no place. Rather, the desired goals for one who is held accountable for wrongs against others or against the environment are repentance, self-reform, reparation, and reconciliation as described in Duff's (1996) communicative punishment theory.

Communicative punishment aims to bring offenders to understand why they are being censured and accept that censure as justified. First, repentance involves recognizing a need for reform and self-reform. Second, a remorseful understanding of past wrongdoing involves recognizing the need to make reparations—a form of payment to those offended. Third, intrinsic to a concern to make reparation is the desire for reconciliation. Fourth, forgiveness is believed to be an important human attribute and essential to ethical practice (Arnold 2000). Punishment is based primarily on a feeling of revenge rather than forgiveness and can only, at best, serve as a function to satisfy that emotion (e.g., Walker 1991). The ethos of punishment often fosters violence and encourages hate rather than forgiveness, kindness, and love. Punishment, violence, and hate serve to eliminate people's choices.

As Tam (1996) recognizes, communicative punishment is not easy to carry out and offers no guarantees. For example, repentance involves the remorseful acceptance of guilt, and this cannot be induced simply through pointing out that someone is guilty if that someone has not felt any remorse up to that point. Equally, self-reform is a process, which some wrongdoers will undergo only with the help of some kind of external pressure or influence. Social pressure, of course, can be powerful. As Auerbach (1983) suggests, law (and subsequently, punishment) begins where community ends. He further notes that the way people dispute depends on how well they relate. If the relationships are intimate, caring, and mutual, conflicts will be resolved quite differently than when relations are hierarchical and competitive. "Selfishness and aggression are not merely functions of individual personality; they are socially sanctioned or discouraged" (Auerbach 1983, pp. 7-8). We suggest that social advancement requires an increasing reliance on values over laws, as well as minimizing the use of punishment by striving toward systems of repentance, self-reform, reparation, and reconciliation.

Rewards do in fact differ from punishment, but it is their similarities that are of interest here. Rewards are extrinsic motivation and in most cases constitute behavioral control of some over others, intended or not. Basically, the notion is, "If you do this, you'll get that," which amounts to a manipulation for compliance. If your goal in education is student compliance, then rewards work very well, though often not as well as punishment. On the other hand, if your goal in education is self-determination for your students, then rewards fail miserably.

Five points are made in support of this contention. First, in virtually all cases, rewards are given by the powerful, those with authority, to control the less powerful, their subordinates. Kohn (1993) states, "The point to be emphasized is that all rewards, by virtue of *being* rewards, are not attempts to influence or persuade or solve problems together, but simply to control" (p. 27, italics in the original). Both rewards and punishments flourish in asymmetrical power relationships, creating or exacerbating that imbalance. Consider rewards within the structures of domination. Who praises whom and why? Kohn notes that almost universally children desire approval, and people in authority positions must be careful not to exploit this for their own purposes. Rewards, even the "social reward" of praise, can have negative effects, especially on females under the current systems of male domination (Kohn 1993).

These arguments against praise may be surprising to the many instructors accustomed to using it, and requires further comment. Praise, like choice, is far more complex than generally thought (see Brophy 1981, Delin and Baumeister 1994 for informed discussions). The general finding concerning the motivational effects of praise is that it may be generally (but not always) effective for increasing motivation and effort; the major exception is "when praise takes on the character of external control and therefore undermines motivation" (Delin and Baumeister 1994, p. 237) or when students are already intrinsically motivated.

Second, when all learning situations are considered, the important comparison is not between rewards and punishment, but between intrinsic and extrinsic motivation. We have already discussed the concept of intrinsic motivation and need only add here that intrinsic motivation has long been understood as the more valued and generally the more effective for bringing about desired behaviors, in almost all cases (e.g., Montessori 1964; Piaget 1970)—that is, behaviors that are most beneficial to both the individual and society as a whole, and when self-determination is a goal.

Third, we emphasize that rewards are capable of stifling intrinsic motivation. While this does not always occur, the fact that it can should make one seriously consider whether or not to use rewards with students, including those with disabilities. Rewards may be successful at changing our actions, but they also may change our reasons for the actions and our attitude toward those actions and ourselves. The question then is not whether rewards are effective in changing actions, but what changes and why. The research cited previously indicates that rewards are most effective for those who lack competence and confidence. The more rewards are used, the more they seem to be needed.

Fourth, institutionalizing the teaching-learning situation is not easily accomplished and requires considerable effort for success, if in fact it can work at all (e.g., Illich 1971). If the primary goal of society is to maximize education for all people, including those with severe disabilities—and we believe it should be—then the task is monumental. Rewards and punishments are attractive because they are in many ways much easier than teaching and good management. In today's private as well as public institutions of education, there are often many obstacles to overcome in creating an optimal teaching-learning environment. Thus, anything that makes the task easier, regardless of the consequences, is tempting.

Fifth, the philosophical assumptions supporting behaviorism extend back to antiquity. But two of the most frequently cited contributors are Thomas Hobbes and John Locke. Hobbes proposed the need for a higher authority for the purpose of enforcing moral and socially responsible actions, usually by means of rewards and punishments. Accepting Hobbes' assumptions, though not to the same extreme, John Locke (1690/1999) suggested that a strong government is essential to establish and enforce the laws needed to maintain social order. However, it is necessary to point out that Hobbes' "state of nature and social contract are, of course, anthropological and historical fictions" (Ophuls 1997, p. 31).

Learned Helplessness

The concept of "learned helplessness" originated from the work of Seligman and his colleagues (Overmier and Seligman 1967; Seligman 1975). Peterson, Maier, and Seligman (1993), noted that "[a]s it was first articulated, the learned helplessness model hypothesized that experience with uncontrollable events leads to difficulties in motivation, cognition, and emotion. Mediating this effect is a person's expectation that responses and outcomes are independent" (p. 141). Bloom and Reichert (1998) suggested that helplessness, along with sickness, pain, and separation and loss of a relationship, is among the four "great evils" of the human condition. They further note that "[h]elplessness evokes shame, a feeling so overwhelming, so paralyzing and disabling, that it must be defended against. One reaction to helplessness is the loss of agency, a perpetual dependent turning toward external authority for rescue, a pervasive sense of powerlessness" (p. 145). Another reaction is anger and a willingness to seize power, which can escalate into rage, fury, and a profound desire to seek revenge and defeat the shame.

There are many explanations for the phenomenon of learned helplessness. Seligman (1975) reported that learned helplessness is depicted by motivational deficits (failure to initiate activities), errors of cognition (failure to learn remediative actions), and emotional problems (depression, heightened anxiety). Learned helplessness is influenced by the belief that both success and failure are outside one's own control. The phenomenon of learned helplessness is a pattern of responses learned over a period of years (Floor and Rosen 1975).

Learned helplessness has been shown to occur in people who are most vulnerable to acts of domination. These groups include young children who are abused, people with mental retardation, and those with severe and prolonged emotional pain. Breggin and Cohen (1999) believe that helplessness is at the root of nearly all disabling emotional reactions. However, overcoming feelings of helplessness is possible. The obvious approach from the ETA model is to assist the person in empowerment. This is often not done in the authoritarian systems, which largely characterize institutional therapy. Well-intended instructors sometimes have an overreaction of sympathy and provide assistance that fosters dependence rather than independence on the part of the student. Opportunities for decision making and problem solving need to be provided on a daily basis and starting at a very early age. Physical activity could be integral in the provision of decision-making and problem-solving opportunities for all individuals, including those with severe disabilities.

Laws and Rules

It is a common belief that laws are the backbone of justice, freedom, and democracy. We want to present an alternative view. We begin with the distinction between responsibility and obedience. Often the behavior outcomes are the same, in certain ways, when a person is acting responsible and a person is being obedient, and therefore the two words are often equated. But the following common definitions of these words illustrate important differences:

> **responsible**—Legally or ethically accountable for the care or welfare of another, or involving personal accountability or ability to act without guidance or superior authority.

> **obedient**—Obeying or carrying out a request, command, or the like; submissive to control; dutiful.

Consider the following question: Is driving 75 miles per hour being responsible? (In the United States, this speed, which is comparable to about 120 kilometers per hour, is considered very fast.) Whether driving this fast is responsible depends, necessarily and sufficiently, on only three general things: (a) one's driving competence, (b) one's goals, and (c) the driving conditions (e.g., road, car). The question does not depend on rules or laws, contrary to popular belief. This is so because regardless of one's driving competence, to be morally responsible, one should always drive for safety and for courtesy when trying to achieve the ultimate goal of going from point A to point B. Efficiency can also be an important goal especially if others may be depending on one's getting there at a certain time or as soon as possible, as in the case of an emergency.

Driving a car at 75 miles per hour will certainly get one there quickly, relatively speaking. Is it a safe speed? Apparently people in parts of the western United States believe so, because some of the speed limit laws there are 75 miles per hour. If visibility and the roads are good and the traffic is not too heavy, driving 75 miles per hour is safe for many people and in some places legal. One can also find those same driving conditions in places where the speed limit law is 55 miles per hour. Consider the case of a competent driver who, in this latter situation, has a very important appointment, that is, needs to drive efficiently and feels safe at 75 miles per hour. So she drives the speed limit of 55 miles per hour but arrives too late to carry out the task. Is she being responsible or obedient? Consider the definition of *obedient* just cited and definition 2 of *responsible*. Being responsible requires critical thinking, but being obedient requires almost no thinking. In the latter case, one only has to know the rule or command and know how to carry it out. To be a critical thinker one must question all things (be critical) and analyze all the information one has available (think). To be a responsible critical thinker, one must make a decision and act on it. If one is free to decide and act, then one must also be accountable for that action. Gandhi pointed out that freedom without responsibility leads to social "blunders." We would also suggest that responsibility without freedom leads to obedience, which in its extreme is slavery, or it leads to revolution.

Laws and ethics are not the same. Ethics depend on values, freedom (choices), and responsibility, which differ from laws in the following ways. Laws, rules, and techniques are written not only with predetermined outcomes, but also with predetermined "means" or procedures. The expected outcome of a speed limit is safety, and the predetermined means is a quantitatively measured driving speed (see Ellul's 1967 discussion of technique). In contrast, safety as a value has no predetermined means; rather one drives at whatever one determines is a safe speed for oneself under the circumstances. Safety as a value is context sensitive, but requires responsible people. Safety as a speed limit law is not context sensitive and does not require responsible people, only obedient people.

Laws are necessary and justified to the extent that people do not take responsibility for their actions, which may result in innocent people's suffering the consequences. However, responsibility is best learned when it connects actions with both their intended and unintended consequences rather than through simple obedience to laws. Responsibility and values are learned and sustained best in close-knit communities through informal interactions and through democratic processes. Laws by contrast are established formally and enforced by authority, which can become coercive, especially in hierarchical or authoritarian organizations and regimes. In hierarchies, laws are made by the rulers or the elite and used to control the majority. In corporate liberal ideology, it is believed that control of the masses by a few elite is natural and necessary. When this ideology is popularly accepted it becomes a self-fulfilling prophesy and is one reason for the abundance of laws in the United States.

If people are more responsible, fewer laws will be necessary, as was expressed by Grant Gilmore (1977, p. 111). He suggested, "The better the society, the less law there will be. In heaven there will be no law. . . . The worse the society, the more law there will be. In hell there will be nothing but law and due process will be meticulously observed." In a hierarchical authoritarian system there is an abundance of laws. In a true democracy where a major societal goal is self-determination for all there will be few laws, and behavior will be constrained by values. Since it is not likely that a perfect society (as heaven is envisioned) will be created soon, some laws are necessary. In a true democracy, laws will be created by consensus and not by a legislative process dominated by economics.

Implications for Instruction

Although the research is not extensive, the results are unequivocal. When given choices, students, including those with severe disabilities, are more productive (e.g., Berk 1976), more active and attentive (Dattilo and Rusch 1985), and more self-confident and self-directed (Berk 1976). These findings are consistent with those in the social psychology literature, which shows that the degree to which people can control their environment and can make choices is positively related to their health, morale, self-esteem, and level of functioning (e.g., Glass and Singer 1972; Langer and Saegert 1977; Wolk and Telleen 1976; see also Monty and Perlmutter 1987; Moos 1981). Thus, acknowledging preferences, teaching choice as a decision-making process, and teaching choice as freedom and responsibility are advocated for all persons, including those with severe disabilities (Guess, Benson, and Siegel-Causey 1985; Newton, Horner, and Lund 1991; Shevin and Klein 1984).

Persons with severe disabilities are particularly vulnerable to having their choices limited by others, though perhaps unwittingly, even by people who are trained and experienced in this profession (e.g., Vaughan

1993). Since choices are limited and helplessness is inadvertently taught, "it appears to be important to expand the concept of leisure to encompass fundamental behaviors involving some expression of choice" (Dattilo and Rusch 1985, p. 19). We would emphasize that this applies to almost all activities.

The four steps of the applied ETA model and the way in which each step is to be implemented are found elsewhere in the literature (Balan and Davis 1993; Burton and Davis 1992; Carson, Bulger, and Townsend, this volume). In this chapter, we focus on and expand the second step of the applied model that we refer to as "providing choices." We begin by noting that *when* choices are given is more important than even the fact of giving choices. Unless the choices are given prior to instruction, some of the benefits of choice, such as empowerment and information about the students, are lost. The emphasis is on giving the students a feeling of control over their situation and at the same time assisting them in understanding responsibility and accountability as discussed in this chapter.

Choices are offered at four different levels. The first two levels are the most important and must be understood and implemented from the perspective of the general task categories, which are based on skills and game strategies as listed in figure 3.3. The essential student choices are made between or within these general categories. It is these categories that provide the appropriate choices.

Figure 3.3
General Task Categories

A **general task category** is a broad classification of motor skills based on the functional goal and criteria and the type of skills and games strategies included. The nine general task categories are as follows.

SKILLS

1a. Locomotion on land—translating from point A to point B. Skills include rolling, crawling, creeping, tumbling, cruising, walking, running, hopping, galloping, skipping, climbing, and jumping.

Criteria: efficiency, velocity, distance, spatial accuracy, temporal accuracy, and accuracy of movement form

1b. Locomotion in water—translating from point A to point B. Skills include dog paddle, human stroke, breaststroke, sidestroke, butterfly, jumping, and diving.

Criteria: efficiency, velocity, distance, spatial accuracy, temporal accuracy, and accuracy of movement form

2. **Object manipulation**—acting upon or using small objects and implements for a wide variety of task goals. The hands are used primarily, but tasks may be achieved with the feet, mouth, or other body parts. Skills are numerous and include writing, drawing, coloring, cutting, hammering, painting, juggling, dressing and undressing, threading, sewing, and weaving.

   Criteria: efficiency, spatial accuracy, temporal accuracy, and velocity

3a. **Object propulsion**—the projection of an object away from the body with the use of a limb, an implement, or both. Skills include throwing, kicking, striking, rolling, heading, shooting, and dribbling.

   Criteria: velocity, distance, spatial accuracy, temporal accuracy, and efficiency

3b. **Object reception**—the act of stopping, securing, or impeding a moving object with use of the body or body parts or an implement. Skills include catching, trapping, tackling, and blocking.

   Criteria: temporal accuracy, spatial accuracy, and efficiency

4. **Postural maintenance and orientation**—holding a steady postural position or changing to a new position but not translating. Skills include sitting, standing, turning, twisting, bending, pivoting, and hanging.

   Criteria: efficiency, spatial accuracy, temporal accuracy, and accuracy of movement form

GAMES

5. **Strike, run, and field**—propelling an object and then locomoting as rapidly as possible to designated location(s) (one or more bases) before the opponents can receive the object. The receivers must secure the object or secure and propel it at the striker/runner or at a receiver standing at a base before the runner reaches that base. Games include baseball, softball, and kickball.

6. **Goal games**—opponents attempt to score a goal by propelling an object into a goal, net, or basket or other container at their end of a playing field or court marked by boundaries while attempting to prevent the opponent from doing the same at their end. Games include basketball, soccer, field and floor hockey, lacrosse, and water polo.

7a. **Net games (individual)**—attempting to propel an object over a net, stretched across a field, court, or table, in such a way that it lands within the marked boundary and so that the opponent does not successfully return it. Games include tennis, badminton, and table tennis.

7b. Net games (team)—attempting to propel an object over a net, stretched across a field, court, or table, in such a way that it lands within the marked boundary and so that the opponents do not successfully return it. Games include volleyball.

8. **Wall games**—propelling an object off the wall and onto a marked court in such a manner that the opponent cannot return it in the same way. Games include racquetball, handball, and squash.

9. **Target games**—propelling an object toward a stationary or moving target using an implement or a hand without any opponent interference. Games include archery, bowling, and golf.

The first level of choice allows students to select across all general task categories and thereby choose the task goal itself. Choosing the task goal means having the environment structured by the instructor, the students themselves, or both. The instructor structures an environment conducive to participation in any of the general task categories. This may mean having a number of stations or a wide variety of equipment and settings available. In the second instance, the students structure the environment through their choice of equipment and its setup. Then they select their own task goal by choosing the game or activity. A variety of equipment must be made available to the students from which to choose. Providing students the choice of task goal is often very useful for instructors who want to discover more about the students' preferences or for students who appear unmotivated regarding physical activity. Of course the social as well as the physical environment is important here. The social environment includes using students as role models, giving encouragement, and showing enthusiasm and interest in the activity and environment and the students.

The second level of choice is made within the general task categories as the students choose one of several possible skills or strategies through which to accomplish the task goal. Giving choices at the skill or game strategy level means that the students have selected a task goal or understand the task goal provided for them, but are not told or shown how to achieve the goal or which strategies to follow and how to execute them. Rules and conditions, which might affect strategies and skills, may also be included as choices for students at this level. Importantly, level 2 structures the environment to specify the task goal. Here the environment may be set up to elicit a "preferred skill" or a "preferred game" chosen by the instructor, or it may be open to any skill or game that might achieve the goal specified by the instructor. The instructor can then establish a movement problem in keeping with the preferred skill or preferred game. In the category of target games or object propulsion, goals or targets of any type are set up, objects to propel at the goals or targets are provided, and the students are instructed to get the object in the goal or to hit the target. At this level, the instructor may provide formations and other conditions. The idea is to establish a task goal to be achieved or a movement problem to be solved and allow the students to devise or discover solutions for themselves.

The third level is giving a choice of movement form, which simply means not demonstrating the skill or strategies prior to the students' performance. Fourth, the instructor or coach may specify the task goal(s) and preferred skills or strategies and allow the students to choose relevant task variables, which include such things as objects, implements, surfaces of support, distances, and game rules. Once the goal has been established and the skill or game chosen, students may be allowed to choose one or more objects or implements that they wish to use.

The first two levels of choice provision are the most important and are essential if students are to become self-determined in physical activities. The benefits of providing choices in physical education, sport, and leisure are many (see figure 3.4). Besides these immediate benefits in physical activities, choices given here contribute to the overall achievement of self-determination, which is at the heart of democracy. Contrary to popular belief, social control is far more prevalent than democracy in Western nations. Thus, providing choices in physical activities is paramount as part of the overall movement to democratize society.

Figure 3.4
Benefits of Choice in Physical Education

- Provides valuable information for the instructor or assessment administrator
- Allows more time for teacher observation and reflection
- Establishes a link to intrinsic motivation
- Helps promote positive affective outcomes
- Provides some autonomy and empowerment for students by giving them some control over their environment
- Connects the movement activities with cognition or knowledge
- Encourages the discovery of the most effective and efficient movement form for each individual
- Encourages creative problem solving
- Reduces behavioral problems by reducing tension and frustration

KEY POINTS

- Choice is a very important concept that affects people in many ways.
- Seven different aspects or levels of choice are conceptualized and described.
- Choices are intentionally and unintentionally taken away from people in a variety of ways.
- Groups of people particularly vulnerable to having their choices taken from them include those with disabilities, the elderly, children, and women.
- Choice is central to the ETA model. It is the second step of the ETA applied model.
- Providing choices in instructional settings benefits both the students and instructors.

Summary

In this chapter we conceptualized choice in its broadest sense, thus elevating its importance. Given that choice is fundamental to human existence, instructors and scientists alike are encouraged to make it more central to their activities. Decision making is essential for subjects in applied research as well as for learners in other movement settings. Choice is discussed from the perspective of complex systems, as a constraint, as possessing skills, as having power, as making decisions, as part of intrinsic motivation, and as the essence of self-determination and freedom.

We also discussed the importance of understanding the limitations and the elimination of choice. Thus, we considered structures of domination, behaviorism, and other forms of social control and linked them in particular to instructional settings. We then provided details of how this knowledge and understanding can be applied to instruction in human movement and enumerated the benefits of these practices.

Perception-Action Judgments in Children With Learning Disabilities

Jill Whitall, PhD, Sarita Sanghvi, MPT,
and Nancy Getchell, PhD

In 1991, Allen Burton wrote an article with Walter Davis titled "Ecological Task Analysis: Translating Movement Behavior Theory into Practice" (Davis and Burton 1991). In that article Davis and Burton offered a new approach to task analysis that was based on the ecological theory of perception and other complementary theories. They proposed that Ecological Task Analysis was applicable to instruction, assessment, and also applied research in movement performance (see prologue). The purpose of the present chapter is to focus on the third corner of this triumvirate and illustrate how ETA drives applied research. In the last section we suggest general future applications for research based on ETA.

Children with learning disabilities (LD) are an increasing proportion of the school-age population, representing, for example, over 2.8 million public school students in the United States who obtain some form of special education for their LD (U.S. Department of Education 2002). In addition to specific academic problems, these children have been documented to have problems with motor skill acquisition and proficiency (Lazarus 1989). One suggestion has been that they are inefficient in motor planning. However, motor planning in this context is not well defined; does it include all three stages of a standard information-processing model (i.e., perception, decision making, and motor programming)? Many studies have looked at perceptual abilities, decision making, and motor programming either separately or through use of a combined reaction-time measure (e.g., Bull and Johnston 1997; Facoetti et al. 2003; Pihl and Niauro 1982; Woodard and Surburg 1999). In general, this approach provides examples of processing differences in children with LD but no further understanding of motor planning, in part because the focus is often on either reading or solving math problems rather than movement per se.

One can take an alternative view of motor planning by adopting the ecological or perception-action approach first suggested by J.J. Gibson (1966) and later expanded specifically to motor development by, among others, E.J. Gibson (1982), Newell (1986), Konczak (1990), and, of course, Davis and Burton (1991) with their ETA model. In this view the three-stage concept arising from an information-processing approach is misleading. Children know their bodies, and the translation from perception to action can be a direct rather than an indirect (multiple stage) process. One question arising explicitly from the ETA approach, then, is whether children with and without LD actually differ in the way they use their perceptual judgment to relate task and environmental constraints to their own capabilities. At the same time it will be possible to see whether both groups demonstrate an invariant relationship between task and environmental constraints and their own body constraints.

One previous study addressed a very similar question in children with mental retardation (Block 1993). Children with and without mental retardation were asked to judge whether they could jump over various lengths of mat using a standing long jump—that is, whether they could assess or perceive the affordance of the mat and judge the critical point of their jumping ability. Subsequently the children demonstrated their longest jump so that the accuracy of their decision making could be assessed. The two sets of children were equally accurate in judging their jumping, although the children with mental retardation were less able jumpers overall. This suggests that the perception-action coupling for this particular task did not depend in any way on cognitive decision-making abilities that did differ between the groups. In another study, Block (2002) found that typically developing male children from 3 years of age were as accurate as adults in judging a jumpable distance, although in general the latter tended to underestimate their ability while the former overestimated their ability. In a related study, Savelsbergh and colleagues (1994) also found no differences between typically developing participants and participants with Down syndrome in type of grasp in a task in which cubes were scaled from either small to large or large to small.

The main purpose of our more recent study, described here, was to investigate whether children with LD could also judge the limits of their motor ability as well as typically developing (TD) children using a similar perception-action paradigm. The choice of task was a simple activity of daily living, namely the goal of stepping over an obstacle. We followed the general process of ETA as described by Burton and Davis (1996): We established a task goal of stepping over an obstacle, allowed participants a choice of movement solutions (in this case determining perceived action boundary), and then manipulated a task variable by raising or lowering the obstacle height. Given the results for the children with mental retardation, we hypothesized that children with LD would also be capable of making accurate judgments but that these judgments would take a longer time to make. A secondary purpose was to add to the literature on affordances by assessing some possible predictors of the perceived ability to step over an obstacle. We consider this a preliminary study; our intent in this chapter is to illustrate how researchers can test the principles of the ETA approach through sound methodology.

Methods

Our participants were six children with LD and six TD children matched for age (±4 months), gender, and race. Children with LD were identified and referred through the Comprehensive Evaluation Unit in the Department of Pediatrics, University of Maryland, and TD children were identified through word of mouth. The age range of the participants varied from 5 to 10 years. None of the children were diagnosed with attention deficit disorder, attention deficit/hyperactivity disorder, or developmental coordination disorder. Children with LD had a diagnosis of either language-based or general LD. Typically developing children 8 years and under were checked for unidentified LD using the Screen (Hresko, Reid, and Hammill 1988) and for mental retardation using the McCarthy Scales of Children's Abilities (McCarthy 1972). For those above 8 years we relied on the reports from parents of their normal intelligence and nonidentified LD.

We constructed a "stepping-over" apparatus with two wooden stands (30 inches [76 cm] apart) and a bar (< 0.5 inch [< 1.3 cm] diameter dowel) that balanced on struts sticking out behind the stands. The struts could be adjusted up and down at 1 inch (2.5 cm) intervals. A cardboard screen was placed in front of the apparatus between trials so that the participant could not see whether the bar was being lowered or elevated.

The procedures began when participants and their parent or caregiver entered the laboratory. The participants were allowed time to become familiar with the experimenters while the parent or caregiver signed a consent form approved by the University of Maryland's Institutional Review Board. Anthropometric measurements of height, thigh, and lower leg length (in inches) were then taken using a measuring tape; and hip, knee, and ankle active range of motion was assessed using a goniometer (in degrees). To determine perceptual judgments, participants stood in front of the apparatus at a distance equal to their height (a relative, not an absolute measure, consistent with ETA principles). The screen was removed, and the participants were asked to judge whether they could step over the bar without hitting it. Instructions to each participant were "Tell me whether you can step over the bar at this height by saying yes or no." There were no instructions regarding how quickly they should make the decision. Initial bar height was adjusted relative to the participant's leg length, and subsequent bar heights were changed according to a specific protocol. Next, actual height of clearance was determined. The participant was allowed to step over the bar at his or her perceived height of clearance. The bar was then adjusted to establish the actual maximum height of clearance without the participant's demonstrating a change of stepping-over pattern (e.g., twisting his or her body).

Although the ETA approach dictates that the goal for an intended task is primary and that relationships of the body parts may differ with respect to accomplishing that goal, we reasoned that the perception-action judgment was probably made *in relation* to how the child would normally step over an obstacle, not how that goal might possibly be attained through unnatural contortions. The perception and action protocols were both videotaped from a sagittal view using a Panasonic camcorder (recording at 30 hertz). Subsequently, the participants undertook the short form of the Bruininks Oseretsky Test of Motor Proficiency (BOTMP) to establish general motor performance ability (Bruininks 1978). Participants were given a prize and small monetary compensation after the session.

The collected variables of interest were the BOTMP score, the perceived action boundary, the actual clearance height, and the three anthropometric and flexibility measures. We estimated the perceived action boundary by calculating the distance that was halfway between the last "yes" and first "no" bar height. We subsequently calculated the difference between perceived and actual height for data analysis. Using the videotape, we also determined the time taken to make the decision of yes or no from removal of the screen to subject's beginning to say yes or no. We ran paired t-tests between the groups on BOTMP scores and perceived, action, and difference step heights and decision times. Next, we ran a multiple regression analysis using all participants on the perceived step height with the anthropometric and flexibility measures as predictors. Alpha was set at 0.05 for all statistical tests.

Results

The BOTMP scores of the LD ($M = 42.0, SD = 14.0$) and TD ($M = 54.2$; $SD = 10.6$) groups were significantly different. This suggests that children with LD had poorer general motor ability than their TD counterparts. The perceived action boundary, actual clearance height, and difference score judgments are presented in table 4.1 for both groups. None of the

Table 4.1 Mean of Perceived, Actual, and Difference in Maximum Clearance Height for LD and TD Children

Height	LD	TD
Perceived	16.8 (2.7)	18.1 (6.2)
Actual	17.3 (1.6)	18.0 (1.8)
Difference	0.5	0.1

Note. Height is in inches; standard deviation is provided in parentheses.

comparisons reached significance. This suggests that children with LD were capable of making the same kind of accurate judgment about what height they could step over as their TD counterparts.

The decision times in milliseconds for judging bar clearance of the LD (M = 2260 msec, SD = 26) and TD (M = 1980 msec, SD = 59) groups were significantly different. Children with LD took longer to make their perceptual decisions on bar clearance than the TD participants. Regarding a performer-scaled predictor of perceived step height, across all participants, the strongest and only significant predictor was participant height.

Discussion

In this study we investigated the capacity of children with and without LD to judge their ability to perform the simple motor task of stepping over an obstacle. We followed the procedures of ETA by establishing a perceptual and action goal, providing decision and movement choices, and manipulating task parameters, all with the purpose of investigating perception-action mapping. We found that the two groups of children were equally capable of making accurate judgments about their actual clearance height. The ability to match perceived action boundary and actual clearance height was present for those with LD despite the fact that these children had poor general motor ability. However, the children with LD did take longer to make these judgments. In addition, we noted that height was the only significant predictor of perceived action boundary in this group of twelve 5- to 10-year-olds.

All Children Can Accurately Judge Their Ability

The finding that both groups of children could accurately judge whether they could step over an obstacle supports the ETA principle that a mover can perceive the limits of an action soon after the ability to perform the action is acquired. These results are also consistent with a number of previous studies on children that have shown good perceptual judgment on the part of the children in their ability to detect a jumpable horizontal distance (Block 2002), when a height afforded sitting or stepping over (Pufall and Dunbar 1992), or when an obstacle afforded going over or under (Burton 1990). As noted earlier, our study was most similar to Block's in that we presented various conditions visually to the children and asked them to verbalize their capabilities. The absolute differences between perception and action capability were small at < 1.2 inches (3 cm) compared with Block's ranges of 4.9 to 4.7 inches (about 12 cm) for different age groups of children. One reason for the lower difference could be that the action of stepping over an object is a more practiced, common, and simple movement compared to the standing long jump. Thus, the children in this study would have learned to step over an object before doing a true standing long jump and would have had far more practice, resulting in a more finely tuned affordance map.

Another potential explanation for the differences may be related to body scaling versus action scaling. If the tasks were scaled on some critical action variable (for example, dynamic force production), then the differences between the groups in the body-scaled measure might disappear in light of the more relevant action-scaled measure. At the same time, Block's study, which included adults, does not suggest that years of experience is an influential factor for accuracy of judgment. One could make the argument, however, that adults are likely to have less recent practice with a standing long jump (e.g., stepping over a puddle) and that their intrinsic affordance capability is therefore detuned for the specific standing long jump task. A second possibility is that the stepping-over task in the present study was a "height" judgment in the same plane as the body rather than a "depth" judgment as in Block's study. Recent experiments in adults suggest that eye height is a more natural and accurate metric for object height than for object width (Wraga 1999), and perhaps the same advantage applies to object depth (see Maraj 2003 for experiments that combine riser height and depth). Certainly the difference cannot be attributed to being physically nearer the object, because our subjects were farther away than Block's (see Maraj and Domingue 1999 for experiment on this topic).

Height Is a Predictor for Judging Ability

In this study we found that height was indeed the best and only significant predictor for the perceptual judgment of stepping over a dowel.

An earlier study on the similar task of climbing stair risers focused on leg length as the most salient body-related scalar predicting the optimal (comfortable) height for climbing the stairs (e.g., Warren 1984); however, others have included (eye) height too as an important scalar (e.g., Mark 1987; Mark and Vogele 1987). More recently, studies by Meeuwsen (1991) and Konczak, Meeuwsen, and Cress (1992) demonstrated that body-scaled information was not the only relevant factor in making perceptual judgments of maximum climbable stair riser height (more akin to the present study). Using older subjects, these researchers demonstrated that factors such as hip flexibility and leg strength also contributed to the accuracy of perceptual judgments. That is, the subjects whose constraints had changed from an optimal level in adulthood were aware of their limitations and took these into account, consciously or subconsciously, when making their judgments. In our study we would not have expected that these factors would be important, because children are still growing into their capabilities, not losing them. However, we did take flexibility measures and entered these into the regression analysis as a check.

Children With LD Are Less Motorically Able and Slower to Make Judgments

Group differences between the children with LD and the TD children were found on two measures. First, the scores on the short BOTMP were different. As expected, children with LD showed poorer motor performance—slightly below average—while TD children were within an average range. This is not surprising, given that one of the warning signs of LD is difficulty in motor skills. However, the two groups were equally good at making the perceptual judgments. This suggests that perceptual affordances, at least for this motor task, were not a major contributing factor for general poor motor performance in the children with LD as measured in the BOTMP. In addition, all participants succeeded in the task; that is, they were able to step over the dowel. That suggests, in relation to the ETA, that this particular task scales into the range of "easy." However, the groups differed significantly in the time taken to reach the correct decision. This suggests that the longer decision time to make the perceptual judgment for the children with LD may be a contributing factor for poor motor performance in certain tasks.

Taking this one step farther, one can speculate that tasks requiring quick reaction time may cause an increased likelihood of error in the child with LD because there is not enough time to precisely map the perceptual cues to movement ability. The slow decision time may also be indicative of a general slowness of the central nervous system that results in reduced, delayed muscle recruitment and less-tuned coordination. In tasks that do not require speed or quick reactions, it is plausible that children with LD may not be that different from TD children (as was true with this study). This hypothesis needs to be tested. If these children have inferior performance in tasks without time constraints, some other motor performance factor may be involved; or alternatively, children with LD may not take the time to precisely map perception and action and tend toward impulsivity. If the latter is true, one might ask why the children in this study were not impulsive. One answer might be that they were deliberately asked to make a decision and, given that none had a diagnosis of attention deficits, they complied with the instructions as given.

This brings up an interesting notion based on the concept of ETA. One would expect that for this particular task, the critical value for obstacle clearance might be body scaled—some ratio of participant height to obstacle height. In fact, it appears that for this task, a temporal action-scaled variable (decision time) may be the critical point on which to scale. That is, in order to make the task more difficult, we would not change the participant/object height ratio but rather scale down on decision time. We would expect the LD group to have a lower critical value above which their actions would result in a greater number of perceptual and motor errors.

Application of the Results

So, what have we learned from this study that will influence teaching and clinical decision making? First, on the basis of our results for the BOTMP and decision-making time, educators and clinicians should expect to see below-average motor performance and perhaps a general slowness in children with LD, even if they are not diagnosed with movement problems. This notion is supported by a study on gross motor coordination and LD (Getchell and Whitall 2003) in which the investigators examined LD children with and without movement difficulties and determined that lack of diagnosis of movement difficulty does not imply lack of differences from TD children.

Second, knowing that children with LD can make accurate decisions about movement capabilities, movement educators should encourage LD students to take their time and not rush their movements in teaching situations in which reaction time and speed are not important. Again, the ETA model suggests that decision time may be the control variable for certain tasks. The critical value after which LD children switch patterns (perhaps from successful to unsuccessful) is likely to be sooner (e.g., happen faster) than in TD children. Therefore, by giving LD children more decision time, a movement educator may provide a broader range of values near the optimal decision time value and a greater opportunity for successful movement. Third, in situations in which quick reactions (and movements) are needed, LD children may be less successful in terms of perception-action mapping and therefore be less successful at performing the task than TD children. However, children with LD know the body in which they live, and they should be gradually encouraged to improve by being challenged to do things a little faster, longer, and harder in a manner consistent with the ETA approach. That is, progression should be based on relative performer-scaled dimensions rather than absolute external dimensions (see Davis and Burton 1991; Burton and Davis 1996). The important point here, as with any child, is not to overchallenge them and cause failure, which will lead to more frustration in movement situations.

Future Directions Related to the Results

Finally, where does this preliminary study lead us? One limitation of the study, related to the small sample size, was that the group with LD was not completely homogenous in diagnosis, although none had attentional problems or a specific diagnosis of movement problems. It would be useful in the future to look at perception-action capabilities in well-controlled studies in children with different types of LD, including the primarily movement-based developmental coordination disorder, as separate groups. The difficulty of finding truly homogenous groups, however, is well recognized given the high existence of comorbid conditions. Nevertheless, larger homogenous groups and the use of individuals as the unit of analysis are desirable directions.

Another direction is to build on the findings of the study. For example, one of the strengths of our study was to test the actual action as well as the perceived action, in contrast to some of the earlier perception-action studies (e.g., Warren 1984). Following the ETA model, the next step in understanding these perception-action relationships is to scale on one or more control variables in order to determine both optimal and critical boundary values for task performance. It would be interesting to look at more challenging perception-action situations for TD and LD populations to see if, when, and under what constraints (e.g., task complexity or experience) the ability to judge accurately will break down. Plausible hypotheses in such experiments can arise from two facets that are unique to our perception-action study: (1) the measurement of decision time and (2) the independent measurement of movement ability through the BOTMP. For example, one hypothesis is that the more complex or less practiced task will demonstrate an even larger difference in decision time between LD children and TD children, suggesting that the optimal decision time value for LD children is higher. A related hypothesis is that children with LD will reach a critical boundary value of decision time sooner than TD children, which will switch them from successful to unsuccessful actions in less time. Still another hypothesis is that children who score especially low on movement tasks that require coordination, rather than speed or visual-motor skills, will show inaccurate judgments earlier than those who score higher. These hypotheses are based on the idea that it may take longer to "acquire" an accurate perception-action link for complex tasks requiring management of multiple muscle-joint combinations.

Future Research Directions Employing ETA

The study we have discussed here illustrates an application of the ETA principles to conduct research that addresses the capabilities of children with LD. It is clearly not a definitive study, but it begins to address both an applied research question (how do children with and without LD differ in perception-action judgments?) and a more basic research question (is there a performer-scaled predictor of the critical point in this particular task?). The former has direct implications for understanding and interacting with the population of children with LD, and the latter provides more empirical support for the principles behind the ecological approach as outlined by Davis and Burton (1991).

What are future directions of applied and basic research specifically related to the ETA principles? Perhaps some would argue that these kinds of experiments are now passé. Certainly there have been many basic research experiments with a focus on detecting performer-scaled dimensions to predict critical points of movement transitions (e.g., Carello et al. 1989, for reachability; Mark and Vogele 1987, for sitting and stair climbing affordances; Diedrich and Warren 1995, Turvey et al. 1999, and Getchell and Whitall 2004, for gait transitions). These examples are all in adult populations. There has also been much work on perceptual judgments in infancy related to performer-scaled dimensions (e.g., Newell, McDonald, and Baillargeon 1993, for grip affordance; Adolph, Eppler, and Gibson 1993, for crawlability; Ulrich, Thelen, and Niles 1990, for stair climbing affordance; Gibson and Schmuckler 1989, for locomotor affordance). Two populations that have received less attention in this regard are children (notable exceptions include Newell et al. 1989b, for grip affordances; Beak, Davids, and Bennett 2002, for tennis racket affordances) and the elderly (notable exceptions include Konczak, Meeuwsen, and Cress 1992).

Thus, one suggestion is that children and elderly populations could be studied more intensely, particularly with regard to establishing developmental trajectories of the relationships between performer dimensions and task and environmental constraints that reflect growing up and aging. This would not be a trivial project. Choosing a relevant task or tasks that are kept constant over a cross-sectional study (or a longitudinal one) can demonstrate whether critical performer-scaled dimensions change over time, and if so when and how. Konczak and colleagues (1992) have already demonstrated that elderly persons appear to accurately perceive their own strength and flexibility in relation to the critical climbability of stairs whereas younger adults apparently need only use a simple scalar like eye height (Warren 1984). In this regard, the experimenter needs to be very thoughtful and thorough in measuring meaningful and relative or related dimensions of the performer. As Block (2002) points out, simple body-scaled information is not always the best predictor of a critical point giving a true dimensionless ratio that is constant across all body proportions and ages. He argues that a "biodynamic" measure such as the movement performance itself (e.g., maximum jump) embodies the dynamics of the jump and the true action potential of the mover and may be a better fit for the prediction of a critical perceptual judgment (see also Carello et al. 1989; Mark and Vogele 1987).

Equally if not more importantly, these experiments can be used to study specific special populations and in particular those with disorders of the nervous system. In addition to children with LD, there are several developmental populations in which movement ability is delayed or altered, and again the questions asked can determine (a) whether perceptual judgments are equal to those in TD children, (b) whether the same performer-scaled dimensions are relevant, and (c) whether changing the complexity of the task or environment has a differential effect on the special population. These types of studies would provide valuable information on the components of tasks, scaling of different task parameters, environmental elements, and individual characteristics. This, in turn, could serve as a road map for movement educators and physical therapists, providing a task-specific route to remediation or proficiency in the given task. For example, if particular control parameters can be identified for activities of daily living, a therapist could assist a stroke patient in his or her rehabilitation by scaling all parameters to the "easiest" value and slowly increasing these values as the individual improves performance.

Finally, an emerging trend in developmental motor control research is to look at how short-term adaptations to changing visual-motor (e.g., Ferrel-Chapus et al. 2002) or force field (e.g., Konczak, Jansen-Osmann, and Kalveram 2003) environments are accomplished. The idea is to begin to understand motor learning, or at least processes that might underlie motor learning such as tuning the visual-motor system to the task attractor landscape—the process of identifying task-specific invariant information. Without discussing the intricacies of this line of work we can hypothesize, based on the notions put forth by ETA, that attunement would be easier to "learn" if the relevant dimensions of a task scaled to the performer were determined first. Our work with LD children suggests that although the relevant dimensions may be the same, the process by which they learn this visual-motor tuning or, more generally, sensorimotor tuning, may be different than in TD children.

PRACTICAL APPLICATIONS

- One can expect children with LD to have poor motor skills in general even if they are not specifically diagnosed with motor problems.
- For motor skills that do not require quick judgments (closed skills), children with LD should be encouraged to take their time since they appear to know their own capabilities as well as TD children.
- For motor skills that require quick judgments (open skills), children with LD are more likely to perform poorly and probably need to build up to speed more gradually than TD children.

Summary

In conclusion, we again applaud the work of Davis and Burton (1991; Burton and Davis 1996) in bringing the concepts of Gibson and the ecological approach to perception-action into the realm of those who assess, teach, and conduct applied (and basic) research through ETA. Our study was certainly influenced by these principles and our knowledge of the work done in this area by Burton, Davis, and others. In fact, we think that ETA provides not only a solid but an essential model for understanding movement development and learning in the diverse populations we interact with daily. From our perspective we will always consider the relationships and linking between performer, task, and environment as well as concepts such as optimal and critical points, even when our research questions are not specifically testing or using these concepts.

5

Manipulating a Control Parameter in Overhand Throwing

Dan Southard, PhD

The human body can be characterized as an open system made up of many components that are free to relate to one another. The components and their relationships create multiple degrees of freedom and numerous possibilities for completing motor activity. The complexity of the system affords the mover flexibility in accomplishing motor tasks. However, the same flexibility increases the difficulty for instructors of motor skills when attempting to individualize instruction. Task analysis is a process utilized by instructors of motor activity to help manage system complexity and individualize instruction. The process involves the identification of components of a skill and ordering them from easy to difficult (Herkowitz 1978b). Traditional task analysis is based on the assumption that breaking skills into sequential parts helps one to understand their development, which aids in the formation of effective teaching-learning strategies. The problem is that the task goal for components of a skill can be substantially different from the goal of the task itself. This raises questions regarding positive transfer of learning when the practice task is different from the actual performance (Magill 2001).

An alternative to traditional task analysis is Ecological Task Analysis (Burton and Davis 1996; Davis and Burton 1991). Ecological Task Analysis was originally intended for children with special needs. However, ETA is grounded in Gibson's concept of affordances (Gibson 1977, 1979) and dynamic systems theory (e.g., Guckenheimer and Holmes 1983), which makes it applicable to any person teaching or learning a motor skill. An affordance is the opportunity or potential for action that a specific environment affords an individual. The ecological point of view dictates that the goal for a given task must be expressed in terms of invariant intended outcomes and not in terms of components or specific body parts (Davis and Burton 1991). A dynamic system is any system whose elements organize to cause change over time (Crutchfield et al. 1987).

"Self-organization" accounts for the formation of new motor patterns through the interaction of constraints on the system. Constraints that limit motor behaviors may be explicitly defined by the goal of the movement or implicitly defined by the nature of the organism and the environment in which the movement is performed (Newell 1985, 1986). One may derive instructional strategies by changing relevant dynamics of a movement to gain insight into the formation of motor patterns. The dynamics of the system are the principles that serve to influence and regulate patterns of movement rather than neural activity alone.

Determining the relevant dynamics of a task that instigate and direct changes in pattern is not easy. New movements emerge following scalar changes in any one of the constraints related to the environment, the individual, or the goal of the movement. The variables that can lead to changes in pattern when scaled to a critical value are termed *control parameters*. The control parameter does not dictate how the pattern should change but rather sets up the conditions for change to occur. The collective action of elements that appear to govern the system's behavior is termed an *order parameter* (Haken 1977). Order parameters reflect the change in pattern by allowing the system to organize within the context of constraints. Constraints eliminate certain configurations and allow the order parameter to self-organize components toward a particular pattern called an "attractor state" (Abraham and Shaw 1982). For example, one of the control parameters for the development of throwing patterns has been shown to be velocity (Southard 1998), and the order parameter is the open kinetic link principle (Southard 2002). When lower-level throwers scale up on velocity, their pattern progresses toward an optimal state. Each change that occurs takes further advantage of the open kinetic link principle or order parameter.

Contrary to traditional task analysis, ETA suggests a shift away from the instructional strategy of breaking skills into components followed by instruction, practice, and feedback. Rather, ETA suggests that learners be provided the goal of the task and be allowed to choose their own movement form. The choice of form need not be a conscious one but may be guided by the task, environmental, and individual constraints. Changes in motor patterns that accompany the learning of skills may occur spontaneously when control parameters are scaled to a critical value. Following ETA logic, it may be that learners would benefit more from changing a control parameter than from practicing a specified component of a skill.

The importance of choice or self-discovery is emphasized in the ETA model for instruction. Allowing choices in movement pattern may provide clues to the intrinsic dynamics of the movement and minimizes verbal instruction without distracting the learner from the overall goal of the task (Davis and Van Emmerik 1995b). One way to offer guidance without compromising self-discovery is to encourage the learner to scale up on a known control parameter. We know that this strategy will lead to a change in motor pattern, but will practice without scaling up on a control parameter result in similar changes? If practice alone results in a qualitative change, will the change be according to the known order parameter and existing constraints? To address these questions, the task of interest should be a relatively novel skill in which the control and order parameters have been identified. Selecting a relatively novel task helps control for past experience as an intervening variable.

Throwing with the nonpreferred arm satisfies the conditions for addressing the questions. Order and control parameters for throwing have been identified. The use of adult participants makes it possible to control for the confounding factors of practice and maturation. Finally, throwing with the nonpreferred arm may be considered a novel task (Fetz and Jaeger 1995; Ning et al. 1999). In fact, throwing is so "one-sided" that hand preference itself is often determined by a series of tasks that includes identification of the limb with which individuals prefer to throw (Gabbard 1998). Incidences of "mixed lateral preference" for throwing are rare.

The purpose of the study discussed in this chapter was to determine changes in throwing pattern of the nonpreferred arm as a result of (1) practicing while scaling up on a control parameter and (2) practicing without scaling up on a control parameter. The results should provide kinesiologists with information concerning why motor patterns change, as well as insight into the nature of self-discovery of motor patterns that is important to the ETA perspective.

Methods

Peak velocity and relative timing of the throwing arm were used to document coordinative changes. Data concerning the lower body (e.g., leg activity) was not recorded for this study.

Participants

Forty university students (ages 20-25 years; 19 males and 21 females) voluntarily served as participants for this study. Participants preferred throwing with the right hand and had no physical limitations that would prevent the development of a mature throwing pattern. Twenty-two percent of the males and 10% of the females indicated that they had practiced throwing (baseball or softball) through high school. No participants indicated that they were currently participating in an activity that required practicing a throwing motion. Each participant was required to read and sign a university-approved consent form prior to participation.

Procedure

It is not known if changes in throwing patterns resulting from practice are different according to the level of performer. Consequently, skill levels for this study were grouped into four categories.

Determining Skill Level

Participants were placed into one of four throwing levels depending on the degree to which they utilized the open kinetic link principle to execute an overhand throw with the preferred hand. The open kinetic link principle (order parameter) allows the upper limb to conserve angular momentum during a throwing motion. Ideally, as the more proximal segments rotate and create angular momentum, their less massive distal neighbor lags behind. Because the distal segment is less massive than its proximal neighbor, the distal segment increases angular velocity as the proximal segment slows down in order to conserve angular momentum. The process proceeds in sequence from the trunk to the hand, with each distal segment increasing velocity in an attempt to conserve angular momentum. This whiplike action occurs only if the mass of the distal segment is less than that of its proximal neighbor and the distal segment lags behind its proximal neighbor. Considering that the upper limb is naturally tapered proximal to distal, the variables important to determining if a throwing pattern has changed are segmental lag and differences in segmental velocity. An increase in the number of segments experiencing distal lag and positive velocity differences would indicate that the performer is utilizing the order parameter to make progress toward what Thelen and Smith (1994) refer to as a global attractor state (i.e., a throwing pattern in which the order parameter is maximized). In ETA terminology, through a determination of segmental lag and velocity differences, the participant's performance on the task can be assessed across a set of dimension values.

Participants were placed in skill level 1 when they exhibited simple arm extension with little or no segmental lag. Throwers were categorized as skill level 2 when they displayed hand lag but no forearm or humeral lag. Skill level 3 throwers displayed hand lag and forearm lag, but lacked humeral lag. Skill level 4 throwers displayed maximum use of the order parameter (kinetic link principle) by displaying hand lag, forearm lag, and humeral lag. Following designation of skill level, each participant was randomly placed into either the practice with increasing velocity condition or practice without increasing velocity condition.

Care was taken in the placement of participants so as not to overload either condition with a particular skill level. See table 5.1 for numbers of participants by condition.

Data used to determine throwing classification were collected with a Watsmart Motion Analysis System at a sampling rate of 200 hertz. Two infrared detectors (cameras) were mounted on tripods. The tripods were raised to a height of 2.2 m (2.4 yd) and spaced 3 m (3.3 yd) apart. The arrangement allowed for a data collection area of 2 × 2 m (2.2 × 2.2 yds). The system was calibrated using a frame of known dimensions. Calibration was completed at the throwing height of each participant. The range of spatial error was from 1.10 to 2.21 mm with a mean error of 1.87 mm that translates to approximately 0.21 m/sec for a high-velocity throw (40 m/sec).

Infrared-emitting diodes (IREDs) were placed on the fingernail of the third finger, ulnar styloid, lateral epicondyle, greater tubercle of humerus opposite the glenoid fossa, and spinous process of the first thoracic vertebra. The power source for the IREDs was placed at the waist of the participant and secured with a self-adhesive wrap. Wires from the power source to the IREDs were routed about the subject so as not to distract participants during data collection. A representation of IRED placement is shown in figure 5.1.

Each participant was allowed warm-up exercises for the shoulder, elbow, and wrist joints prior to data collection. Participants were required to throw a ball with a circumference of 21 cm (8.3 in.) and a mass of 100 g (2 cm [0.8 in.] smaller and 20 g lighter than a regulation baseball). There was no requirement for accuracy, but participants were encouraged to throw toward a pad that extended from floor level to a height of 2 m (2.2 yd) and was 3 m (3.2 yd) wide. Five trials were completed

Table 5.1 Number of Participants Within Level by Gender and Conditions

Gender	Level 1	Level 2	Level 3	Level 4
Practice with velocity				
Male	1	1	3	4
Female	2	4	3	2
Practice without velocity				
Male	0	2	3	5
Female	3	3	2	3

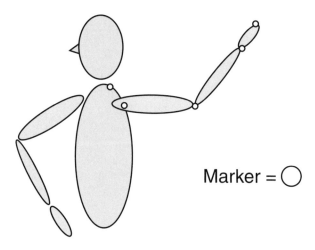

Marker = ◯

Figure 5.1   Representation of infrared-emitting diode placement for each segment.

at a preferred velocity. The five trials were digitized to determine placement within a throwing level. Preferred velocity was used to determine throwing category, since previous work (Southard 1998, 2002) indicated that throwing patterns of less skilled throwers may resemble those of skilled throwers at higher-velocity throws.

Data Collection

The apparatus and procedures for collecting data were identical to those for determining throwing level. The Watsmart system was calibrated for each participant. The range of error was 1.51 to 2.48 mm with an average of 2.07 that translates to approximately 0.26 m/s for high-velocity throws. A JUGS radar gun provided immediate information to participants concerning velocity of throw during data collection.

Participants in the practice with velocity condition were encouraged to increase throwing velocity and to throw at maximum speed for each trial. A radar gun (JUGS) provided immediate feedback concerning performance. The idea was to vary a task constraint (velocity of throw) while stabilizing environmental and performer constraints. Participants in the practice-only condition were required to maintain velocity across trials and sessions. Participants in the practice-only condition were given direction regarding the velocity of throws. If their velocity exceeded 25% of their maximum velocity (nonpreferred hand), they were required to slow down; if it was less than 25% of their maximum velocity, they were required to speed up. Generally, participants were able to maintain a constant velocity at 25% of maximum without problems. Participants in the practice with velocity condition were given their velocity after each throw and encouraged to increase velocity. No augmented information other than velocity of throw was provided to participants in either group.

Analysis

Temporal lag and differences in peak velocities were dependent measures for this study. Temporal lag was determined by the difference in time to peak angular velocity for each segment relative to its proximal neighbor. Differences in angular velocities were determined by subtracting the peak velocity of the distal segment from the peak velocity of its proximal neighbor. Three-dimensional angular velocity of segments (angular movement of a segment in any plane of motion) was determined by the angular movement of vectors formed by two IREDs. Angular displacement of the vectors was determined relative to the same externally defined reference point. IREDs on the first thoracic vertebra and the greater tubercle of the humerus defined the vector representing the trunk. The humerus was defined by IREDs on the greater tubercle of the humerus and the lateral epicondyle. The forearm was defined by IREDs on the lateral epicondyle and the ulnar styloid. The hand was defined by IREDs on the ulnar styloid and the fingernail of the third finger. The degree of lag (lag was in milliseconds) was determined by the relative position of the segment at peak velocity. A positive value indicated that the distal segment lagged behind its proximal neighbor, and a negative value indicated that the proximal segment reached peak velocity before its proximal neighbor. The time to peak velocity for each segment was determined from a common starting position (initial movement of any segment beginning the throw). Differences in peak velocity were measured in radians per second. A positive value for differences in peak velocity would indicate that the distal segment was moving faster than its proximal neighbor, and a negative value would indicate that the distal segment was moving slower than its proximal neighbor. Digitizing was accomplished with commercially prepared software designed for the Watsmart system.

Statistical analysis served to quantitatively determine changes in motor patterns. An alpha level of 0.05 was used for all statistical measures. A three-way multivariate analysis of variance (MANOVA) was performed on the dependent measures of segmental lag (hand, forearm, and humerus) and differences in peak velocity (hand-forearm [H-F], forearm-humerus [F-H], and humerus-trunk [H-T]). A significant MANOVA was followed by univariate analysis of variance (ANOVA) to determine dependent measures responsible for significance. The Huynh-Feldt epsilon (H-F epsilon) was applied to degrees of freedom to account for violation of sphericity assumption. A Scheffe post hoc procedure was used to determine mean scores responsible for significant ANOVA.

Results

Results for temporal lag and velocity differences are presented in separate sections. A third section combines results for temporal lag and velocity differences relative to the use of the open kinetic chain.

Temporal Lag

A condition × level × session MANOVA for dependent measures of hand, forearm, and humeral lag indicated significant main effects for condition (Hoteling's T = 0.40), $F(1,1278)$ = 168.50, $p < 0.001$; level (Hoteling's T = 0.32), $F(3,1278)$ = 42.29, $p < 0.001$; and session (Hoteling's T = 0.63), $F(9,1278)$ = 29.52, $p < 0.001$, with a significant condition × level × session interaction (Hoteling's T = 0.13), $F(27,1278)$ = 20.59, $p < 0.001$. Follow-up univariate ANOVAs (condition × level × velocity) indicated that all three dependent measures were responsible for significant main effects and interaction. H-F adjustment (ε = 0.61) did not affect levels of significance. See figure 5.2 for representation of means for three-way interaction.

Post hoc results for the significant three-way interaction indicated the following trends in the data. Humeral lag was experienced earlier when velocity was increased with practice. Figure 5.2 indicates that for all levels, the humeral lag changed from negative to positive at an earlier session when the performer scaled up on velocity. For level 1 the humerus did not reach a positive value until session 10. Level 2 performers (practice only) did not experience consistent humeral lag during the 10 sessions. That is, there was not humeral lag for more than one consecutive session. Forearm lag was consistently positive across sessions, levels, and conditions, with greater positive lag experienced by lower-level practice-only participants. The first segment to experience positive lag (not considering the forearm, which was consistently positive) was the hand. Participants who increased velocity with practice experienced hand lag earlier in sessions than those in the practice-only condition. Figure 5.2 indicates that the hand experienced positive lag at session 2 for level 1 throwers who scaled up on velocity, but not until session 6 for practice-only throwers. Interestingly, the higher-level throwers (levels 3 and 4) experienced distal lag (hand and forearm) in the first session. However, hand lag did not occur again for level 3 and 4 throwers until after it occurred for the lower-level throwers. The only group that did

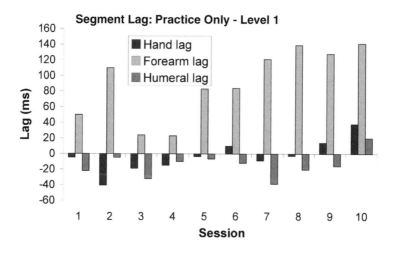

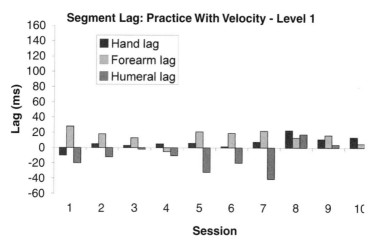

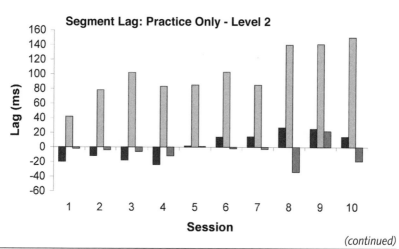

(continued)

Figure 5.2 Graphs representing condition × level × session interaction means for segmental lag. Positive lag values are required for throwers to take advantage of the open kinetic chain.

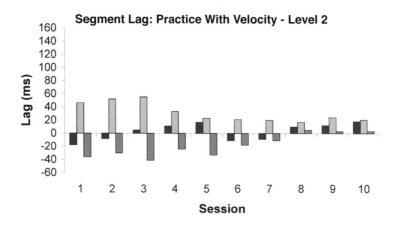

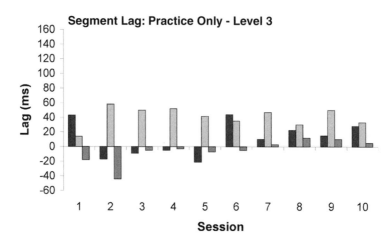

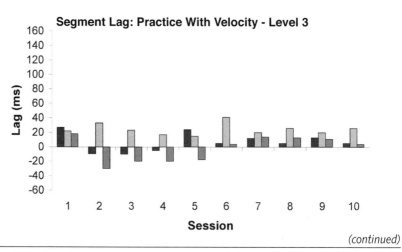

(continued)

Figure 5.2 *(continued)*

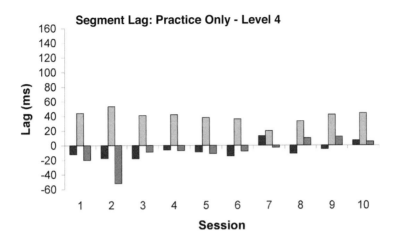

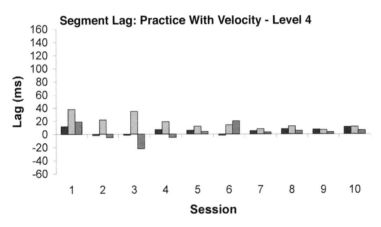

Figure 5.2 *(continued)*

not take maximum advantage of the order parameter (positive lag for each segment) by the 10th session was the level 2 practice-only group (note that the humerus changes from positive lag at session 9 to negative lag at session 10).

Differences in Peak Velocity

A condition × level × session MANOVA for dependent measures of differences in peak velocity (H-F, F-H, H-T) indicated significant main effects for condition (Hoteling's $T = 0.31$), $F(1,1278) = 44.87$, $p < 0.001$; level (Hoteling's $T = 0.24$), $F(3,1278) = 60.17$, $p < 0.001$; and session (Hoteling's $T = 0.20$), $F(9,1278) = 17.07$, $p < 0.001$, with a significant condition × level × session interaction (Hoteling's T = 0.20), F(27,1278) = 5.68, p < 0.001. Follow-up univariate ANOVAs (condition × level × velocity) indicated that all three dependent measures were responsible for significant main effects and interaction. H-F adjustment (ε = 0.65) did not affect levels of significance. See figure 5.3 for representation of means for three-way interaction.

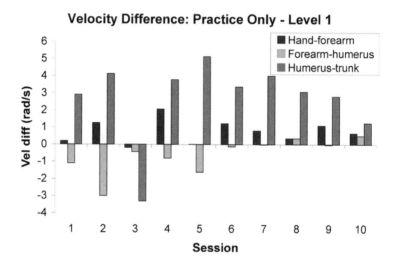

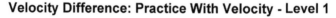

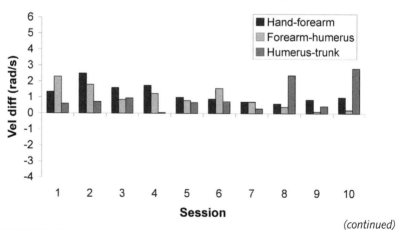

(continued)

Figure 5.3   Graphs representing condition × level × session means for differences in segmental velocities. Positive velocity differences are required for throwers to take advantage of the open kinetic chain.

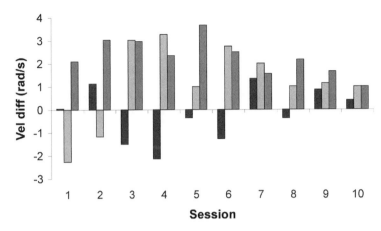

Velocity Difference: Practice Only - Level 2

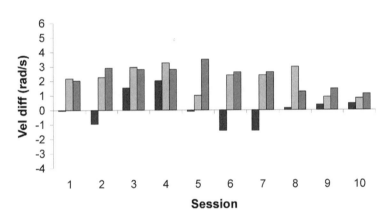

Velocity Difference: Practice With Velocity - Level 2

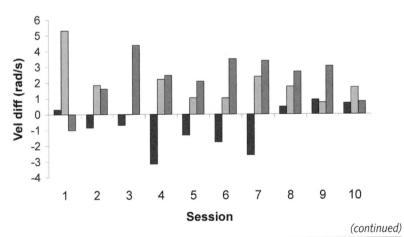

Velocity Difference: Practice Only - Level 3

(continued)

Figure 5.3 *(continued)*

Velocity Difference: Practice With Velocity - Level 3

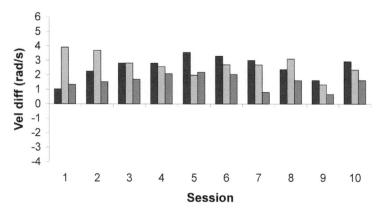

Velocity Difference: Practice Only - Level 4

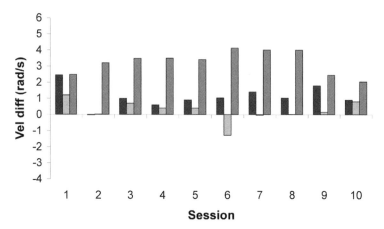

Velocity Difference: Practice With Velocity - Level 4

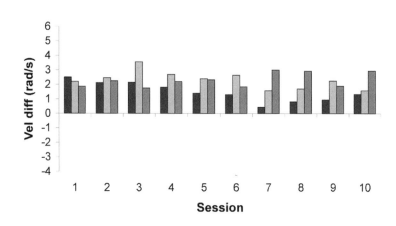

Figure 5.3 *(continued)*

Post hoc results for the significant three-way interactions indicated the following trends in the data. The practice with velocity condition was consistently positive with the exception of level 2 throwers, who experienced negative hand velocity differences for sessions 2, 5, 6, and 7. Throwers in the practice-only condition experienced negative velocity differences at all levels, with the majority of negative values occurring in the earlier practice sessions for levels 1, 2, and 3. Throwers in the practice-only condition were the only participants to experience negative velocity differences for all dependent measures. Finally, the higher-level throwers (levels 3 and 4) displayed more positive values than their lower-level counterparts (levels 1 and 2) across conditions.

Temporal Lag in Combination With Velocity Differences

Distal lag is necessary for the upper limb to take advantage of the order parameter (kinetic link principle) and conserve angular momentum. However, distal lag alone is not necessarily indicative that the limb is taking advantage of the kinetic link principle. If distal lag results in the conservation of angular momentum, then the angular velocity of the more distal segment should also increase relative to its proximal neighbor. That is, whenever there is positive lag represented in figure 5.2 there should also be positive velocity differences for corresponding segments indicated in figure 5.3.

Examination of results from segmental lag and velocity differences indicates that early positive forearm lag (sessions 1 and 2, levels 1 and 2) did not result in the transfer of angular momentum because such lag was not accompanied by a positive velocity difference. The velocity differences for the level 1 throwers (practice only) were negative for the forearm in sessions 1 through 5, and in sessions 1 and 2 for the level 2 throwers (practice only). Note also that positive lag of the hand for levels 2 and 3 (practice-only condition) did not result in an increase in velocity until later sessions.

Discussion

The procedures utilized for this study fit well with two ETA perspectives regarding instructional strategy. First, the learner should be allowed a period of choice or self-discovery before being given verbal instruction or demonstration (Burton and Davis 1996). Allowing the participant a choice in the selection of motor pattern may provide clues about the intrinsic dynamics of the task (Davis and Van Emmerik 1995b). For this study the task was defined in functional terms (throw at constant velocity or throw with increased velocity) rather than the performer's being provided with components of the task to be practiced in a specific sequence. Second, a known control parameter was manipulated (Davis and Van Emmerik 1995b) to determine the effect on motor pattern. Scaling up on a control parameter allows the performer a period of self-discovery while helping to determine links between task goals and performer constraints. Such links can help establish information relevant to the control and coordination of the movement. Instruction may then proceed relative to the natural development of the skill.

Data from this study indicate that as the task dimension of velocity (control parameter) is increased, the motor system takes advantage of the kinetic link principle (order parameter for throwing). Changes in pattern (distal lag and velocity differences between adjoining segments) occurred as a result of practice with the absence of instruction or any augmented information concerning throwing technique. Furthermore, when participants practiced and scaled up on a known control parameter (velocity of throw), patterns changed significantly earlier than when participants maintained a constant throwing velocity. For this study, increasing a task dimension (control parameter of velocity) assisted the learner in moving toward an optimal performance. It should be noted that while lag is a prerequisite to taking advantage of the order parameter, lag alone may not be indicative of a global state. The data indicate that higher-level throwers achieve total lag earlier and have segmental lag values significantly less than their lower-level counterparts. In addition, the lag times for participants scaling up on velocity were significantly less than for those with constant velocity. It appears that not only lag but also the "degree of lag" is an important indicator that throwers have reached a global pattern.

Self-discovery could be an important part of learning to throw. Consider that during scaling up on the task variable of velocity, throwing patterns in this study developed in a sequence from distal to proximal. That is, the hand was the first to demonstrate distal lag, followed by the humerus (the forearm experienced distal lag throughout practice and therefore did not change). Since the system self-organizes in a sequence counterintuitive to the use of the order parameter (distal to proximal rather than proximal to distal), proximal to distal instruction may not complement the "natural" development of throwing.

The fact that level 3 and 4 throwers demonstrated distal lag of all segments in the first session, followed by the slower development of hand lag (compared with levels 1 and 2), lends support to a distal to proximal sequence for the development of throwing skill. When questioned about throwing strategies, the higher-level throwers (3 and 4) reported that they attempted to mimic their dominant throwing arm patterns during the first session. This statement is supported by the lag data (see figure 5.2), particularly for those participants increasing velocity of throw. The penalty of going against the distal to proximal change to positive lag may have been delayed lag of the most distal segment—the hand. It appears that scaling a control parameter (velocity of throw) enhances the development of a skilled throwing pattern and may assist the learner and instructor in discovering the boundaries of motor performance.

Further studies are required to determine conditions that cause change for various motor skills. The "natural" development of motor patterns should help determine appropriate instructional strategies that encompass the interaction of environment, task, and individual constraints. When control parameters are determined, different instructional strategies can be compared with self-discovery. For example, experimental conditions could be created that permit investigation of pattern change with and without instruction during scaling up and not scaling up on a known control parameter.

INSTRUCTIONAL STRATEGIES

- Instruction may not be necessary for motor pattern change.
- Performers may scale up on relevant task variables or control parameters to improve performance.
- Scaling up on control parameters allows performers to develop skills within individual constraints.

Summary

Throwing patterns change without instruction and are guided by a collective variable (order parameter). Intrinsically based instruction or augmented information is not necessary for skill levels to improve. These results support the ETA applied model, which encourages learners to discover a movement form that best fits their individual constraints relative to the task goal and context conditions. Instructors and coaches may assist learners and athletes with this discovery by manipulating the relevant task variables (step 3 in the ETA applied model).

In the study discussed in this chapter, the control parameter was identified as velocity of throw. When throwing velocity was manipulated, the motor system adapted by taking advantage of the order parameter (kinetic link principle). In the language of ETA, throwing velocity is a goal condition that can be manipulated by the instructor or coach. Such manipulation resulted in an increase in skill level. Thus, from a practical standpoint, instructors and coaches are encouraged to be cognizant of control parameters as relevant task variables that help initiate changes in motor patterns. Such manipulations allow time for, and assist in, self-discovery as is consistent with the ETA applied model.

Enhancing Instruction Using Ecological Task Analysis

Geoffrey D. Broadhead, PhD

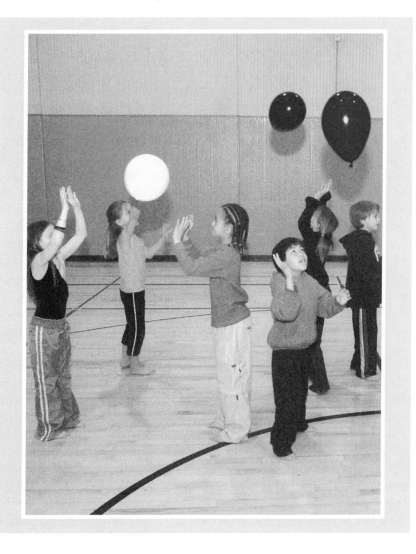

The chapters in part II illustrate first and foremost that the Ecological Task Analysis model has wide application as an empowerment approach to learning. The model has been used with individuals in school, health care, and sport settings; with those who develop typically and also those with disabilities; and with average performers as well as elite athletes.

Perhaps one of the reasons the ETA model has not found widespread use in physical education and sport is that it has not been found to be as user friendly as first anticipated. This issue is addressed extremely well in several chapters and also in the Epilogue.

Decision-Making Process

Kidman and Davis (chapter 6) emphasize the importance of empowerment and student decision making, introducing the topic of empowerment in coaching. Participant empowerment and decision making are central to ETA, but run counter to traditional ways of thinking in which the coach has an authoritarian role. The authors enumerate differences between empowered athletes and disempowered athletes, as well as an empowering versus a disempowering coach. They also report results of an elaborate case study by the lead author about establishing quality team culture. Within what is termed the value of "oneness," which is the stated preferred culture, the objective was to see how empowerment could work during a full season of volleyball. Although no quantitative measures were taken, the persons involved in the case study outlined their thoughts concerning the process and outcome of empowerment in coaching. Interestingly, the team members together developed goals and objectives that were not related to on-court skills or strategies.

Student decision making in physical education, as part of the implementation of the ETA model, is the subject of the Carson, Bulger, and Townsend chapter (chapter 7). While the student-centered approach is supported, the starting point is the "traditional" teacher-directed methodology. Rather than an indiscriminate use of student involvement, Carson and her colleagues promote a more balanced approach. They suggest that a sequence of stages be followed in order to develop students' responsible decision making, catering to inter- and intra-individual student differences. Teachers, acting as guides rather than directors of student activity, provide alternative solutions from which students are invited to choose their path to achieving the task goal.

Ways of ensuring student accountability, including use of peers to observe, record, and guide, are suggested.

Incorporating Elements of Tradition Into the ETA Model

The authors of two of the chapters integrate the ETA model into their own or another established teaching model. Mitchell and Oslin (chapter 8) use the four tenets of ETA to draw parallels with their own work on the Tactical Games model (TGM). Their version of TGM greatly clarifies the idea of teaching games by emphasizing the context rather than physical skills per se. However, the enhanced benefits of combining a focus on strategies with a focus on skills show the futility of an either/or debate, other than as a way of clarifying and discriminating between the two emphases. In describing the links between task goal and the constraints of the performer and the environment, Mitchell and Oslin use a fairly traditional method of task analysis, which is different from what is advocated in the ETA model.

Hutzler (chapter 9) outlines the development of a model that seeks to extend the ideas of the ETA model. His focus is on the need to improve inefficient movement patterns by seeking adaptation strategies ("ecological interventions"). Hutzler emphasizes that manipulations made to previously chosen movement patterns increase the effectiveness and efficiency of the adaptation and simultaneously decrease unnecessary adaptations. Some may see this adaptation strategy as limiting student choices, which is a central idea of the ETA model. Several examples of ineffective and inefficient movement patterns are described in support of the model (Systematic Ecological Modification Approach; SEMA), as part of its development and testing. It can be said that by identifying errors in relation to preferred movement patterns, the SEMA model may be less flexible than the ETA model.

Including Individuals Who Are Different

Three chapters demonstrate the inclusiveness of the ETA model by ensuring that it caters to individuals who are different from those who develop typically. Taylor, Goodwin, and Groeneveld (chapter 10) outline decision-making opportunities for learners with disabilities.

In their experience with the ETA approach, these authors found two major barriers to its implementation in settings for students with disabilities. One is that teachers in the field are entrenched in the directed approach. Without a history of student choice in pedagogy, greater personal commitment and more intense professional preparation are required. The other barrier "relates to our own knowledge and understanding of the interactions of task dimensions and participant characteristics and the necessary role they play in presenting an environment that encourages choice making from any and all participants."

Strategies for overcoming these barriers are given, as is a rationale for using choice with students with disabilities. These authors argue that a prime reason for presenting a choice instructional model is to simultaneously decrease undesirable responses while increasing desirable responses. They cite evidence to show that many students with disabilities can learn to select from a range of choices and thus can establish a wide repertoire of motor skills. The authors suggest that "creating opportunities for choice making in instructional settings requires numerous instructor and learner conditions to be in place." As one example, they advocate the use of "ETA simulations" to help achieve this. They give special emphasis to the needs of those students who function at the lowest levels, and stress the importance of peers in the instructional process of such children.

Mullally and Mullally (chapter 11) address the goal of improving the efficiency of compensatory strategies in pediatric physiotherapy. They provide detailed, insightful, and often colorful case studies to elaborate each of the four tenets of the ETA model. Thus, when structuring the social and physical environment, the authors emphasize the importance of the process by which the task solution is attempted. When choice of movement solution was encouraged, improved mobility resulted after a child's own movement preferences were sought. For children with and without disabilities, choice appeared to encourage intrinsic motivation, which was of considerable help to therapists. When providing instruction, Mullally and Mullally place importance on the increased efficiency of dyadic training, particularly with respect to the element of partner competition and use of peer observation. Drawing on their own experiences in therapy in Ireland, the authors promote the role of the therapist as a team member in what they call distributed intervention. This new role for therapists is similar to recent developments in the supervisory role of adapted physical education specialists in the public schools of the United States.

Citing the relative importance of the "immediacy of the situation and the task at hand" over individual structures in influencing performance, Vermeer (chapter 12) discusses a number of possibilities for individuals with various neurological impairments. He mentions that in health care settings it is important that intervention provides specific assistance to those whose capacity to apply experience in new settings may be weak. Vermeer focuses on the expectations of society for actions to fit a prescribed format, that is, normalization. Such strictures are thought to impose undue complications on some individuals with disabilities. Thus the environment does not change to suit the traits of individuals; it is the individuals who have to make the change. From this, Vermeer introduces the notion of providing "support" and offers examples of what is needed in various health care settings. By inference, the conclusion is that with a better-educated and -informed society, accommodations to individuals might be achieved.

Emphasizing
the Cognitive Element of ETA

Wall, Reid, and Harvey (chapter 13) offer a "knowledge-based approach" (KB approach) to explaining movement, which extends the ETA by emphasizing the importance of knowledge in a way the original ETA did not. Five types of knowledge about action are described as affective, declarative, and procedural knowledge and two metacognitive knowledge bases: metacognitive knowledge and metacognitive skills. Like ETA, the KB approach places emphasis on different learning environments. The authors discuss three progressively more challenging environments—instructional, practice, and competitive—and their importance for different populations. This classification of environments seems to be an important addition to the general task category classification of ETA (chapter 3). The authors claim that the KB approach is sensitive to the role of cognition in influencing movement competence. This claim appears to rest largely on the different degrees of knowledge about movement rather than level of cognitive functioning per se. It is perhaps the flip side of an early view of perceptual-motor theorists like Kephart (1971), who theorized that cognition has a motor base.

Summary

In conclusion it is important to note that from these chapters, it is readily apparent that it is not straightforward for practitioners to translate the four steps of the ETA model into the instructional process. In describing what they have accomplished, the authors have demonstrated that there are many more possibilities for evaluation and extension of the model than might have been implied by Davis and Burton when they first proposed the ETA model. It is hoped that scholars will independently, or through the influence of this book, seek to develop their own ideas for investigation and, of course, disseminate them widely.

CHAPTER 6

Empowerment in Coaching

Lynn Kidman, PhD, and Walter E. Davis, PhD

Coaching is a dynamic process that involves interactions for the purpose of enhancing athlete performance. Among the many reciprocally related elements that coaches need to consider in a sporting environment, the most important are the athlete, environment, and task (athlete performance). This idea of reciprocal relationships in coaching is consistent with the Ecological Task Analysis model. Ecological Task Analysis was "designed to gain insight to the dynamics of movement behavior by examining interacting constraints (both limitations and enablement) of a performer, environment, and task" (Burton and Davis 1996, p. 287). A major premise of ETA is that there are many possible solutions to a movement task as determined by the mutual interaction of the performer and the environment. One implication of the ETA model for practice is that the performer should first be given choices in selecting the appropriate solution rather than being told what to do and how to do as occurs in most traditional teaching models. Likewise, in the performance and participant coaching environment there has been a major paradigm shift from a "prescriptive" to an "empowerment" approach in which athletes share in decision making and contribute to their learning, based on their goals and intents of action (Lyle 2002).

Coaching has traditionally focused on prescription, in which coaches use a "do as I say" approach to learning and performance. Traditional coaching has not really focused on the athlete, environment, or task. Coaches simply tell athletes what goal to achieve and which game plan to run. In contrast, empowerment in coaching, as in ETA, focuses on enabling the athletes to take responsibility for their own performance. Thus, empowerment is an evolving paradigm that challenges the traditional practices in coaching in which coaches hold total power and control over the athletic environment. Empowerment coaching utilizes steps similar to those of the ETA model (Burton and Davis 1996): (a) establishing mutual goals and directions (e.g., coach and athletes), (b) allowing athlete choice and control in the sporting environment, (c) manipulating variables within the sport environment to facilitate athlete performance, and (d) providing instruction.

Sport should provide an opportunity for participation in which the growth and development of the individual, rather than the sport jock, are a priority. Lombardo (1987) suggests that to develop the whole person, sporting environments should be enjoyable as well as promote learning. Coaching using an empowerment approach ensures that both these objectives are met, as will be demonstrated in this chapter. Empowerment is a form of coaching that will develop thinking people, as it promotes athlete problem solving. When coaches use an empowering style of coaching, athletes gain and take ownership of knowledge and understanding of sport and their own lives. When athletes take ownership and responsibility for their learning, their performance can be greatly enhanced. The premise of empowerment coaching is that athletes have a capacity to learn from their experiences if they have been "actively involved in determining and evaluating these experiences" (Cross and Lyle 1999, p. 39).

This chapter highlights some current qualitative research on how coaches employ coaching. It addresses the benefits and challenges of an empowerment style of coaching. The chapter includes a discussion of various attributes of empowerment coaching and reflects on an approach known as Teaching Games for Understanding. The importance of the development of a team culture is discussed, followed by an excerpt from a case study of a high school team's establishment and maintenance of vision, goals, values, and strategies. The case study provides a practical example of athlete success using an empowerment style of coaching.

What Is Empowerment Coaching?

Although the term *empowerment* has many interpretations, at a general level it may be thought of as a process by which people gain control over the decisions affecting their lives. According to Giddens (1984), power, as a relationship between agents, is the utilization of resources to act on the world in such a way as to make a difference. This notion of power suggests that there are resources (including the agency of others) that may be utilized to enhance one's self at the expense of others and thus to dominate them. A person with more power can co-opt or appropriate power from others (Eskes, Duncan, and Miller 1998). Contrarily, there are resources (including those given freely by others) that may be utilized to enhance one's self but not at the expense of others. This is power through enablement (Davis and Strand, this volume). Persons with more power can also act in a manner that enhances rather than appropriates the power of others.

In a well-known quote, Ginott (1972) had this to say about teachers,

I am the decisive element in the classroom. It is my personal approach that creates the climate. It is my daily mood that makes the weather. As a teacher I possess tremendous power to make a child's life miserable or joyous. I can be a tool of torture or an instrument of inspiration. I can humiliate or humor, hurt or heal. In all situations it is my response that decides whether a crisis will be escalated or de-escalated, and a child humanized or de-humanized. (p. 15-16)

Coaches, the same as teachers, have the power to determine directions and actions of athletes, the team environment, and performance. It is power they could use to dominate. On the other hand, coaches can use their power as enablement and thus empower athletes. Giving athletes choices, opportunities for decision making, and control over their own destiny is at the heart of empowerment coaching.

Coaches often highlight the importance of gaining trust and respect from their athletes (Potrac 2004; Shogan 1991, 1999). As Shogan (1999) states, " . . . the imperative of teamwork requires that athletes and coaches trust each other, even though coaches often exercise more power on teams than do athletes" (p. 81). In an empowerment model of coaching, this trust must be mutual and is largely dependent upon the coach. Mutual trust and respect between coach and athlete do not mean sameness. Athletes must trust their coaches to make suggestions and decisions and ensure athlete responsibility in the best interest of the team. Athletes trust coaches to be knowledgeable and prepared and to provide a safe and supporting environment (Shogan 1999). Through mutual trust, athletes take responsibility for their and the team's learning and performance, which enhances the team environment. In turn, coaches trust athletes to be serious about their performance goals and the goals of the team. Empowerment (power through enablement) promotes a shared, dynamic power relationship between athlete and coach. Empowerment is a pedagogical strategy that will enhance the trust and respect that so many coaches suggest are important to athlete performance.

A coach who is coach-centered—that is, who coaches for him- or herself, uses power to dominate, and considers athletes (whether consciously or unconsciously) as only a means to an end—is a disempowering coach. This approach is more likely to meet the coach's goals and less likely to meet athletes' goals. A coach-centered coach is one who totally directs and prescribes every aspect of the sporting environment and thus disempowers the athletes.

On the other end of the continuum (see table 6.1), an athlete-centered coach is one who tends to empower and use many tools and methods of enablement. This coaching approach is similar to the ETA applied model, in which students (athletes) make choices and contribute to the direction and mutual goals of the student and teacher (athlete and coach). An athlete-centered approach promotes a sense of belonging and provides opportunities for athletes to have a role in problem solving and a shared approach to learning (Arai 1997; Freysinger and Bedini 1994).

Table 6.1   Practices That Characterize Empowering and Disempowering Coaches

An empowering coach	A disempowering coach
Motivational climate • Provides a safe and confirming environment • Encourages wairua (being one) • Promotes athlete independency • Gives athletes responsibility to encourage accountability for their actions • Trusts athletes to live by the values created by the team • Promotes a positive learning environment	**Motivational climate** • Expects a conforming environment • Bases team culture on the coach's direction • Promotes athlete dependency • Uses threats or punishment to coerce athletes into following coach's expectations • Insists that athletes abide by coach's rules • Promotes fear of failure
Athlete centered • Is empathetic and values all athletes' contributions equally • Accepts each athlete as a unique individual • Listens to athletes and takes them seriously	**Coach centered** • Treats the team as one entity rather than as individuals • Does not accept athletes' opinions • Speaks to athletes, rather than listening to their opinions
Values • Is open and honest • Is flexible • Reinforces values and morals through facilitation of team's goals • Acts as a role model • Recognizes the role of sport in the larger society	**Values** • Is not open and tells white lies • Is inflexible • Has a "winning at all costs" attitude, thus promotes unprofessional ways of seeking an advantage • Tells athletes to act one way and acts another • Promotes the role of sport as the most important aspect of athletes' lives

An empowering coach	A disempowering coach
Enables learning	**Instructs**
• Makes each athlete feel capable of succeeding	• Promotes authoritarianism and "one size fits all" philosophy
• Is purposeful and provides meaningful learning opportunities	• Coaches to win, rather than develop or educate athletes
• Asks open-ended questions	• Asks redundant and closed-ended questions
• Encourages problem solving and critcal thinking	• Tells athletes answers and provides feedback of what to fix
• Encourages athletes to ask questions and seek knowledge	• Discourages athlete questioning
• Provides athletes with appropriate choices and opportunities for decision making	• Makes decisions for athletes and the game play
• Uses mistakes as a learning opportunity	• Criticizes athletes for mistakes
• Asks athletes to evaluate coaching practices	• Does not ask for athletes' evaluations of coaching practice
Psychological, physical, and emotional needs focus	**Physical needs focus**
• Stresses intrinsic value over extrinsic rewards	• Stresses extrinsic rewards over intrinsic values
• Promotes healthy attitude toward sport and competition	• Does not monitor psychological or emotional needs, focuses on physical
• Assists athletes in analyzing their individual and team actions and feelings	• Ignores athletes' feelings and needs
• Gets to know each athlete as an individual	• Gets to know only athletes who are important to the coach

One of the main advantages of using empowerment in coaching is that athletes are motivated to learn and have a greater understanding and retention of both tactics and skills (cognitive, psychological, emotional, and physical) that are so important to success in sport. A coach who empowers his or her athletes facilitates the athletes' learning, but does not control it. Athletes are required to be self-sufficient in their performance and option taking while participating in their sports; an empowering approach encourages athletes to become self-aware and self-directed (see table 6.2). Such an approach allows athletes to be self-responsible and make informed decisions, and emphasizes individual growth and change.

The style of coaching that is promoted here is an alternative to traditional, disempowering coaching styles because it gives athletes more ownership of their sport and of their life in general. Empowerment provides athletes opportunities for decision making, a cognitive process

Table 6.2   A Comparison of Empowered and Disempowered Athletes

Empowered athletes	Disempowered athletes
• Set their own goals and have an intrinsic desire to reach them • Enjoy their sport • Show enthusiasm • Develop self-efficacy and confidence in their ability and are enabled to control results produced by their skill and effort • Understand that they contribute and take responsibility for their learning and direction • Are accountable for their actions • Are resourceful and innovative • Feel that they are important because of coaches' actions toward understanding them (e.g., listening, empathy) • Understand that there is a mutual trust and respect • Cooperate to enhance mutual goals and directions • Are more coachable because they have freedom and choice • Are highly committed to achieving levels of excellence • Are willing to engage totally in what they believe in	• Have their goals set for them • Feel as if they don't have a say in any direction • May lack enthusiasm • Are treated as a means to an end • Make no decisions • Talk back when they've had enough • Often compete "robotically" • Can display anger and stubbornness • Listen to the coach's way • Often have a disrespectful attitude • Are defensive when challenged • Get easily frustrated • Are not listened to • Feel that there is no respect or trust from the coach • Are not encouraged to be individuals and therefore show uncooperativeness • Lack ability to make informed decisions

that coaches often suggest is missing in athlete development (Kidman 2001). The lack of decision making results mostly from the fact that coaches often model their coaching styles on those practices used by the coaches they had when they were athletes.

Empowerment coaching builds a committed partnership between the athlete and team and the coach. In this partnership, the coach acts as a facilitator or catalyst for athletes' optimal performance. When the goals of the athletes and coaches are mutual and teamwork is enhanced, the chances for achieving positive outcomes, including winning, increase. An empowering coach helps athletes learn and enables them to understand how to exceed their current limits. The coach nurtures involvement and autonomy in athletes (Usher 1997).

The empowering approach does not suggest that the coach should give full responsibility to athletes. Rather, coaches should exercise their leadership, guiding athletes by setting up problems to solve and allowing them to take their own responsibility for their sport participation and performance. Clearly in some situations, with some athletes, coaches need to be more prescriptive, but the aim should always be to encourage self-reliance.

A number of successful coaches base their style on an empowerment approach that encourages athletes to become self-aware of skill execution and tactical play. These coaches include Wayne Smith, All Blacks assistant rugby coach; Rick Charlesworth, ex-Australian women's hockey coach; Don Tricker, New Zealand Black Sox coach; Wayne Bennett, Brisbane Broncos rugby league coach; and Phil Jackson, Los Angeles Lakers coach. Much of what these coaches focus upon is athlete problem solving as a key to holistic athlete development (physical, psychosocial, cognitive, and moral).

Many people practice coaching without really understanding the process. Comparable to the ETA model (Davis and Burton 1991), the coaching process is dependent on the complex dynamics between coaches and athletes, their individual attributes, their desires and ambitions, and the training and competition context surrounding all this. Empowerment coaching considers all these complexities, but with an emphasis on the development of the athlete.

Coach Questioning

One way of helping athletes learn to problem solve is for coaches to pose meaningful questions. It is not simply a matter of asking questions; effective coach questioning requires purposeful questions phrased in a way that encourages the athlete to respond. Stimulating questions are an extremely powerful means to inspire athletes and enhance intrinsic motivation (Butler 1997; Kidman 2001). Questioning also engages athletes on a conscious level and enhances their concentration, and thus their intensity. This "intensity" transfers well into game situations in which the pressure is great.

Because coach questioning is not as prevalent as direct coaching, athletes may be reluctant to respond to posed questions. Once athletes become more accustomed to this practice and see that it gives them ownership for their learning, they will be more accepting of the questions and become more cognitively involved in the sport environment.

Among advocates of a prescriptive coaching approach, there is a perception that coaches who ask questions do not know the answers themselves. Indeed, coaches may find it difficult, and at times daunting, to design questions that generate high-level thinking from the athletes.

Yet to create situations in which athletes learn best, coaches must listen to their athletes' responses, then redirect, prompt, and probe for better or more complete answers. This all demands an in-depth understanding of the game, the athlete, and the context in which the approach is applied. As Wayne Smith suggests,

> To truly empower athletes to take responsibility for their learning, use game specific activities, ensure that they have fun and use questioning for them to become self-aware . . . I believe at the élite level, the questioning approach really tests your knowledge and in particular your eyes and technical nous. (Kidman 2005, p. 245)

Athletes will make an ever-increasing effort and will enjoy problem solving if given the opportunity. Generating their own solutions empowers athletes and gives them more self-awareness, which enhances their performance, as is well documented (Metzler 2000; Ravizza 1993; Schempp 1982). For example, athletes who take ownership will remember, understand, and apply the content more effectively than those who are told what to do, when to do it, and how to do it. Solving problems through coach questioning enables athletes to explore, discover, create, and generally experiment with a variety of movement forms, skills, and tactics or strategies of a specific sport. When athletes are enabled to problem solve, long-term learning is enhanced (Thorpe 1990). Mark Norton (Riccarton High School volleyball coach) reiterated the usefulness of solving problems when he said,

> . . . the problem solving stuff was about them experiencing situations where certain team cohesiveness and tactical strategies were required. The questioning that followed allowed them to discover the strategies that would work in similar future situations. When the same or similar situations arose in the game context, they identified them as problems they had already faced and knew ways of solving them. I don't think I had to call a time out and say you have to do this and this. Often I would call the time out because they needed a break, but they more often than not did all the talking and problem solving. (Kidman 2005, p. 56)

Coaches should test out their questioning strategy in each particular situation and adapt it to meet the purpose of the training session and athletes' needs and expectations. Sport and physical activity offer relevant contexts to involve athletes in high-level thinking. Coaches are often surprised and excited by how much athletes really do know and how easily they self-learn.

Teaching Games for Understanding

Teaching Games for Understanding (TGfU), the original model for a games approach to learning, has been adapted and modified in various contexts and can be found under various names, including Play Practice (Launder 2001), Tactical Games model (Griffin, Mitchell, and Oslin 1997), and Game Sense (Australian Sports Commission 1997). The commonality of all these games approaches is that the game is used for athlete learning of the skills and techniques and their tactical understanding of the sport. The TGfU model sets up games as problem-solving activities. As a full chapter devoted to the Tactical Games model is included in this volume, only the relationship to empowerment coaching is discussed here.

Teaching Games for Understanding advocates student problem solving and is thus consistent with an empowering style of coaching. The model was developed as a result of Rod Thorpe and David Bunker's observations of children in physical education classes, which led them to conclude that children learn well in game situations. Developed from "educational gymnastics" and originally designed for children, TGfU has been adapted by many coaches to suit players on different levels of many sports, from children through to high-performance teams. Teaching Games for Understanding challenges the traditional training program in which the game is often saved for the end of a training session (and often used as a reward for good behavior). Instead, purposeful games are the essence of the training program. This approach enables athletes to learn about the game and practice skills and technique within the context of a game rather than separately from it. Learning in context provides a sound understanding of the game and opportunities to apply skill and technique in pressure situations. When athletes are allowed to play or practice, undistracted by coaches telling them what to do and where to go, they are more productive in terms of learning in context, and motivation is enhanced through challenges, social interactions, and decision making (Kidman and Hanrahan 2004).

Rod Thorpe (2001) suggested that TGfU was a reaction to "traditional instruction" in two ways. He and his coauthor, Dave Bunker, could not understand how one could expect children to learn if they were not involved in the learning process and did not understand what they were trying to do. Moreover, as sport psychologists, they could not continue to accept an approach in which children lost the motivation to play and improve. According to Thorpe,

> We wanted an approach that we felt youngsters could contribute
> to, know what they were doing and where they were going. We

found most children pre-12 years of age wanted to "play", so we wanted to capture and keep this personal (intrinsic) motivation. We wanted to challenge and we wanted improvement and we realised we could not achieve any of these things if we continued to deliver a technical model, suitable for the average, using a "prescriptive" style. (p. 25)

The ability to use an understanding of the rules, strategies, tactics, and most importantly, "of oneself to solve the problems posed by the game or by one's opponents" (Launder 2001, p. 36), is the basis for TGfU. It is understanding in action and the ability to respond or make decisions, even while new events are happening, and applying game sense—"reading the game."

Teaching Games for Understanding fits into the empowering philosophy because it enhances athletes' motivation and thus intensity of performance through athlete problem solving. Athletes' effort is increased because of meaningful challenges. These challenges also create opportunities for athletes to respond to pressure situations inherent in sport competitions. Achievement is also enhanced as TGfU enables athletes to do something well, to problem solve, and to take ownership for their own learning. Of course, enjoyment is definitely enhanced because games are fun. Through games, athletes share success and failure; they learn how to trust each other and to know each other's ways of competing and making decisions, thus enhancing team culture.

Developing Team Culture

One major way to encourage self-reliance is the pursuit of quality team culture through which athletes gain responsibility for establishing and maintaining a direction for the team. Team culture is a major philosophical underpinning in empowerment coaching and is defined as the ability to bring individuals together for the pursuit of a common goal (Yukelson 1997). Team culture is a multifaceted process in which mutual goal pursuit informs the quality of the team's functioning and operation. Without quality team culture, success, learning, and often winning, are difficult. Thus, a major challenge for coaches is to bring athletes together for learning and success.

It is important to define success within an empowering coaching approach. A sport environment focus should be on success, not on winning. That is, striving to win is more important than actually winning. An athlete can win without performing well and can lose even if the performance has been outstanding.

Unfortunately, winning is often equated with success and defined as the result of a competition. Winning, based on a comparison with others, is a major outcome of sport competition and thus important and valued. However, success is a measure of athletes' learning, enjoyment, performance, and personal growth, all of which may be achieved with or without winning. As an example, Wayne Smith suggested that his most successful season was in his first year of coaching the Canterbury Crusaders:

> It was a brilliant year, the best year of rugby I'd ever had in my life, either playing or coaching. We didn't even make the semi-finals, but we built a lot of self-esteem. We had players who, in interviews at the start of the season, said they didn't feel they should be on the same field as Auckland. Just getting them to the point where they could hold their heads high, where they knew they understood the game better than most players around the country was satisfying. We were starting to do something special and we knew it. It was a process of building self-confidence and belief. It was very rewarding and enjoyable. (Kidman 2001, p. 19)

In any competition, it is difficult to win if athletes do not experience success and there is no quality team culture, athlete-centered environment, or balance in their lives. Success as athlete learning, enjoyment, performance, or growth is often overlooked with a "winning at all costs" attitude. With a "winning at all costs" attitude, sport participation degenerates into a means to an end as athletes' needs are ignored and the pursuit of excellence is sabotaged (Boxill 2003).

There is an important Maori word we use in New Zealand that encompasses the notion of team spirit: *wairua,* which means "oneness." It refers to a spirituality that contributes to an individual's well-being. The word encompasses all that is positive about team culture (i.e., values and attitudes, respect and trust, caring and concern for others). Without wairua, the quality of team culture is diminished and therefore the chance of success is limited.

Some of the coaches identified previously have suggested that wairua is the key to any team's success (see Kidman 2005). Ensuring wairua includes constructing team standards and having spiritual appreciation. Quality team culture helps to fulfill the psychological and social needs of the athletes (Liu 2001). In team culture, according to Liu, all members voluntarily have a "common faith, valuation view, morality, spirit pillar, ceremony, intelligence factor, and entertainment life" (p. 28). Jerry Lynch (2001) suggests that the "root of true cohesion is selflessness, willingness to see that the team goal is greater than the goal of any one athlete" (p. 77). To ensure wairua, enabling athletes to make decisions on team direction enhances selflessness and benefits the team vision, goals, values, and strategies as it allows for self-responsibility.

It is important to note that each team is unique, with the individuals having unique attributes as well as some commonalities with other athletes. Teams also participate in an ever-changing context. Thus, teams may develop their own unique culture. What works for one team does not necessarily work for another team. The empowerment approach to coaching takes uniqueness into account by focusing on the nurturing of athletes and enhancing the positive aspects of each environment in which they participate.

It is clear that establishing a mutual direction and goals for a team enhances athlete and team performance (Carron and Dennis 1998; Kidman 2001; Liu 2001; Yukelson 1997). The purpose of establishing a vision is to formulate season goals so that all athletes strive for the same purpose. Values serve the purpose of establishing "rules" for the team and form the basis for setting up strategies to meet team goals. It is important when establishing the vision and goals that the athletes are included in decision making so that they take ownership and assume responsibility for monitoring themselves.

Case Study:
Establishing Quality Team Culture

This section presents an account of action research conducted with the Riccarton High School boys' volleyball team, 2003-2004, by the lead author of this chapter. The purpose is to illustrate the process of establishing a vision, goals, values, and strategies and reinforcing these elements throughout the season. The action research study, based on the coach, used Yukelson's (1997) components of team culture (i.e., unity of purpose, individual and team accountability, teamwork, open and honest communication, positive atmosphere, and mutual trust), which were trialed with the team and maintained and reinforced through the coach's empowerment approach. To study the effects of these components, I acted as a participant observer for the volleyball season and conducted two interviews each with the coach (Mark Norton) and two players (Luke Russell and Simon Kidman) during and after the season. I took on the role of "manager" to become part of the team and its process. I attended every training session and every game and went to the national tournament. The team culture, athlete learning, and coach's approach were followed and analyzed and are reported using "confessional tales"

(Sparkes 2002). This chapter includes only an excerpt from the full case study (see Kidman 2005).

Before the season began I met with Mark to discuss the process of working together and my role as a researcher. Mark explained that he was a physical education teacher at the school with a passion for volleyball. He had been a New Zealand volleyball player until 2003. Mark had coached the school's volleyball teams for the previous five years and had decided to learn more about an empowerment approach. He already used many practices of empowerment, but for this season, he expressed an interest in establishing wairua

> . . . to create a positive, enjoyable and meaningful experience for the kids to be involved in. I want the team and the team mission to become a focus in the boys' lives. I also want to create good volleyballers and a team that plays quality volleyball. I suppose I like to use volleyball and physical activity as a vehicle to teach the kids about themselves, other people and how to effectively interact and function with others. That's how I treat my teaching of Physical Education also. Volleyball, a game hugely reliant of team work and one's team mates lends itself to do this superbly. At the end of the day, if the kids have developed into better people, then I've been successful (Kidman 2005, p. 46).

Eighteen boys, ranging in age from 15 to 18 years old, trialed for the team. They formed a squad of two teams. Mark said,

> We wanted to have all the boys playing in the top grade, because I thought to improve at all, they needed to be playing the top volleyball, even if they were out of their depth a little. So, I split up what I thought was the leadership and ability and I tried to make two even teams, so they both would be able to hold their own, not necessarily win, but hold their own (Kidman 2005, p. 48).

An "A" and a "B" team were chosen in the second half of the season, but Mark indicated that making the A team was still an option for those chosen for the B team until two weeks before the Canterbury Championships. The boys and Mark decided that the criteria for selection to the A team should be skills and value contribution, considered equally.

The players were initially skeptical about this squad system. As Luke said, "I think the older guys didn't respect the younger guys that much because we thought that they sort of just mucked around all the time." Luke changed his mind after he saw how hard everyone on the squad worked. He said,

I think it was really good keeping that huge squad and all training together. I think it brought everyone's level up quite a lot. That made it better when we did split up because we played the Bs and they actually challenged us. If we just split up into As and Bs, then the As would waste the Bs every time we played them and it wouldn't do them or us any good. But having close games, made the Bs positive about things because they were beating us. It makes us all step back and see that we had to work a bit harder (Kidman 2005, p. 49).

At the end of the season, Simon also valued the squad system; he said, "It makes you work harder because you want to get to the top team and have more fun trying to do that. It makes you attend [training]" (Kidman 2005, p. 49).

Mark was keen to try this empowerment approach in several different ways and used many of the empowerment practices listed earlier (see table 6.1). However, the focus of this case study excerpt is only on the process of establishing the vision, goals, values, and strategies and the creation and maintenance of wairua.

First, to establish the goals and direction with the team members, Mark gave each boy a homework book for writing down decisions made during team training sessions. To establish both dream and performance goals, Mark asked, "If you were at the end-of-season dinner and had to make a speech and talk to everyone about the sort of team that we are, what would be the things that you would like to be able to say?"

Because of the size of the group, I didn't see much interaction at first; and it was obvious that due to comfort and confidence, the seniors had more to say than the junior members, who were hesitant and waited to see what their role in the whole process would be. The squad at first was quite curious about the idea of giving this input; even though Mark had been their coach in previous years, they had never been through the process of contributing to the direction of the team. Initially, they didn't understand or know their roles. As this was Mark's first attempt at such a process, there seemed to be a fair amount of experimenting and "going with the flow" (which in itself fits an empowering philosophy).

As would be expected of someone new to the empowerment approach, Mark found it difficult to allow athlete decision making, but he was consciously aware that he had to let the athletes speak and make these decisions if they were going to become owners. I noted that quite a few of his questions and statements were leading, but ultimately the team decided that the main mission goals were these:

- To win 6 of 10 Monday night games (with the squad system)
- To win the Canterbury Champs (once the A team had been selected; the boys decided that this would be two weeks before the champs)
- To achieve top 10 at the Nationals
- To achieve a semifinal spot at the Nationals (a dream goal)
- To be an exciting team to watch
- To become known as the team that never gives up; is the tightest; is mentally tough

Mark next explained that the boys needed to establish some values to live by and provided them with a list of 30 values from Jeff Janssen's (2002) book, *Championship Team Building.* He asked them to pick six values they considered to be important for the team, write down why they were important, and provide a definition of each value to enhance mutual understanding.

At the next training session, Mark divided the 18 boys into small groups (composed of one senior player and two junior players) and asked them to collate all of the athletes' values and prioritize the top six within the small group. Once each small group had prioritized their values, Mark wrote these values on a whiteboard and the whole group discussed their meaning. Mark facilitated the discussion and contributed his ideas as well.

I thought this process was particularly difficult for Mark, as he had his own preferred values for the team. Even though his views were also included, he seemed to "bite his tongue" several times to ensure that a decision was the boys'. A coach's power can often supersede what the athletes want, but Mark concentrated on enabling the athletes to contribute to major decisions. He realized that his role was to facilitate and follow through with the consensus of the team. Just as the boys had to come to a consensus and go with the majority, so did Mark. "Social power" in this process was also evident, as Mark was a physical education teacher for many of the players. However, in my interviews with the athletes, they both suggested that the goals and values were the players'. Luke said, "We were the ones that made the values. Because they came from us, we respected them a bit more than if they were just given to us and someone says, 'This is how you've got to act.' It wouldn't have been the same." Simon said, "The coach was in on it, but the kids did most of it. It's better because the coaches just don't make rules and the kids have things to say, so it's better to listen to everyone."

After much discussion and some debate, the team came up with six values for the volleyball team. These were respect, communication, cohesion, enjoyment, invulnerable, and commitment (all worded and defined by the boys). Once these values were decided on, the next step in the process of establishing vision and values was to come up with strategies to meet the goals. This time Mark asked the boys to think about strategies needed to ensure that the values were practiced. The same process was followed; the boys were placed into small groups for a discussion and then brought back into the whole group to make the decision. To achieve their goals and live the values, they committed to the following:

- Talk constructively at appropriate times
- Take care of things outside volleyball so we can enjoy the game and our season
- Respect each other at all times
- Attend all trainings, physically, mentally, and socially (be intense)
- Remain positive no matter what
- Always demonstrate positive winning posture
- Always be there for my teammates

By about the fifth training session, the team had established the goals, values, and strategies for the season. The process was enjoyable to watch. I had often wondered how this age group would react to such a process, but the enthusiasm on the part of the boys (once they knew that Mark was going to follow through and monitor their decisions) highlighted to me that this age group reveled in the process. As the boys were the main decision makers, they ensured that the values and strategies were followed when striving for their goals. In other words, they owned the team culture.

Once the vision, values, goals, and strategies were established, it was decided that the team needed one short, precise mission statement that could be used to represent the team. After much discussion and about two training sessions later, the team came up with "Binding Together to be Better (B3)." The boys also decided they needed a symbol that represented the vision, goals, and values of the team and chose a glue stick because they saw it as a tool that "binds them together to be better." Mark bought three-sided glue sticks to match the B3 vision statement. The boys wrote their names and the values on the glue sticks and carried them everywhere as the symbol of their volleyball campaign.

As a result of this process, the boys created a tight group who were well known within their school. To show their commitment (one of the values), they hung the glue sticks around their necks to wear around school and to volleyball. Teachers and other students came to "idolize" the glue stick. Simon told this story:

> In a way, the year 9's respected us because we were wearing these glue sticks. An example was that last term we were sitting in the hall and a member of the team had a Stage Challenge Practice and they put all their gear down, including the glue stick. The year 9 kid went up and grabbed his glue stick and put it on and was walking around during lunchtime and they thought he was cool. The glue stick really helped us. It wasn't just at volleyball, but at school everyone respected and thought we were awesome (Kidman 2005, p. 52).

In a similar vein, Luke said,

> [The glue stick] was good, that was a way to reinforce the values. It brought all the values together. It was the way for our season and stuff. It reinforced it a bit more. It was really cool to see people wearing them at school. Everyone knew we were a team as well. Everyone knew that we are a pretty good team and that we were pretty close (Kidman 2005, p. 52).

The boys carried the glue sticks everywhere, including into classes and external exams. The boys then decided that if someone was caught without the glue stick, that player or coach would get a slit in his or her eyebrow (i.e., a shaved line through the eyebrow) as another symbol of the values. The boys also decided that if they failed to communicate (e.g., to tell the coach they couldn't make it to training), they would get a slit. Most boys were happy to take the slit for the team, but some had some cultural issues about it. Mark set up a team discussion, and the boys changed the system. By this time, not much coach monitoring was occurring because of the boys' ownership of the values.

Another part of this process was the creation of a poster that included all of the boys' photos and listed the vision, goals, strategies, and values. At an official signing-off ceremony all the team members signed the poster as a type of contract to strive for the goals and adhere to the values created. This "contract" proved to be another binding element, as when issues arose, the boys and Mark always referred to the poster, saying, "You signed that you agreed to these values." As the athletes self-managed the direction of the team, the coach's role was instructing and focusing on the values.

The poster also proved to be binding when one of the boys did not live up to the values. When this incident was raised in front of the team, a discussion followed, which demonstrated athlete decision making. The team expressed its concern about his well-being but believed that the values were important and that if someone wasn't living up to them, he didn't belong on the team. So, the team decided that the boy had agreed to the contract but was not living the values, so he must be asked to leave. Mark was given the responsibility to inform him, which proved to be another learning experience.

For the season, the boys achieved all but one of their goals. They won Canterbury Championships and placed fifth at Nationals. At Nationals, it was evident not only to the boys and to the coach, but also to opposing and observing teams, that the wairua felt by the boys enhanced their play. The skill level of the team was considered lower than the standard of many others, yet they still managed to beat higher-skilled teams. The boys, the coach, and outsiders attributed their success to the wairua they had created, symbolized by the glue stick. Many a player and coach from other organizations wanted to know about the glue sticks. This became quite a talking point at the Nationals and then back at school after the Nationals.

Reflecting on the season, Mark, Luke, and Simon commented that this volleyball season was one of the most successful sport seasons in which they had participated. They indicated that the success did not come from winning (e.g., Canterbury Championships), but from meeting all their goals (except placing in the semifinals at Nationals, the dream goal) and exceeding their expectations. Luke said, "Bringing the team together, having [everyone] on the team contributing and everyone knowing that they are useful and being positive about it." Simon noted, "Because we knew each other, we knew how we played, we worked out a good game plan and we knocked off bigger teams because we didn't get down and we just played as a team." They believed that the team achieved the value of cohesiveness, which made the season enjoyable (one of the values).

Enabling athletes to make decisions highlights the natural expectations of any team. The athletes in this case chose the direction of the team, and therefore they took on the role of self-monitoring, which enhanced wairua. With respect to reinforcing the values and the symbol of the glue stick, Mark said, "I think it gave them complete ownership and I think when they had that sense of ownership, they were prepared to do more, were prepared to work harder, and were prepared to sacrifice other things. . . ." This self-responsibility led to athletes' taking ownership of preparation and performance, a foundation to the empowerment approach.

INSTRUCTIONAL STRATEGIES

- It is important to shift coach instruction from telling athletes what to do to enabling athletes to take responsibility for their performance. This actually improves athletes' performance.
- Sport, like physical education, is about growth and development of the individual.
- Teaching Games for Understanding is a problem-solving approach in which athletes use a game to answer questions.
- Developing a quality team culture is essential to enhancing athletes' performance and this can best be done by involving athletes in decisions about the team's vision, goals, and values.

Summary

If a coach is dedicated to enhancing athlete performance and developing athletes as people, he or she can offer athletes a profound, enjoyable, positive, and successful experience. Our athletes deserve good coaches, dedicated to athletes' betterment and to the development of confident, motivated, successful, and happy people. This dedication is embedded in the values and principles of an empowering philosophy. This power through enablement helps athletes to achieve success through self-reliance, self-fulfillment, and self-awareness.

CHAPTER 7

Enhancing Responsible Student Decision Making in Physical Activity

Linda M. Carson, EdD, Sean M. Bulger, EdD,
and J. Scott Townsend, EdD

The promotion of lifelong physical activity has been recommended as a contemporary mission for the physical education teaching profession (Pate and Hohn 1994). Practicing physical educators would be well served to provide an instructional environment that contributes directly to the development of the cognitive, psychomotor, affective, and fitness characteristics that will enable a child to maintain a physically active lifestyle throughout adulthood. Corbin (1994) suggests that physical education students must acquire the necessary problem solving, self-evaluation, and decision-making skills if they are to effectively progress along a developmental continuum from a state of dependence to independence regarding their own physical activity behaviors. Accordingly, physical education professionals should employ instructional methodologies that facilitate the development of these higher-order cognitive skills as a natural consequence of the teaching-learning environment.

The proposed benefits associated with the provision of meaningful decision-making opportunities for physical education students include enhanced self-responsibility, increased self-motivation, heightened levels of engagement, and the achievement of higher-order educational objectives (Balan and Davis 1993). The purpose of this chapter is to extend the application of Ecological Task Analysis for teaching practitioners by suggesting a systematic approach to decision making. We recommend teaching strategies that will acquaint students with components of ETA as well as formalize and structure the opportunities for student

---

The first paragraph in this chapter and the section "Implementing ETA in Physical Education" are reprinted with permission from S.M. Bulger, J.S. Townsend, and L.M. Carson, "Promoting Responsible Student Decision-Making in Elementary Physical Education, *Journal of Physical Education, Recreation and Dance* 7 (2001): 18-23.

decision making. Furthermore, the benefits associated with the use of learner-centered instructional environments in physical education are presented, along with practical guidelines for (a) making the transition from teacher-directed to learner-centered instructional models, (b) establishing a physical environment that facilitates responsible choice, and (c) encouraging a high degree of student accountability within a learner-centered physical activity setting.

Role of the Teacher in an ETA Approach

The movement from teacher-directed to learner-centered instruction remains a highly significant trend across educational levels and disciplines. While there is no uniform agreement on a definition of the term *learner-centered,* Paris and Combs (2000) propose five characteristics that exemplify the teacher's role in a learner-centered instructional environment: (a) The teacher is focused on the individual needs of the learner; (b) the teacher promotes active learner engagement; (c) the teacher is a guide, rather than a director; (d) the teacher facilitates learning through interactive decision making; and (e) the teacher is a reflective practitioner. Advocates suggest that the teacher's role in a learner-centered environment represents a significant departure from the more traditional role of teacher as "transmitter of knowledge that is so deeply rooted in the American schooling tradition (Brooks and Brooks 1993)" (Paris and Combs 2000, p. 3).

In an effort to assist teachers with this difficult transition, educational theorists have recommended a number of curricular and instructional strategies (e.g., Grace 1999; Manning 2000; Vars and Beane 2000) that are intended to help practicing teachers move from teacher-directed to learner-centered classroom environments. These strategies reportedly afford students more meaningful opportunities to actively engage in their own learning. This trend is also evident in the physical activity literature, which presents alternative instructional models like Sport Education (Siedentop 1994), ETA (Balan and Davis 1993; Burton and Davis 1996; Davis and Burton 1991), and the Tactical Games model (Griffin, Mitchell, and Oslin 1997) that require students to assume a more significant role in the determination of the teaching-learning environment. While there is some evidence to support the position that students are capable of this type of responsible decision making (Lydon and Cheffers 1984; Martinek, Zaichkowsky, and Cheffers 1977; Schempp, Cheffers, and Zaichkowsky 1983) and critical thinking (McBride 1989, 1999; McBride and Bonnette 1995) in relation to their own learning in physical education, additional research is needed to further delineate the benefits and liabilities associated with the use of learner-centered instructional approaches in comparison to traditional, teacher-directed models.

Direct instruction is a widely recognized model of teaching that has received a considerable amount of support in the literature regarding its effectiveness in a variety of educational contexts (Brophy and Good 1986; Housner 1990; Rosenshine and Stevens 1986). When using a direct instructional approach, the teacher typically exhibits the following behaviors: (a) communicating clear lesson objectives; (b) engaging the students in a progressive series of learning activities that allow for a high rate of success; (c) employing a variety of teaching strategies, such as modeling and instructional cueing, to explain the lesson content; (d) asking frequent questions to monitor student comprehension; (e) providing continual performance-related feedback; and (f) reteaching the lesson content as needed (Housner 1990). McBride (1999) summarizes the role of teacher and student during a physical education lesson that is delivered using direct instruction:

> Today, most physical educators (and many other teachers) use the traditional demonstration/replication instructional model, whereby they control most, if not all, of the class decision making. The teacher first identifies the skill or concept to be learned, breaks it down into component parts (teaching points), explains how to execute the assigned task, and then provides a visual demonstration. The students take this information and may work with a partner, go to a learning station, or simply practice the skill by themselves. The teacher circulates, observes learner performance, and provides corrective feedback. (p. 218)

Despite the substantial amount of empirical support concerning the effectiveness of a direct model of instruction, critics have argued that "direct instruction may not be as effective if the teacher's intent is to promote affective, social, or higher order cognitive growth in children" (Housner 1990, p. 221). McBride (1999), for example, maintains that teacher-centered learning environments in physical education offer few opportunities for students to think critically about their own learning. McBride goes on to suggest that teachers can restructure the learning environment in a physical education class to actively promote critical thinking among students by (a) assuming the role of facilitator rather than director, (b) using a variety of cooperative learning strategies, and (c) encouraging students to think reflectively about their cooperative learning experiences.

Ecological Task Analysis has been proposed as a learner-centered approach to movement skill instruction and assessment that incorporates critical thinking and decision making as defining characteristics of the teaching-learning environment (Balan and Davis 1993; Bouffard, Strean, and Davis 1998; Davis and Burton 1991). A primary goal of the ETA model is to individualize instruction by providing learners with increased opportunities for making choices regarding the learning activities in which they are engaged. Balan and Davis (1993) theorize that the encouragement of this type of learner decision making in physical education serves a number of instructional purposes: providing self-motivation; developing decision making, self-monitoring capabilities, and other cognitive skills; encouraging the discovery of the most appropriate movement form for each individual; and empowering students by giving them some control over their environment, which enhances autonomy and individuality and provides a general feeling of belonging. A more productive and cooperative instructional environment can be established when students are provided with choices regarding their own learning (Monty and Perlmutter 1987).

In a teacher-directed model of instruction, "the teacher chooses the task goal, the skills, and the movement form. The emphasis is on directly changing the movement form through verbal explanation, demonstration, and passive movement" (Balan and Davis 1993, p. 54). Furthermore, a direct instruction model of teaching is based on the assumption that there is one proper movement pattern, and that the most effective way to achieve it is to prescribe a series of highly structured tasks that will facilitate the student's development toward the desired outcome.

The ETA model represents an alternative to traditional task analysis. As a hybrid of indirect and direct instruction, ETA accounts for the complex interactions among the task, environment, and learner through the provision of instructionally valid choices. The contemporary conceptualization of human movement production suggests that there is a dynamic interaction among these three areas and that the consequence is a particular movement outcome (Newell 1986). The ETA model suggests the following four basic application steps to allow the performer to identify what the optimal movement form is for a particular task goal and environmental condition with little direct instruction from the teacher: (a) establish the task goal by arranging the physical and social environment, (b) allow the learner to initiate his or her own learning by providing choices, (c) manipulate the task and environmental variables to facilitate continued progress, and (d) provide instruction based on observations made during the previous lesson segments.

Implementing ETA in Physical Education

In order to understand how the ETA model is applied in a school-based physical education setting, the reader must conceptualize how a typical lesson transpires. Bulger, Townsend, and Carson (2001) described the components of an ETA designed lesson for an elementary physical education class and suggested the use of task sheets to help students to document their decision-making. ETA is an integrated model for instruction and assessment in which the teacher systematically facilitates student learning by (a) establishing the movement problem or task goal, (b) providing choices, (c) manipulating task variables and direct instruction, and finally, (d) evaluating results (Balan and Davis 1993).

Presenting a Task Goal

Prior to the lesson, the teacher determines a task goal that contributes to the student's ability to achieve the designated learning outcomes of the school physical education curriculum. The teacher should initially present the task goal as a broad outcome that requires the learner to use discovery strategies to self-determine the movement form or skill that produces the most success. It is essential that the teacher provide each learner with the opportunity to pursue a personal goal that is dependent upon individual ability level and perception of success.

Providing Choices

The process of learning is facilitated in the ETA model by the arrangement of the teaching-learning environment to reflect the stated task goal, and elicit a preferred movement form. During this phase of the lesson, the students are provided with a specific movement problem that they need to solve. The teacher's responsibilities during this portion of the lesson are to observe student choices and skill performance, and to identify the task dimensions that should be manipulated to provide further challenge and refinement of the preferred skill.

Manipulating Task Variables and Direct Instruction

In order to further challenge students who are achieving a relatively high rate of success, and/or assist students who may be struggling during skill practice, the teacher can vary the task goal and environmental conditions accordingly. The teacher can begin to manipulate the task as a whole class or individually to further refine student decision-making and skill practice. By using high inference techniques such as rating scales, checklists, and intuitive assessment (Treanor 1996), the teacher is able to monitor the student choices that are being made, and manipulate specific dimensions of the environment (e.g., people, time, space, and/or equipment) in order to promote continued student learning.

Having provided students with ample time to discover the movement form they can use to successfully accomplish the task, the teacher then presents instructions or cues to help shape the students' performance towards the preferred movement form. The teacher also provides specific instructions to those students who have not discovered the preferred skill as a result of the previous manipulation of the task dimensions. The teacher can use modeling or physical guidance at this point in the lesson as well. These teacher-student interactions are often characterized by the use of evaluative, corrective, and congruent feedback (Rink 1998).

This manipulation of task dimensions can be augmented by the provision of direct instruction and skill feedback concerning the actual quality of the movement. The critical concept is to afford the learner the opportunity to discover the intended movement solution, while shaping performance toward the preferred movement form through the careful manipulation of both the task and environment.

Evaluating Results

It is important for the students to finish the lesson with perceptions of success. With this in mind, the teacher returns the students to the optimal condition, the movement pattern and associated task dimensions that resulted in the highest degree of success for each individual. The students are then given the opportunity to practice the skill and environmental condition that combined to produce the highest rate of success regarding the lesson goal. Hopefully, the success that the students experience will stay with them through subsequent lessons. The teacher should use this instruction-free component of the lesson to gather additional information on (a) the choices that students are making, (b) the students' level of skill performance, and (c) the areas in need of continued intervention. Additionally, we suggest that the teacher monitor for comprehension during the closure of the lesson by asking students questions regarding the types of choices they made and the levels of success that they experienced. The students should leave feeling successful and also understanding the task goal they were attempting to accomplish.

Practical Implications
for Teaching Physical Education

While the previously discussed benefits provide a relatively sound ratio-nale for the inclusion of student choice in physical education, teachers must maintain an appreciation of the associated liabilities and concerns as well. McBride (1999) encourages teachers to provide a gradual transition to more learner-centered instructional approaches. Lydon and Cheffers (1984) agree, suggesting that teachers exercise a considerable degree of caution when making the transition to a more student-centered learning environment.

The indiscriminate use of student decision making is a potential area of concern (Blumenfield and Marx 1997). Understandably, the teacher must continually maintain the delicate balance between student choice and the need for direct guidance. Fortunately, the ETA model's flexible design encourages student choice within a teacher-determined learning environment that may, in fact, include teacher intervention with direct instruction.

Strategies for Teaching Students
to Make Responsible Decisions

In order to foster responsibility and decision making in students and avoid overwhelming them, it is important to introduce the ETA model systematically into an instructional environment. The use of teaching strategies that would allow students to make gradual adaptations to ETA would be advantageous for both teacher and students. Several instructional approaches can be used that would guide students in the decision-making process and help make the experience more productive. In order to provide students with time to learn how to make appropriate decisions, we suggest that teachers take an experimental-progressive approach to planning and implementing ETA.

Experimental-Progressive Approach

An experimental-progressive approach (Townsend et al. 2003) to planning and implementing ETA is a systematic strategy for introducing choice to learners. The following guidelines characterize this approach to imple-menting the ETA: Teachers should (a) choose task goals that they are comfortable with and have the resources to accommodate, (b) start with a single class, (c) select a few choices at a time to introduce to the learners, and (d) introduce more decision-making responsibili-ties and involve more classes as students become accustomed to the initial strategies selected for implementation in the ETA lessons. The key to success is to systematically introduce decision-making responsibilities to the students, affording them ample opportunities to adjust to the transition of taking on increased responsibilities for self-management. The use of the experimental-progressive approach increases the likelihood of success for the teacher, the students, and the ETA model itself.

Additional strategies can be used in combination with the experimental-progressive approach. In fact, these strategies dovetail nicely with the progressive nature of systematically guiding students to be better decision makers. Examples of strategies include intratask variation, teaching by invitation, and the use of task sheets. Each of these strategies adds another layer of decision-making responsibility to the students' repertoire for self-monitoring.

Intratask Variation

Intratask variation is defined as a strategy involving the teacher who modifies the task parameters to meet the needs of a particular learner or a small group of learners (Graham 2001). This strategy allows teachers to monitor a student's performance and systematically introduce choices to students by adjusting the difficulty of the task. For example, the teacher may observe an individual or a small group of students who are experiencing a low level of success striking a small ball with a small implement. The teacher can suggest, to those students only, selecting either a larger ball or a larger implement, which should increase their rate of success. The parameters that the teacher modifies make the students aware of other options and their relative effect on task success. This strategy is inherent in the third step of the ETA model, manipulating the task variable. So while this strategy is part of the model, it can also be used to introduce the types of choices students make.

Teaching by Invitation

Another strategy that allows students to begin taking on more responsibility in the decision-making process is teaching by invitation. This strategy allows for the teacher to provide students with several options, which they select from based on their ability and interest (Graham 2001). The strategy allows the teacher to begin introducing a variety of choices to the students while still maintaining some control over the types of choices they make. As an example, a teacher may set a task goal of hitting a small target positioned at a low level. The teacher may provide the students with options for selecting the prop or piece of equipment to accomplish this goal: a softball, a playground ball, or a beach ball. The students are afforded the opportunity to select which piece of equipment they feel will best accomplish the task goal. This instructional strategy is inherent in the second step of the ETA model, providing choices. The limitation here is that the teacher needs to have multiple pieces of equipment to accommodate student choices. It may happen that all students in a practice area select the same type of equipment to meet the demands of the task. The physical learning environment should be able to accommodate for this occurrence.

Task Sheets

When students have developed an awareness of the types of choices that are made available to them, as well as a level of responsibility that encourages appropriate decision making, task (or recording) sheets are effective tools for promoting choice and visually displaying a selection of choices. The use of task sheets permits the teacher to introduce and initially limit simple choice options and gradually provide students with more numerous and complex choices.

Figure 7.1 illustrates a task sheet that provides students with a structured approach for making decisions in a variety of dimensions related to skill performance. The student choice task sheet also enables the teacher to assess and evaluate the students' progression toward the task goal. We recommend that teachers systematically introduce the various dimensions of the task sheet through use of the teaching by invitation strategy mentioned earlier. To maximize the success of such a strategy, we suggest that the following set of guidelines be followed in training students to take an active role in their own learning: (a) explain the task sheet and its purpose, (b) clarify how the task sheet works through demonstration, (c) check for student understanding of how to use the task sheet by directly questioning students and allowing for student demonstrations, (d) provide students with multiple guided and independent opportunities to practice using the task sheet, (e) provide more practice by increasing the complexity or amount of information being collected, (f) offer more feedback, and (g) hold students accountable for accurate data collection. Using this systematic process for introducing and using the student choice task sheet increases the meaningfulness of the process for the students and teacher.

We have pointed out how important it is to gradually and systematically introduce the ETA model to students. The use of teaching strategies that would acquaint students with the steps of ETA, as well as formalize and structure the opportunities for student decision making, can be empowering and motivating for students. To give students time to learn how to make appropriate decisions, it is suggested that teachers plan

Directions: Make any choice of skill activity to attempt, but record what choices you make by putting an "X" in the appropriate square. In the boxes marked "choice," fill in any other choice that relates to that section that you do not see but would like to try. Choose from five or more of the areas.

Task	Type of equipment						Target change		Body moving				Presence of others			Distance from target			Height of target			Movement form						Amount of force			
	Bean bag	Yarn ball	Yellow foam ball	Small plastic ball	Large ball	Choice:	Nonmoving target	Moving target	Standing still	Walking	Running	Choice:	Alone	With a partner	Choice:	Close to a target	Medium distance	Far away	High-level target	Medium-level target	Low-level target	Kick	Catch	Throw	Strike	Bounce	Choice:	Small amount	Average amount	Great amount	Self goal
1		X					X		X				X				X			X				X						X	
2																															
3																															
4																															
5																															
6																															
7																															
8																															
9																															
10																															
11																															
12																															

Figure 7.1 Student choice recording sheet.

Reprinted, by permission, from S.M. Bulger, J.S. Townsend, and L.M. Carson, 2001, "Promoting responsible student decision making in elementary physical education," *Journal of Physical Education, Recreation and Dance* 72(7): 21.

for and implement ETA in a progressive fashion utilizing a variety of strategies that individualize instruction for the learner.

Strategies for Establishing a Student-Centered Physical Environment

Whether environment is considered to be instructional strategies that will be implemented, or the props and equipment needed for instruction (Goodway, Rudisill, and Valentini 2002), or the physical and sociocultural setting (Haywood and Getchell 2005) in which practice will take place, the context is a profoundly influential component of the dynamic constraints model.

Physical education manuals often include discussions about the learning environment with regard to safety, class size, grade level, skill range, management protocols, equipment selection and placement, student formations, and other elements (Rink 1998; Graham 2001; Gallahue and Donnelly 2003; Sanders 2002). While each of these context variables contributes to the characterization of the teaching-learning environment, and while we do not want to diminish the significance of any single contributing component, our discussion here will be limited to structuring the physical environment to facilitate responsible decision making by students. As stated earlier, the process of learning is facilitated in the ETA model by the arrangement of the teaching-learning environment to reflect the stated task goal and elicit a preferred movement form. In a jumping-for-distance lesson, for example, the teacher might select and arrange the props and accompanying equipment to encourage, though not mandate, jumping. Depending on the size of the class and the dimensions of the space, many teachers find that practice stations, with a few children positioned at each, offer an efficient use of space and equipment. The planned environment for the jumping-for-distance lesson would most likely include ropes, a series of taped lines on the floor or on a mat, hoops or poly spots, and a single hurdle apparatus made from short traffic cones and a wand or cardboard tube, this latter serving as the hurdle. These environmental constraints indirectly guide the learner's decision-making process and skill practice toward the preferred movement form.

During this phase of the lesson, the students are provided with a specific movement problem that they need to solve. For example, students might initially be asked to figure out the best way to get from one place (location) to another place (location) using only one movement form. Without any additional verbal explanation and without direct guidance from the teacher, and utilizing the equipment selected and clustered by the teacher, the students might try hopping from poly spot to poly spot, or jumping over the hurdle, or jumping over ropes or lines. The students are free to select and arrange the equipment. The teacher's responsibilities during this portion of the lesson are to observe student choices and skill performance and to identify the task dimensions that should be manipulated to provide further challenge and refinement of the preferred skill. As the teacher employs the next step in the ETA model, manipulation of dimensions of the task or environment, students have new options and choices and new opportunities for success and challenge (Balan and Davis 1993).

When the teacher alters some dimension of the task, there may be a corresponding alteration of the movement pattern selected by the learner, that is, a critical point at which a preferred pattern is forced to change as a result of modified task demands (Davis and Burton 1991). For example, in the jumping lesson and still without direct instruction from the teacher, increasing the distance between props (ropes, lines, poly spots) will likely, at some specific distance (different for each child), change the child's hop on one foot to a jump with two feet; and as the distance increases further, the child may demonstrate a preliminary crouch and arm swing to gain the force production required in the task challenge. Likewise, when jumping from one location to another, the student who was demonstrating consecutive small jumps to get from point A to point B may significantly alter the movement form when the new challenge is to get to point B in the least number of jumps possible. With a V-shaped rope on the floor, when children jump over the ropes from positions where the ropes are close together, most select movement patterns that require minimal force production. However, as a child chooses to jump from positions where the two ropes are progressively farther apart, there will be a juncture (again, different for each child according to experiences and capabilities) at which the demands of the task may push the child to a critical point of change in the jumping pattern to include force production and momentum-enhancing movements.

The choice recording sheet (figure 7.1) provides a matrix of options, both stated and open-ended, to help guide the learner's choices. It offers variety within a set of conditions. Classifying skills or conditions from simple to complex is not new. It has been done for many years in physical therapy, industry, athletics, and classrooms. Physical education teachers have used the Developmental Task Analysis matrix offered by Herkowitz (1978b) to assist them in selecting equipment and task variables. Herkowitz (1978a) further suggested modifying the equipment to help increase success rates of basic skill practice. Popular physical education texts (Gallahue and Donnelly 2003; Graham 2001; Rink 1998) support the notion of modifying equipment, especially if the learner's movement patterns are becoming more ineffective or inefficient as a result of the use of regulation equipment. Modified equipment adds variety and choice options for the learner.

While Herkowitz's (1978b) task analysis framework elaborates on classifying the various dimensions of the task, it fails to address the characteristics of the learner (Davis and Burton 1991). Ulrich (1988) developed a task analysis matrix that not only addressed task conditions but also included environmental context variables such as informal play, structured play, and testing conditions. While this was an extension of the earlier model proposed by Herkowitz (1978b), the Ulrich (1988) model also failed to address the characteristics of the learner as part of the matrix and teacher decision making. The ETA model is designed to accommodate the learner's unique characteristics, limitations, and abilities by honoring the student's adaptations and solutions to the movement problems. Providing choices within a framework of conditions that will allow the student to reach the criterion for success is the key to effectively creating, modifying, and monitoring the teaching-learning environment.

Establishing Student Accountability Within the ETA Model

The ETA model of instruction provides students with choices in determining the movement forms and learning activities that they will engage in to accomplish a stated task goal. Additionally, the teacher must carefully arrange the teaching-learning environment to promote responsible student decision-making and skill practice. While it seems reasonable to allow students the opportunity to exercise their decision-making skills in a well-established physical education environment, we suggest that the transition for students who are accustomed to a teacher-directed model of instruction be gradual. Consequently, teachers may need to offer students additional instruction, guidance, or structure (or some combination of these) in order to promote responsible decision making during this transitional period.

The term *accountability system* is frequently used with reference to the instructional practices that teachers use to establish and maintain student responsibility for task involvement and outcome achievement in order to establish an effective student-centered teaching-learning environment (Siedentop and Tannehill 2000). Teachers should consider building an accountability mechanism into the lesson's instructional format. A variety of authentic, formative assessment techniques can be employed to monitor student progress and provide a basis for the continued refinement of the learning process. Sample formative assessment techniques include rating scales, checklists, self-evaluations, and written logs. An accountability system may represent the most efficient and least restrictive instructional strategy for providing students with guidance at the same time that they are being encouraged to use their individual decision-making capabilities.

One type of formative assessment tool that seems to fit most effectively and efficiently into the ETA model is the student choice recording sheet provided in figure 7.1. The teacher can use this type of recording system to focus the students' attention on the various types of choices that they will be asked to make throughout the entire lesson. Requiring the students to record the choices they make during the lesson holds them accountable for performing the tasks and identifying the choices that they made throughout the lesson. In this situation, the students are responsible for practicing the skill and collecting data regarding their own learning. While the sample recording sheet incorporates student decision making across a number of different task dimensions (e.g., type of equipment, location, direction moving), it can easily be simplified or expanded in accordance with the students' developmental readiness. Three instructional purposes are associated with the use of this type of student choice recording sheet during an ETA lesson: (a) providing the students with a structured approach for making decisions, (b) enabling the teacher to assess and evaluate the learners' development and progression toward the task goal, and (c) providing an accountability mechanism to encourage student adherence to the stated task.

Lesson Structure

One of the limitations associated with the use of a student-centered model of instruction like ETA is that students who are suddenly confronted with a number of choices may not have the knowledge, ability, or experience to make appropriate decisions regarding their own skill practice. Some students may have a relatively shallow repertoire of personal experiences to draw on during this decision-making process. By providing the students with a checklist of optional skills and task dimensions initially, the teacher can complement the students' ability to make appropriate decisions. We recommend that the teacher introduce this type of recording sheet by explaining or demonstrating (or both) for the students what each of the different choices looks like. When providing a demonstration of the sample choices, the teacher enables the students to view the outcomes that particular choices may have. In figure 7.1, the example used is (a) throwing at a (b) nonmoving target, (c) standing still, (d) alone, (e) from a medium distance, (f) at a medium-level target, (g) with a yarn ball, and (h) using a great amount of force. Students would be unlikely to understand that they are making decisions on that many levels or task dimensions without some type of guidance from the teacher. If the students are not successful at first, they can manipulate one or more task dimensions to see if they can increase their rate of success. When a student sets a goal (e.g., hit the target three out of five times) and either successfully reaches it or falls short, he or she can then manipulate the dimensions of the task to further modify its complexity. Accordingly, the recording sheet affords the students the opportunity to analyze the effectiveness of their own decision making. It also allows students to evaluate the choices that they have made and the effects on their skill performance.

Student Assessment

Using a student choice recording sheet also helps the teacher assess the ability of the learner to choose appropriate tasks. The ETA model enables students to individualize their learning and to progress at a highly personalized rate. This is valuable for the learner but makes assessment using traditional methods extremely difficult for the teacher. Allowing students to record their choices will provide the teacher with important assessment information at the lesson's conclusion. As with any student recording sheet, such as rating scales and checklists, the teacher needs to move through the learning environment continually spot-checking to ensure the accuracy of recordings. Contingencies in the form of checkpoints can also be built into the recording sheet as a system of checks and balances. Every third recorded task could have the criteria of needing to be checked off by a peer, with every five tasks requiring the teacher's evaluation and approval to move on. Students may not progress any further until the teacher observes them successfully performing the selected task. This will maintain the integrity of the data and allow the teacher to make sure students are engaged appropriately. This information can be used to evaluate individual levels to see where the students are in relation to the learning objectives. The teacher can be freed up during instruction to observe student performance and to manipulate the task dimensions individually, as well as for the whole group.

The recording sheet provides the teacher with a structure for delivering feedback and discussing related task dimensions with students. If students are aware of the various task dimensions used in the class, it will be easier for the teacher to communicate variations or adjustments in those dimensions to the learners following observation. The sample recording sheet has eight different categories with a total of 26 options and a few variables left blank for students to have added choices (see figure 7.1). It is apparent that the number of task variations is endless, and the student is not really limited when the teacher formalizes and structures the available choices. The presentation of a few categories or dimensions (three to four) in a systematic fashion keeps the student and teacher from being overwhelmed in the experimental-progressive approach. After the initial presentation of dimensions, subsequent lessons can be used to introduce other dimensions that add complexity to the original tasks. In addition, the recording sheet leaves blank areas within selected categories so that students can select a dimension not included on the recording sheet.

Accountability Mechanism

Finally, the choice recording sheet provides an accountability mechanism that contributes to increased student motivation and learning. This type of authentic assessment technique can be fully integrated with the instructional step of the ETA model. If the tasks that the students are selecting are aligned with the goals of the lesson, then the students should be practicing with increased interest. Because students are motivated by success, they can select their own criteria for achieving the goal. We all perceive success in a variety of ways. While success on a skill for the teacher may be 7 out of 10 trials, a low-skilled student may feel successful if he or she completes 4 out of 10 attempts. The primary educational goal is that the students experience a level of success that encourages them to continue to engage in learning activities outside of the gymnasium. So success, when guided by the teacher's manipula-

---

INSTRUCTIONAL STRATEGIES

- Ecological Task Analysis provides a conceptual framework for planning, instruction, and assessment in a learner-centered environment.
- Teachers should gradually introduce students to increased decision-making responsibility by using proven instructional strategies such as teaching by invitation.
- Assessment strategies such as task choice recording sheets can be used to help guide student decision making, establish accountability, and monitor student learning.

tion of task dimensions and instructional feedback, should result in the development of self-motivated and self-regulated learners.

Summary

Ecological Task Analysis is an alternative instructional model that incorporates frequent student decision-making opportunities as a defining characteristic of the teaching-learning environment. To embrace ETA, teachers must make the transition from a teacher-directed to a learner-centered instructional model. Recent studies (Sweeting and Rink 1999; Goodway, Rudisill, and Valentini 2002; Condon and Collier 2002), have demonstrated that both models improve performance. Direct instruction has ample support as a strategy for improving motor skills (Kelly, Dagger, and Walkley 1989; Housner 1990; Silverman 1991; French et al. 1991). Direct instruction may be useful when the content is skill oriented and when efficiency of learning is the teacher's goal; but when teacher objectives also include cognitive and affective domains of learning, direct instruction may not be the best choice despite its efficiency (Rink 1998).

While direct instruction involves the reproduction of specified movements and behaviors, indirect, learner-centered instruction can be conceptualized as involving production strategies because of the learner's role in experimentation, problem solving, and self-discovery (Gallahue and Donnelly 2003). Although indirect instruction has not been studied as extensively, there is empirical support for it (Sweeting and Rink 1999; Goodway, Rudisill, and Valentini 2002; Condon and Collier 2002). As we discussed, some practicing teachers have difficulty making the transition from teacher-directed, reproduction strategies to learner-centered, production styles for creating the teaching-learning environment. Physical education texts have included learner-centered approaches and have encouraged teachers to use a number of instructional strategies, such as teaching by invitation, intratask variation (Graham 2001), environmental design (Rink 1998), child-designed tasks, task teaching, convergent and divergent inquiry (Graham, Holt-Hale, and Parker 2001), and self-check and guided discovery (Gallahue and Donnelly 2003).

The appeal of the ETA model, and perhaps an overlooked enhancement to helping teachers make the transition we have discussed, is that it combines indirect and direct approaches into one instructional model. One of the unique features of ETA is that it promotes the production of movements first, nurtured by experimenting with options. After a learner has had ample time to experiment, then selects and practices a skill that achieves the goal, direct, specific instruction is used to refine the skill pattern and foster the reproduction of movements that are considered to be more mechanically efficient and effective. Ecological Task Analysis provides a framework for planning lessons that invite participation, decision making, and problem solving. Once learners have been guided to their self-selected optimal level of performance, direct instruction is utilized to refine or extend student learning (Balan and Davis 1993).

Not only do teachers have to transition into new and different responsibilities when implementing the ETA model, but so do the learners. Consequently, teachers must provide students with some form of instruction, guidance, or structure (or a combination of these) in order to promote responsible decision making during this transitional period. We have shared an example of an accountability system in figure 7.1. The teacher can use this type of recording system to focus the students' attention on the various types of choices that they will be asked to make throughout the entire lesson, particularly when students may not have the knowledge, ability, or experience to make appropriate decisions regarding their own skill practice. This permits a new dimension for the ETA model in that the choices can be limited and graduated from simple to complex. This type of performance-related documentation holds the students accountable for performing the tasks and identifying the choices that they made throughout the lesson.

We have attempted to support ETA as an alternative instructional model to enhance responsible decision making. We offered suggestions for fostering the transition of teachers and students into learner-centered, production-oriented instructional strategies. To demonstrate that ETA is not an extreme departure from traditional direct instruction strategies, ETA was presented as a model that utilizes both direct and indirect styles of delivery. Finally, we offered practical guidelines for establishing a physical environment that facilitates responsible choice, and for encouraging a high degree of student accountability within a learner-centered physical activity setting. The selection and arrangement of equipment and the modification of the tasks are crucially important to the student's problem solving and decision making. Why would we not want a learner to link the consequences of a motor decision, based on trial and error, with the process or product variables of his or her performance? This approach was introduced as a useful instruction and assessment technique in adapted physical education (Davis and Burton 1991). We ask: and why not? In most schools, agencies, and centers, adapted physical education is replete with modifications to equipment, tasks, and rules and includes assistive devices. Adaptive physical educators realized a long time ago that task tinkering would result in desired changes in movement forms.

More research is needed in the following areas: (a) methodological comparisons to contrasting teaching strategies; (b) identifying and sequencing task variables; (c) identifying optimal and critical points for various skills, ages, physiques, and experience levels; (d) determining the most effective accountability systems and strategies; and (e) the role of decision making in the acquisition of skillful movement. More applied presentations are needed at conferences and workshops to inform practicing teachers of the value and benefits of ETA so that when teachers are making their decisions about which instructional strategy to employ, if their goals and objectives include cognitive, affective, and decision-making attributes, this model will receive consideration.

Ecological Task Analysis in Games Teaching: Tactical Games Model

Steve Mitchell, PhD, and Judy Oslin, PhD

The teaching of games in public school physical education represents a complex environment for both teachers and students. It is complex for teachers in that they must afford maximum opportunity for all students to respond to the challenges of game play while managing time, people, and equipment effectively. It is complex for students in that as games players they face a learning environment in which performance success is dependent on factors such as appropriate decision-making abilities, efficient execution of motor skills, and effective movement to respond to the ever-changing demands of game play situations. The concepts underpinning Ecological Task Analysis (Davis and Burton 1991) provide a useful lens through which to view games teaching and learning. Coincidentally, the ongoing debate (beginning in the early 1980s) on games teaching has identified the Tactical Games model (TGM; Metzler 2000; Mitchell, Oslin, and Griffin 2003) as an effective model through which students can learn the complexities of games playing.

Development of the Tactical Games Model

The roots of TGM lie in the work in England of Bunker and Thorpe (1982), whose experiences with undergraduate teacher education in physical education, involving considerable time spent in schools supervising field experiences, led them to conclude that traditional games teaching in schools has done little to educate students about and for games playing. Bunker and Thorpe's conception of Teaching Games for Understanding (TGfU), with its focus on developing understanding of game tactics and strategies, aimed to promote greater interest in learning games, more understanding of game play, and improved ability to play games.

The traditional approach to games teaching is technical and focuses on teaching skills to answer the question, "How is this skill performed?" For example, badminton instruction often develops service, overhead clear, drop shot, and smash by concentrating on specific critical elements of these skills. Though this format *might* improve technique, it has been criticized for teaching skills before students can grasp their significance within the game. As a result, we lose the contextual nature of the skill, and games teaching becomes a series of drills conforming to textbook techniques (Pigott 1982). Commonly used drills often lead students to ask, "Why are we doing this?" or "When can we play a game?" For example, you might hear these questions in a volleyball lesson in which students must pass or set a volleyball against a wall. For many, particularly the less able, the volleyball game is characterized by aimless participation following a breakdown of passing and setting techniques. This situation creates frustration for the student and teacher. It is possible that the only thing many children learn about games is that they cannot perform the necessary complex skills (Booth 1983). In addition, skilled students often perceive isolated drills as tedious and irrelevant to their performance during game play.

Continued work in TGfU led to the approach being brought to the United States in the 1990s, leading to gradual development of the TGM. We believe that TGM can provide an exciting alternative through which students can learn to play games. Our research, and the experience of others, indicate that students find a tactical approach motivational and that teachers find it a preferable way to teach games (Berkowitz 1996; Burrows 1986; Griffin, Oslin, and Mitchell 1995; Mitchell, Griffin, and Oslin 1994; Nevitt, Rovegno, and Babiarz 2001; Turner and Martinek 1992). The purpose of this chapter is to present the TGM as a model complementary to ETA by drawing parallels between ETA's four relevant concepts (Davis and Burton 1991) and components of TGM. To review, the four relevant concepts are that (1) actions are relations, not parts; (2) tasks should be categorized by function and intention, not mechanism; (3) invariant features of a task and variations within a task may be defined in terms of essential and nonessential variables, respectively; and (4) direct links should be established between the task goal and the constraints of the performer and the environment.

At this point it is appropriate to distinguish between what we consider to be *tactics* and what we mean by the term *strategy,* as we use the former term in this chapter. Grehaigne and Godbout (1995) define tactics as "an adaptation to opposition," meaning *what* players should do to respond, offensively or defensively, to the changing demands of a game in progress. For example, novice soccer players who are playing as defenders will stay back in front of their own goal even when the ball has moved to the far end of the field. A more appropriate response to the movement of the ball in this case would be for defending players to move up the field, to at least the halfway line.

Similarly, Bunker and Thorpe (1982), in their original TGfU model, aimed for a higher degree of "tactical awareness" in the learner, meaning an increased understanding of *"what to do"* during game play situations. This recognizes that decision-making capacities are particularly important during game play, but that execution of appropriate decisions made might be limited by physical capabilities. Research does suggest that novice students will acquire cognitive understanding (i.e., knowledge) more easily than physical skills (French and Thomas 1987). For example, in early net games learning, a novice tennis player might be able to see the value of pushing the opponent toward the back of the court but may lack the skill (i.e., the ball-striking abilities) to achieve this outcome.

Our use of the term *tactical* refers to the problems to be solved for players to be successful in game play. In this sense it corresponds quite closely to Bunker and Thorpe's notion of "what to do." In any game there are two fundamental problems to be solved: (a) how to score and (b) how to prevent an opponent from scoring. We view strategy as the sum of tactics used, or the overall game plan. For example, one team's strategy (perhaps in soccer) might rely heavily on a possession game (i.e., a lot of passing) and a low-pressure defense, while another team might emphasize a more direct attacking style of play (more dribbling and perhaps longer passing) and a high-pressure defense.

Actions as Relations, Not Parts

Game playing is relational. Relations exist between teammates and opponents, offensive and defensive demands of play, skills and the application of skills to game play. This section of the chapter addresses these relationships through the lens of literature focusing on TGM and the interweaving components of the game play environment.

Relations Between Opponents

Typically game playing involves two opponents for whom the aim is to score goals or points and to prevent the other from scoring. In an individual activity such as singles tennis or badminton, the relationship between opponents is relatively straightforward, with each player attempting to score against the other and to prevent the other from scoring. As players are added to the game environment, the complexity of relationships increases as freedom to make decisions increases. Doubles play in a net game is significantly more tactically complex than singles play due to the presence of a teammate on the court and the need for the two players to consider each other's actions as play develops. Consider then the additional complexity of adding five teammates in the case of volleyball, or 10 in the case of soccer, in terms of relationships that now exist between both teammates and opponents. With increasing numbers of players come additional complexities to be addressed, related to what a team accomplishes both offensively and defensively. Players need to be more aware of where teammates and opponents are positioned on the field or court, and what various options are available to the player in possession of the ball. Again, these options increase as the number of players increases. Game complexity might perhaps best be thought of as a greater degree of freedom to make and implement decisions about action.

Relations Among Game Components

Relations exist between components of game play such as the game rules, game goals, and tactics and skills used. This is illustrated in table 8.1, which demonstrates how a rule change affects the goal, tactics, and skills of the game. In game 1, teams score by passing the ball among team members for an uninterrupted four passes. This rule emphasizes the tactical problem of keeping possession of the ball, to be solved by passing and receiving skills and by supporting the player who is in possession of the ball. In game 2, players score by shooting into the opponent's goal, forcing players to address the tactical problem of attacking a goal. They need to be able to shoot the ball to be successful in this game. Lastly, in game 3, scoring is accomplished by passing the ball to a teammate who is positioned permanently behind an end line (along which he or she can move). The size of a playing area will also affect tactics and the skills and movements used. For example, using a larger field or court will lead to the need for longer passes and more sophisticated receiving skills. The point here is that relations between game components are such that teachers can affect players' use of skill during game play by instituting simple rule changes.

Tasks Categorized by Function and Intention

Curriculum implications of TGM are driven by a games classification system that categorizes games according to the tactical goals of game play rather than simply by skills used (Almond 1986). This classification is shown in table 8.2. The categorization of games into invasion,

Table 8.1   Effects of Game Rules on Teaching Content

Rules of the game	Goal of game play	Tactical problem to be addressed	Decisions and skills or movements needed to solve the tactical problem
Game 1: 4 vs. 4 (small field) possession game 4 passes = a goal	Offensive goal: to score by keeping the ball	Keep possession	- *Where or when to pass* - Short possession passes - Receive on the ground - <u>Support</u>
Game 2: 4 vs. 4 (small field) game, each team trying to score in other's goal	Offensive goal: to score by shooting the ball into the opponent's goal	Attack the goal	- *When to shoot* - Shooting
Game 3: 4 vs. 4 (small field) game, each team trying to score by passing to a target player	Offensive goal: to score by passing the ball to a target player positioned behind an end line	Attack the goal	- *Passing between defenders* - Penetrating passes - Use of target player - <u>Support</u>

Decisions required are in *italics,* skills required are in regular type, and movements needed are <u>underlined</u>.

net/wall, striking/fielding, and target games aids teachers in curriculum design initiatives while also enabling students to see common elements of seemingly different games (e.g., soccer and field hockey are very similar games despite employing very different motor skills). Brief descriptions of each category follow.

Invasion Games

The fundamental problems to be addressed in nearly all competitive games with opponents are scoring and prevention of scoring. In invasion, or goal (Davis and Strand, this volume) games, teams score by moving a ball (or other projectile) into another team's territory and either shooting into a fixed target (a goal or basket) or moving the projectile across an open-ended target (i.e., across a line). To prevent scoring, one team must stop the other from bringing the ball into its territory and making scoring attempts. Solving these offensive and defensive problems will require similar tactics (similar things that have to be done) even though many of the skills to be used will be quite different from one invasion game to another. In both floor hockey and team handball, for example,

Table 8.2   Tactical Games Classification System

Invasion	Net/wall	Striking/ fielding	Target
Basketball (FT)	**Net**	Baseball	Golf
Netball (FT)	Badminton (I)	Softball	Croquet
Team handball (FT)	Tennis (I)	Kickball	Bowling
Soccer (FT)	Pickle ball (I)	Rounders	Lawn bowls
Hockey (FT)	Volleyball (H)	Cricket	Pool
Lacrosse (FT)	**Wall**		Billiards
Water polo (FT)	Racquetball (I)		Snooker
Speedball (FT/OET)	Squash (I)		
Rugby (OET)	Handball (H)		
Football (OET)	Fives (H)		
Ultimate Frisbee (OET)			

FT = fixed target; H = hand; I = implement; OET = open-end target.

Adapted from L. Almond, 1986, Reflecting on themes: A game classification. In *Rethinking games teaching*, edited by R. Thorpe, D. Bunker, and L. Almond (Champaign, IL: Human Kinetics), 71-72. By permission of R. Thorpe.

while players must understand the need to shoot if they are to score, the striking and throwing skills used to shoot in these two games are very different.

It is true that some games within the invasion games category can be differentiated from others by virtue of unique rules. For example, in football (American), players are permitted to intentionally block opponents from the ball and from other players; this is also the case in basketball, where players can set screens to prevent an opponent from moving either toward the ball or toward a player. Perhaps the most unusual rule of all is in rugby, where players can pass the ball only in a backward direction. Nevertheless, despite these rule variations, the essential principles of these invasion games remain consistent within the category as a whole, these being to move into the other team's space by keeping the ball and creating space, in order to score, and to prevent opponents from moving into one's own space and scoring.

Net/Wall Games

In net/wall games, teams or individual players score by hitting a ball into a court space with sufficient accuracy or power (or both) that opponents cannot hit it back before it bounces once (as in badminton or volleyball) or twice (as in tennis or racquetball). To prevent scoring, players and teams must return the ball before it bounces once or twice.

Striking/Fielding Games

In striking/fielding, or strike and run (Davis and Strand, this volume) games, players on the batting team must strike or kick a ball with sufficient accuracy or power (or both) that it will elude players on the fielding team and give time for the hitter to run between two points (bases or wickets). To prevent scoring in striking/fielding games, the fielding team members must position themselves in such a way that they gather a hit ball and throw it to the base or wicket (to which the hitter is running) before the hitter reaches this base or wicket.

Target Games

In target games, players score by reaching a target with a ball either by throwing or striking the ball. Some target games are unopposed (e.g., golf, bowling) while others are opposed (e.g., croquet); in the latter case one participant is allowed to block or hit the opponent's ball. In opposed target games, players seek to prevent scoring by hitting the opponent's ball to place it in a disadvantageous position relative to the target.

Function and Intention in Operation

Similar game functions and intentions are made explicit through the development of tactical frameworks, which can form the basis for identification of task goals related to game play. Table 8.3 provides an example of such a framework, illustrating the possible tactical breakdown of invasion games for instruction at the elementary level by identifying tactical problems and solutions to these problems. Solutions are in the form of decisions to be made, on-the-ball skills, and off-the-ball movements, and these solutions represent the content of games instruction at the elementary level. This framework provides the "scope" of content for teaching invasion games at the elementary level by breaking down invasion games according to the problems associated with scoring, preventing scoring, and starting and restarting play. The levels of game complexity shown in table 8.4 provide an appropriate "sequence" for this content. Taken together, the framework and levels of game complexity provide developmentally appropriate scope and sequence of invasion games content for elementary children. Ideally, games should be no larger than 3 versus 3 at first, progressing to a maximum of 6 versus 6 in games such as soccer and hockey.

The sequence of learning suggested in table 8.4 is designed to make games instruction developmentally appropriate. We recommend identifying

Table 8.3 **Framework for Invasion Games Content in Elementary Physical Education**

Tactical problems	Decisions and movements	Skills
Offense and scoring		
Keeping possession of the ball	Supporting the ball carrier	Passing and receiving the ball
	When to pass	
Penetrating the defense and attacking the goal	Using a target forward	Moving with the ball
	When to shoot and dribble	Shooting
		Feinting
Transition	Moving to space	Quick passing
Defense and preventing scoring		
Defending space	Marking and guarding	Clearing the ball
	Footwork	Quick outlet passes
	Pressuring the ball carrier	
Defending the goal	Goalkeeping—positioning	Goalkeeping—stopping and distributing the ball
	Rebounding—boxing out	Rebounding—taking the ball
Winning the ball		Tackling and stealing the ball
Starting and restarting play		
Beginning the game	Positioning	Initiating play
Restarting from the sideline	Supporting positions	Putting the ball in play
Restarting from the end line	Supporting positions	Putting the ball in play
Restarting from violations	Supporting positions	Putting the ball in play

levels of game complexity for each games category. These levels will include the learning of concepts and skills across a variety of games. So, at level I, teachers might teach students to keep possession of a ball by passing, receiving, and supporting in soccer, hockey, and basketball. Depending on the length of time spent on invasion games, level I might also include the learning of shooting techniques in these games. Table 8.4 presents three possible levels of game complexity on which the development of unit and lesson plans can be based for teaching invasion games at the elementary level. Notice that we advocate beginning invasion games play with no more than three players per team. This allows for some decision making (should I pass to player A or player B?) but does not force a vast range of possibilities. We have even found 2-a-side games effective because this forces players to make only decisions about passing, shooting, or dribbling. This represents decreased complexity in the early stages of invasion games learning. Note in table 8.4 that game complexity increases as students progress through levels II and III. For example, transition is a more complex tactical problem and is addressed only at level III.

Using a tactical games approach, teachers can plan instructional units that enable students to learn to address identical tactical problems across a variety of invasion games. From table 8.4 it is evident that initial

Table 8.4   Levels of Game Complexity for Invasion Games in Elementary Physical Education

Tactical problems and concepts	Game complexity Level I 3-a-side maximum	Game complexity Level II 4-a-side maximum	Game complexity Level III 6-a-side maximum
Offense and scoring			
Keeping possession	- Pass, receive, footwork - When to pass	- Pass, receive, footwork - Support	
Penetration or attack	- Shooting, moving with the ball (dribbling) - When to dribble and shoot	- Shooting, feinting	- Using a target forward - Shooting - Feinting, change of speed, moving with the ball - Moving to space, quick passing
Transition			
Defense and preventing scoring			
Defending space		- Marking or guarding, pressure	- Clearing the ball, quick outlet pass
Defending the goal		- Footwork (stance) - Goalkeeper positioning	- Goalkeeper shot stopping and distribution, rebounding
Winning the ball			- Tackling and stealing the ball

(continued)

Table 8.4 *(continued)*

Tactical problems and concepts	Game complexity Level I 3-a-side maximum	Game complexity Level II 4-a-side maximum	Game complexity Level III 6-a-side maximum
	Starting and restarting play		
Beginning the game	- Initiating play	- Positioning in a triangle	
Restarting from side and end line	- Putting ball in play	- Positioning	- Quick restarts
Restarting from violations	- Putting ball inplay	- Positioning	- Quick restarts

exposure to invasion games might consist of the concepts of possession, penetration, defending space, and simple starts and restarts in playing a small, modified version (2 vs. 2 or 3 vs. 3) of any invasion game. Although the game can be changed at any time (because the problems addressed are the same regardless of the game being played), the skills taught will be different. For example, skills needed to keep possession in soccer are different from those needed in basketball and hockey. However, the key to this approach is that by learning the same concepts, students will more quickly understand what needs to be done to play invasion games successfully.

Essential and Nonessential Variables

While some aspects of game play are essential, others are less essential and so might be varied in order to maximize student challenge, success, or choice. For example, while in soccer one must use the feet to propel the ball, the type of ball used can easily be varied, as can the size of the goal. In this section of the chapter we discuss the concepts of "primary and secondary rules" (Almond 1986) as a way of distinguishing essential from nonessential features of game play.

Primary and Secondary Rules

In his analysis of games problems, Almond (1986) focuses on the rules of game playing because it is the "rules which provide a structure for the game since they state clearly the nature of the game problem and closely constrain the means available to the player(s) for solving the problem" (p. 73). Almond makes the distinction between what he terms *primary* and *secondary* rules. Primary rules identify how a game is played and how winning is accomplished. Because these rules define the game and distinguish it from other games, they cannot be changed. For example, players must kick the ball in soccer as opposed to throwing it, at which point the game becomes one of team handball. Kicking the ball is a primary rule for the game of soccer. On the other hand, the identification of secondary rules allows teachers to shape a game for instructional purposes. In soccer, these secondary rules might include the size of the playing area, the size of the goal, the number of players on each team, or the number of touches each player is allowed to have before passing or shooting. This use of secondary rules to shape game play is a process otherwise known as game conditioning, a useful tool in games teaching.

Game Conditioning

Game conditioning is really a process of rule modification to ensure that game play in physical education is representative of the mature form of the game, but exaggerated to provide developmentally appropriate levels of cognitive and psychomotor challenge for all students. With reference again to table 8.1, recall the three different ways of scoring in games 1, 2, and 3. In this example, the scoring system represents a secondary rule that has been conditioned by the teacher to encourage players to pass, move, and shoot in different ways. Consider a similar example in volleyball, a net game. By placing conditions on the game that stipulate the use of an underhand toss into the back court, and a minimum of two contacts per side before a point can be scored, the teacher increases the likelihood of intentional use of the forearm pass. Game conditioning is a powerful tool to enable the teacher to place the students in particular game situations that require critical thinking and development of decision-making skills to solve game problems.

The positioning of game conditioning is evident in Mitchell, Oslin, and Griffin's (2003) three-stage TGM (see figure 8.1), this in itself an adaptation of Bunker and Thorpe's (1982) original TGfU model. Figure 8.1 focuses on the essential lesson components of TGM, namely modified game play, development of tactical awareness and decision making through questioning, and development of skill. All parts of the process are important and must be planned so that several things occur:

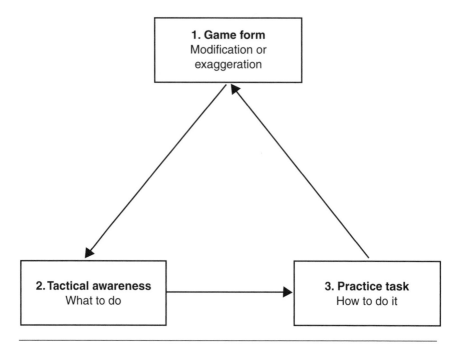

Figure 8.1   Three-stage Tactical Games model.
From Mitchell, Oslin, and Griffin 2003.

- Games are modified appropriately, through application of suitable game conditions, to encourage student thinking relative to the tactical problem on which instruction is focused.
- Questions designed to develop tactical awareness (understanding of what to do to solve a problem) are well thought out. Questions might relate to factors such as time ("when is the best time to . . ."), space ("where is/can . . ."), or risk ("which choice . . .").
- Practice tasks teach essential skills to solve problems in as gamelike a manner as possible.

Direct Links Between Task Goal and Constraints

In TGM, links between task, performer, and environment can be established through the application of a developmental task analysis (DTA) for game play (Oslin and Mitchell 1998). In this section of the chapter we describe the development of a DTA and give an example to demonstrate the thought processes through which a teacher might progress as he or she seeks to adapt game play to suit individual student needs. Though the original conception of a DTA was for the purpose of modifying early skill and movement instruction (Herkowitz 1978b), a DTA can also be useful in linking the task, performer, and environment in game playing to ensure maximally challenging learning experiences for all students. A DTA relative to invasion games (with the game of soccer in mind) in elementary physical education is presented in table 8.5.

Table 8.5 demonstrates how some factors related to the task and the environment can be manipulated to either increase or decrease level of complexity according to the abilities and needs of the students. Factors are presented in the left-hand column, with appropriate modifications to move the task from simple to complex suggested in the remaining columns.

Within a single mixed-ability class, a physical education teacher might develop games of varying complexity according to student need. For example, a simplified game might include only one or two players per team, playing with a small ball in a small playing area, with small goals and no goalkeeper to beat in order to score. Any or all of the factors can be modified according to the needs of the players and the desired focus of a lesson. If a teacher wishes to focus on the possible decisions players must make when in possession of the ball, it would be appropriate to increase the number of players per team and thereby increase the number of possible decisions open to each player upon receiving the ball. The inclusion of a wider goal with an active goalkeeper would also add to the task complexity, since players now would have a wider target but would have to beat an opponent to score (hence perhaps need to shoot at the corners).

Lest we run the risk of oversimplification, we should note that use of a DTA should reflect task goals and the developmental needs of individuals. While the example in table 8.5 might be generally appropriate for a

Table 8.5   Developmental Task Analysis for Elementary School Soccer

Factors to be modified	More simple to more complex		
Size of the ball	Small	Medium	Large
Size of playing area	20 3 10 yards	40 3 30 yards	60 3 40 yards
Width of the goal	6 feet	12 feet	18 feet
Use of goalkeeper	None	Passive	Active
Number of players	1 vs. 1 or 2 vs. 2	3 vs. 3 or 4 vs. 4	5 vs. 5 or 6 vs. 6
Number of required skills	2-3	3-4	4-5

typical elementary physical education class, its use might vary. For example, a teacher who wishes to work specifically on accuracy of shooting might narrow the goal (as opposed to making it wider) in order to present a greater challenge for players, particularly those of higher skill levels. Similarly, for higher-skilled players it might be appropriate to play with more players (more complex) but in a smaller playing area, thus increasing the playing demands relative to time (less available) and skill (more required).

Application of TGM to the ETA Applied Model

In the closing section of this chapter we further address the application of TGM to the individual games lesson, and draw a parallel to ETA and the four-step approach to setting up an ETA teaching-learning environment (Davis and Burton 1991). Figure 8.2 presents a more complete analysis of the thinking and planning processes that a teacher must undertake when using TGM. Major components of the plan are in bold, followed by points for the teacher to consider. An actual sample lesson, focused on net games instruction at the second or third grade level, is presented in figure 8.3.

Figure 8.2
Teacher Thinking and Planning in TGM

Game _____ Lesson number _____ Grade level _____

Tactical problem: What is the tactical problem being addressed during the lesson?

Lesson focus: What is the focus of the lesson, in terms of how the tactical problem will be solved?

Objective: What are the major cognitive and psychomotor learning objectives for the lesson?

Game: What is the modified game that is being played?

> **Conditions:** What conditions will you put on the game to ensure that students have to address the tactical problem?

> **Goal:** What performance goal will you give to the students for the game?

Questions: After this initial game play, what are the questions you might need to ask (and what answers do you anticipate) to help students focus on the tactical problem and its solution?

Practice task: What skill practice is appropriate to help students develop a solution to the tactical problem when they return to game play?

Goal: What performance goal will you give to the students for the skill practice?

Cues: What teaching cues will you use to assist the learner in skill acquisition?

Extension: How might you extend the skill practice to make it more challenging, or easier, for students of varying abilities?

Game: What is an appropriate modified game to help students apply newly learned skills to solve the tactical problem during game play?

Conditions: What conditions will you put on the game to ensure that students use the skills learned to address the tactical problem?

Goal: What performance goal will you give to the students for the game?

Closure: What would make an appropriate closure or discussion for the end of the lesson?

Figure 8.3

Net Games Sample Lesson (2nd grade)

Tactical problem: Playing a competitive game and setting up to attack

Game: Throw tennis (singles)

Lesson focus: Game rules and use of court spaces

Objective: Students will play a game, with appropriate rules, and try to move their opponent to the back of the court.

Game: Throw and catch over the "net." Choose your own ball.

Conditions: All throws must be underhand.

Throw over the net: Ball must bounce only once on the other side of the net. Ball cannot bounce on your own side of the net.

Goal: Try to make your opponent move around the court.

Questions (interjected during game play):

Q. What spaces are there on the court for you to throw the ball into?

A. Front and back.

Q. Is it hardest to make a good throw from the front or the back?

A. Back.

(continued)

Figure 8.3 *(continued)*

Q. So where should you try to make your opponent move to (front or back)?

A. Back. Try to get the ball to bounce close to the back line.

Continue game play.

Q. When you have made your opponent move back, where is the space now?

A. In the front.

Q. So to make it hard for your opponent, where should you throw to now?

A. The front.

Q. Should you throw quickly or should you wait to throw? Why?

A. Quickly. Because your opponent will be farther away.

Continue game play.

Q. When should you stop and restart a rally?

A. Restart a rally if

- ball bounces twice on opponent's side
- opponent throws the ball out of court
- opponent makes the ball bounce on his or her own side
- opponent throws overhand
- opponent catches the ball before it bounces

Note. Set up demonstrations of these scoring rules.

Continue game play.

Closure: Review restart rules.

To better align TGM with ETA, we refer to Davis and Burton (1991), who identified four major steps in setting up an ETA environment. The first step is to select and present the task goal and structure the environment to allow for understanding of the goal. Figures 8.1 and 8.2 show a similar process, apparent in stage 1 of TGM, in which the task and its conditions are presented to students. In the sample lesson in figure 8.3, the teacher sets a task in which students play a throw-catch game over a low net with the goal of attempting to move a partner or opponent around the court space. This goal encourages students to engage in some thinking about how best to accomplish the task goal, leading to step 2 of ETA.

Step 2 of ETA requires the teacher to provide choice of student response to a task in terms of skill selected and perhaps equipment used. Again, the presentation of the game problem in stage 1 of TGM allows students to identify solutions in their own way, as is the case in figure 8.3. In this particular example, the choice of equipment will have an impact on the solutions to the problem presented. By allowing choice of ball to be used, the teacher provides students with the autonomy to make the task more or less challenging. A smaller ball will be more difficult to catch, as will a ball with considerable bounce. A ball with very little bounce will increase the speed of movement required to prevent a double bounce. The provision of equipment choice adds a learning dimension for students. However, as stressed by Davis and Strand (this volume), "Unless the choices are given prior to instruction, some of the benefits of choice, such as empowerment and information about the students, are lost" (p. 78). In figure 8.3, choices concerning equipment and problem solution are given prior to instruction, which in this lesson takes place in the form of questioning, thus maximizing the impact of choice for the students. Interestingly, as suggested in table 8.5, there are numerous factors available to the teacher that can be manipulated to provide for student choice and critical thinking in games playing.

In step 3 of ETA, the teacher and students identify the relevant task dimensions and performer variables. In TGM this is accomplished as the teacher asks questions to encourage thinking about solutions to the game problems. The questions in figure 8.3 are designed to elicit student thinking regarding ways to move the playing partner from the front to the back of the court and then use the space created in the front to effectively win a point. Step 4 of ETA requires that the teacher provide direct instruction in skills and movement forms. The skill practice and game application stages of TGM also focus on practice of selected skills and extend this to application of these skills to game play situations. Though this does not appear evident in figure 8.3, consider teaching the same lesson but requiring students to strike the ball with the hand (definitely a recommended task extension and one that some students might choose to do anyway). This would require formal instruction on striking skills as a means of ensuring that students can maintain a rally, keep the ball in court, and eventually place the opponent in a situation of disadvantage by moving him or her around the court.

INSTRUCTIONAL STRATEGIES

- Modify games with appropriate conditions to emphasize the problem of focus.
- Plan questions to elicit student responses that will demonstrate awareness of skills needed to solve the problem.
- Develop game-like and progressive skill practices.
- Use game conditions to ensure that skills are used appropriately as solutions to the problem in a game setting.

Summary

The chapter provides food for thought regarding the continued need to investigate the implications of using TGM in public school physical education. Certainly the steps of the ETA model suggest the need for researchers to ask questions concerning the impact of goals on performance and motivation of students of all ages, the effects of choice on students' ability to comprehend task requirements and to think critically, and the merits of questioning as a means to facilitate student understanding of game problems and solutions.

In closing, we emphasize that ETA and TGM provide valuable, student-centered alternatives to traditional models of teaching in physical education, particularly in the area of games teaching and learning. The two models reflect each other in providing for student choice and placing an emphasis on critical thinking and skill acquisition within appropriate contexts. We hope this chapter will provide teachers and teacher educators with encouragement to attempt to integrate new models into the processes of curriculum and instruction.

Systematic Ecological Modification Approach to Skill Acquisition in Adapted Physical Activity

Yeshayahu Hutzler, PhD

The process of motor skill acquisition has traditionally been viewed as a gradual change in the organization of movement patterns leading to automatic performance, increased effectiveness, and adaptability (Clark 1995; Magill 2001). The goal of instruction according to this perspective, known as information-processing theory, pertains to identifying errors along this process and attempting to provide corrective input (Adams 1971; Magill 2001; Schmidt and Lee 1999). Numerous studies have manipulated feedback conditions such as internal versus external, process oriented versus product oriented, and concurrent versus terminal. Visual demonstration, such as video feedback (e.g., Morya, Ranvaud, and Pinheiro 2003; Van Wieringen et al. 1989), and verbal feedback (e.g., Messier and Cirillo 1989) are by far the preferred practices of information input among physical education teachers and sport instructors.

However, throughout the history of physical education and sport instruction, other modes of teaching and learning have been successfully implemented that involve manipulation of environmental variables rather than feedback processes. This chapter describes the Systematic Ecological Modification Approach (SEMA), which is designed to identify relationships between the environmental and individual variables responsible for an inefficient movement pattern and to suggest adaptation strategies. The result is a set of ecological interventions that facilitate acquisition of motor skills and movement behavior. Thus SEMA is compatible with and extends the Ecological Task Analysis model. Following a brief theoretical review, a range of selected examples from the SEMA model will help to demonstrate how this approach can be put into units of instruction.

Theoretical Foundation

In this section theoretical frames of reference will be linked to the model proposed in this chapter. Four conceptual frameworks are borrowed from different disciplines—human movement sciences, medicine, and social networking—and linked together.

Action Systems Theory

The principal ecological action system is represented as a triangular structure composed of the individual, the environment, and the task (Newell 1986). Accordingly, individuals possess resources enabling them to cope with environmental challenges while meeting a task goal. The task is a specific relation between an individual and the environment, such as changing a position from one point in space to another, crossing a distance, or catching a flying object. The goal of a task may be purposefully determined by the individual or imposed by environmental stimuli such as teaching, instruction, or therapeutic treatment. According to the ecological view, movement skills emerge due to the three general constraints in the triangle model. Constraints are viewed as boundaries or features that limit the motion of the individual by imposing certain patterns of movement while restricting others (Newell 1986; Newell and Jordan, this volume).

An example of a constraint is restriction to the preferred motor pattern through slinging, casting, or the use of a padded mitten, thereby forcing the use of the affected limb. Modern rehabilitation literature acknowledges constraint-induced therapy as a promising practice aimed at the rehabilitation of limbs affected by central nervous system disorders (Liepert et al. 2000; Taub and Steven 1997). Research has demonstrated significant improvements of motor function in the involved extremity that are attributed to mechanisms described as overcoming or avoiding learned nonuse, unmasking of excitatory central nervous system connections, or use-dependent cortical reorganization (Dromeric, Edwards, and Hahn 2000; Liepert et al. 2000). Further modalities of constraining within physical activity programs are outlined later in this chapter.

International Classification of Function and Disability

The same major components underlying action systems theory (individual, environment, and task) have been addressed in the recent widely accepted International Classification of Functioning, Disability and Health (ICF; World Health Organization [WHO] 2001). This taxonomy provides criteria for classification, assessment, and intervention in health and disability. The ICF addresses three major terms characterizing the range of potential limitations to the interactions of an individual with his or her environment. These include (a) impairment of the affected *body structures* (e.g., lungs, joints, limbs, brain) and *functions* (e.g., respiration, range of movement, muscular strength, motor control, decision making); (b) limitation in *activities* required for daily living, vocational engagement, and leisure time; and (c) restriction of *participation* in socially appropriate activities (WHO 2001). The functions, the activities, and participation are related to the health condition and contextual variables including individual predispositions and environmental factors that could be perceived as facilitators or barriers (limiters). Figure 9.1 shows an extended triangle model including some of the basic variables that could facilitate or limit function, activity, or participation.

Adaptation Theory

In her landmark essay on adaptation theory, Sherrill (1995) acknowledges the ecological orientation as one of the theories underlying the core paradigm of adapted physical activity (APA):

> Our body of knowledge extends beyond skills and fitness to function, the ability to function in mainstream sport and exercise. . . . Now we realize that it is unjust to assess only the individual with a disability. We must assess his or her environment, or ecosystem, and identify the attitudinal, aspirational, and architectural barriers and affordances that interact to impact the learning and practice of physical activity. (p. 34)

At present, the ecological view is an important component of the principles of APA (Sherrill 2004), given that adaptation is a fundamental, interactive, and reciprocal process of change between the individual and the environment. Adapted physical activity entails modifying, adjusting, or accommodating relationships within elements of the ecosystem (Sherrill 2004).

While APA functions well as a service delivery system, its function as a profession and as a scholarly field of study is still being explored (Reid 2003; Reid and Stanish 2003; Sherrill 2004). There is no doubt that service provision by means of activity or curriculum adaptations is the core input that promotes learning and performance under limiting

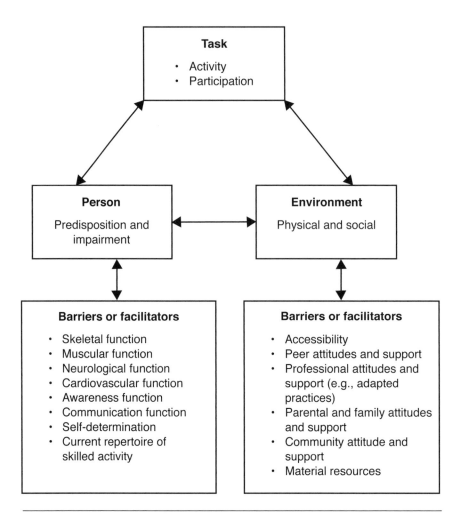

Figure 9.1   Facilitating and limiting variables in an extended ecological model of adapted physical activity variables.

conditions (e.g., Lieberman and Houston-Wilson 2002). However, when movement tasks are taught to individuals with limiting conditions, the typical developmental progression of task criteria often varies. Some criteria do not appear at all, and others may appear but in a different progression and at a slower rate than in participants who are able-bodied. In such a case, most APA professionals would increase variations of their cuing and feedback accommodations (e.g., Block 2000) and increase the breaking up of a task into subtask stations (Block, Provis, and Nelson 1994). A different approach is advocated here.

Dynamic Systems Theory

The work of Thelen and her collaborators (Thelen and Smith 1994; Thelen and Ulrich 1991; Ulrich, Ulrich, and Collier 1992), using dynamic systems theory, provides a set of principles pertaining to the specific relations between the environmental and individual conditions that make movement patterns change. According to this theory, patterns are spontaneously explored and selected by the individual due to contextual criteria known as rate limiters and control parameters. Rate limiters are specific relations limiting the natural selection process, and control parameters are relations facilitating a selection. Thus, the acquisition of motor skills can be interpreted as learning to select preferred patterns through exploration. Burton, Greer, and Wiese-Bjornstal (1993), for example, have adopted this theory to examine the dynamic relations of body and ball conditions in controlling the change in preferred patterns of throwing and grasping. Their exploratory work has indicated that transitions from one- to two-handed grasping were made as ball diameters increased. It thus may be suggested that the relation between ball diameter and hand size can be considered a control parameter for a one-handed grasping pattern. The dynamic systems view of movement skills acquisition (Thelen and Smith 1994; Ulrich, Ulrich, and Collier 1992) can be linked to the practice of ETA (Burton and Davis 1996; Davis and Burton 1991), creating a body of knowledge alternative to that obtained with the conservative information-processing model of movement skill acquisition.

Development of the Systematic Ecological Modification Approach

In spite of the substantial use of an ecological model in the study of motor control (e.g., Piek 1998), its practical application to curriculum planning and instructional design has been very limited. Following on the experimental work of Burton, Greer, and Wiese-Bjornstal (1993), it may be suggested that if the parameters controlling change from noneffective to effective movement patterns are recognized, they can be systematically modified to produce a pattern shift. The development of efficient adaptation and inclusion practices through continuous experimentation with ecological modification was undertaken at the Center for Active Learning and Empowerment. This was a three-year project aimed at enhancing participation in school physical activity, funded by the Israeli National Insurance Institute, Funds for Special Projects (Reiter, Talmor, and Hutzler 2004). In this project, a collection of 25 individual cases was analyzed according to SEMA in different curricular subareas including fundamental motor skills, lead-up games, ball games, gymnastics, dancing, athletics, and swimming (Hutzler 2004). Each case was described using a vignette, a methodological dilemma, a series of potential answers to the dilemma, and a complete analysis and discussion of the case using SEMA (see tables 9.1 and 9.2, p. 187-188). The following are the major elements of this ecological-oriented approach.

• *Identifying task objective.* The ecological perspective maintains that tasks are expressed as anticipated functional outcomes related to an individual and his or her environment (Reed 1988). For example, balancing would mean maintaining a relatively persistent orientation to the environment, while movement skills would assume various changes to this persistent orientation, effecting desired outcomes in the relations between the individual and the environment (Reed 1988).

• *Extracting qualitative and quantitative criteria for task negotiation.* These criteria include mechanically described displacements of the participant's body and task-related objects with respect to environmental demands. Each motor skill has identifiable qualitative criteria that are typically used for assessment (e.g., Ulrich 2000). These criteria are used within SEMA as one way of addressing task goal standards. Other standards are normative performance outcomes, such as distance a ball is thrown and time taken to perform a 100 meter (109 yard) run. In group events, criteria may include behavioral or interaction scores, such as the number of times group members hit a ball during a certain period.

• *Identifying limitation criteria.* These criteria manifest as deficits in the individual's functional abilities and include limitations in the various body systems (e.g., cognitive, perceptual, motor control, muscular strength, and range of motion) required in order to cope with environmental factors such as height of the net, size of the court, and so on.

• *Identifying performance errors under the limited conditions.* Identification of errors is the way most teachers perceive and describe the inability of a student to cope with task criteria. Identification is followed by enhanced instructional cues and feedback practices. However, without a complete ecological analysis, the teacher may be unaware of the individual and environmental constraints leading to the performance errors observed. Thus, his or her instructional strategies may be ineffective or even contraindicated. For example, passing in volleyball usually requires having a steady posture. If a participant fails to pass a ball while moving, he or she might usually be instructed to maintain a static position while passing. However, for individuals with certain conditions, such as cerebral palsy, standing still might be more difficult than being in motion, since persons with this condition may find it easier to achieve dynamic balance than static balance.

• *Detecting task- and individual-related control parameters.* These are typically relations between environmental and individual criteria that can be manipulated to bring about pattern shifts during the acquisition of movement skills in spite of the limiting conditions. Such manipulations are typically operationalized as adaptation suggestions, modifying (a) task criteria, which can mean using a different skill (e.g., moving in a wheelchair instead of running), or specific technical criteria (e.g., extending an arm sideways during a long jump for an athlete with leg amputation, thus correcting for the asymmetric inertia); (b) environmental conditions such as court size, treadmill speed or slope, and so on; (c) the equipment used, such as size of the ball or racket; (d) the game rules, as in affirmative action strategies; and (e) the instruction modalities from verbal to manual guidance (Center for Active Learning and Empowerment 2004; Lieberman and Houston-Wilson 2002; Sherrill 2004). Figure 9.2 depicts a summary model of the SEMA.

Table 9.1 presents an example of each of the modification strategies within SEMA for running, one of the most common tasks in physical education and sport coaching practice; table 9.2 presents modifications for bouncing or dribbling. The examples given in the tables suggest a multiplicity of alternatives for curriculum modification based on (a) identifying relations between the functional capabilities of the individual and environmental context variables and (b) constraining these relationships to achieve shifts in activity patterns. One should remember, however, that sometimes it is more useful to change a task rather than the movement pattern. If the functional conditions of an individual do not permit fast and accurate movements required in ball games, task goals should be changed from a competitive goal orientation to task mastery. The complex demands of attention and performance under multiple task conditions and extreme time pressure are likely to result in failure, disappointment, frustration, and consequently avoidance for individuals with severe cognitive, physical, or emotional limitations.

When the complex of task, individual, and goal relationships is not considered, modifications of task criteria may be oversimplified and may further limit individuals with disabilities rather than assisting them. For example, lowering the basket is a common suggestion for basketball players in wheelchairs (Block 2000; Lieberman and Houston-Wilson 2002). However, this adaptation by itself allows other players to easily screen the basket, making it more difficult for wheelchair users to score.

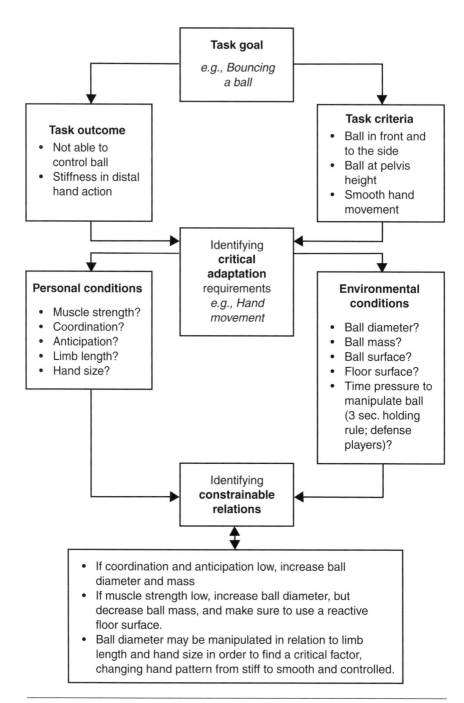

Figure 9.2 A systematic ecological modification approach illustrating bouncing pattern modification.

Table 9.1 Examples of SEMA Applied on a Locomotor Task

Task objective	Task criteria	Performance outcome	Individual limitation criteria	Control parameters (adaptations)
Locomoting fast for 15-50 meters	Both feet off ground	• Can't stabilize trunk while standing upright • Can't raise both feet off ground; runs abruptly with short steps and reduced fluency	• Complete lower limb paralysis • Reduced plantar-flexion strength • Reduced foot clearance (drop-foot) • Reduced hip flexion strength • Reduced stabilization strength • Increased plantarflexion tone	• Change task to wheeling in a seated position (task) • Change surface from stable to rolling (environment) • Use body weight supports (equipment) • Use ankle cuff weights (equipment) • Run on mattresses, use rebound effects (trampoline), obstacles, and direction change (environment) • Increase uphill incline (while using the treadmill)
	Contralateral arm-leg movement	• Can't coordinate arm to leg movement	• Difficulty in dissociating multi-limb movement	• Load hands with weight cuffs (equipment) • Use verbal rhythmic or spatial colored cues (instruction)
	Rolling over ankle joint	• Puts flat foot on floor	• Difficulty in coordinating rolling pattern	• Use rebounding surface (trampoline)
	Hip and knee joints 90° during swing	• Reduced range of motion and clearance above surface	• Reduced stabilization control • Reduced plantar-flexor strength • Depressed mental state	• Run down an incline or increase treadmill speed (environment) • Use rebounding surface (trampoline) • Use obstacles (environment), get more points for higher obstacles (rules)

Task criteria taken in part from TGMD-2, Ulrich, 2000.

Table 9.2   Examples of Individual Case Management Applying SEMA in a Ball Activity Setting (Hutzler 2004)

Criteria	Limitations	Outcome performance	Modifications
Hand contact at waist height	Ineffective proprioceptive control may limit timing and force application.	The ball is not pushed at the proper time and location, and may be pushed either too strongly or too weakly.	Using a larger and more massive ball such as a physio-ball (Fit-BALL) may enhance activation of proprioceptive control. This reduces improper force application.
Ball contactr in front of and external to the leg of the bouncing hand	Spatial perception is inefficient and pushing of the ball is imprecise.	An angled rebound of the ball off the ground leads to losing the ball.	Using a larger ball will make it easier to track its bounce and control the following strike.
bouncing using smooth hand contact	Due to difficulty in precision control, range of movement is frozen (i.e., elbow and hand joints are held at a fixed position).	Due to the larger moment, force regulation of the arm and hand is more difficult, leading to a larger variation of strikes than with hand contact only.	The larger mass rebounded from the floor will be too heavy for an extended arm at the elbow and hand joint, leading to unfreezing joint degrees of freedom.

The task analyzed in this table is bouncing, that is, the continual repeated pushing of the ball to the floor using one hand without losing the ball.

The advantages of using SEMA as an extension of the ETA model can be summarized as follows: (a) increased effectiveness of adaptation, due to a more goal-directed analysis; (b) increased efficiency of adaptation, due to decreased experimentation time; and (c) a decrease in unnecessary adaptations that may inhibit the individual's self-efficacy and socialization. The examples described in this chapter are expected to increase current intuitive use of ecological modification to constrain shifts between proficiency patterns within physical education instruction in general and APA in particular. It is proposed that SEMA follows up on the paradigmatic concepts of Burton and colleagues (1993) by developing them into a well-established analysis of control parameters across fundamental and sport-specific skills.

Selected Practical Examples of Ecological Modification

This section describes a number of established procedures for inducing constraints to selected ecological task categories. These task categories are the functional units identified in motor development literature as fundamental motor skills and in ICF taxonomy as activities. These types of functions were selected due to their importance for movement preservation and improvement across the life span. The specific tasks selected are those for which substantial practical and empirical evidence exists.

Postural and Locomotor Tasks

This section discusses tasks pertaining to maintaining and changing a position on the ground. By means of postural control and locomotion tasks individuals construct their orientation toward the environment, enabling them to pursue physical and social goals required in daily living as well as in exercise, sports, and recreation.

Postural Control

Maintaining postural control (balancing) is defined here as keeping an individual's orientation toward the environment (Reed 1982, 1988). Postural control is most widely used in bipedal standing and sitting. A common practice among dance teachers for controlling standing posture is to ask dancers to hold a book on their head, thus aligning the body through fixating its numerous degrees of freedom. This practice has a long tradition, acknowledged through anthropological observations of the controlled posture of females walking while holding jars on their heads. The Halliwick concept, common in aquatic practice (Lambeck and Coffey Stanat 2000, 2001), suggests using a variety of buoyancy-assisted postures and gravity-induced perturbations called "metacentric effects" for correcting maladjusted postures, thereby facilitating rotation control. The objective is to hold the posture in spite of the perturbation and is achieved through raising body parts out of the water. Muscular activation is required to counterbalance the mass and direction of raised body parts. This procedure is used to activate moderately controlled muscles. Recent clinical experiments in our laboratory have used the FitBALL for modifying sitting postural control. Our data have suggested a greater than 50% increase in achievement of a sacral neutral position in comparison to conventional modes of sitting in children with behavioral disorders.

Walking

Walking is defined as locomoting while keeping at least one foot in contact with the support surface (Davis and Rizzo 1991). Many factors may contribute to an impaired walking pattern, ranging from neuromuscular and orthopedic disorders (Shumway-Cook and Woollacott 2001) to depressed mood (Lemke et al. 2000; Sloman et al. 1982). An unstable surface has been used to induce stepping pattern in infants (Thelen and Ulrich 1991; Ulrich, Ulrich, and Collier 1992). On this basis, Ulrich and colleagues used the treadmill to facilitate walking in infants with Down syndrome and successfully increased their rate of progress in achieving developmental milestones (Ulrich et al. 2001). An increasing number of studies support the use of treadmills, particularly with partial body weight support, to facilitate walking in individuals in postacute phases of stroke (Hesse, Konrad, and Uhlenbrock 1999) and cerebral palsy (Schindl et al. 2000). Further research has established a significantly better outcome with speed-dependent treadmill training compared to conventional treatments (Pohl et al. 2002). Movement velocity and percent of body weight released may be suggested as the control parameters for initiating pattern shift. Another potential equipment modification is strapping ankle weights to an individual's legs. Clark and Phillips (1993) have used such weights in infant walkers, immediately eliciting a more mature pattern of shank-thigh coordination.

Running

Running is defined here as locomoting with both feet momentarily leaving the support surface simultaneously (Davis and Rizzo 1991). As running serves the same goal as walking, that is, locomoting from one point to another, one may ask, why change gaits? Research has revealed that at increased velocities, animals and humans change gaits to conserve energy and to allow for improved dynamic stability (Alexander 1984, 1992). The locomotor control system has been described as a spring-loaded inverted pendulum (Full and Koditschek 1999) representing an action model similar to jumping on a pogo stick. The important factors in such a system are acceleration, leg length, and velocity. Animals change their gait pattern due to a constant relation between these variables called the Froude number (Full 2000). This is a dimensionless measure of speed that is not dependent on individual criteria. Since acceleration in this system cannot be greater than gravity, the Froude number equals speed squared divided by gravity multiplied by leg length:

$$\text{Froude} = \frac{V^2}{g \cdot \text{leg}}$$

Most mammals (independent of leg number) change gait at similar Froude numbers, particularly between walking and running at a value between 2 and 3 (Full 2000). Observing a young child starting to run may help explain some of the reason for gait change. Trying to increase speed with relatively short legs (half the adult ratio to body size), small children increase their cadence until at a certain point, the time at contact does not permit the range of pendulum movement required and if the pattern did not change, the child would fall. In order to prevent a fall, the child switches to a pattern incorporating a time frame with both legs in the air (i.e., running). Table 9.1 lists the many possibilities of specific limitations and a variety of environmental and equipment modifications that might be imposed to shift running patterns. For example, using barriers at a certain percentage of leg length or an uneven terrain may induce improved foot clearance. Using an uphill running surface (on a treadmill or outdoors) poses a constraint to prevent a running pattern with excessive tramping on the forefoot and a limited heel strike, which is quite common in participants with spasticity.

Jumping

Jumping is defined as locomoting by leaving the support surface, from one or both legs, and landing only once (Davis and Rizzo 1991). One common flaw in jumpers with coordination disorders is a stepping-like movement: leaving the surface foot by foot, landing foot by foot, or both. An increased vertical load, achieved either by addition of ankle weights or by use of an incline, may contribute to changing over to the simultaneous bilateral jumping pattern. Another common flaw that reduces jumping distance is the lack of full extension of the arms up and forward during the flight phase. A hanging ball to be touched during flight is often used in order to correct the deficient pattern. Experimental designs are warranted to compare conservative curricular approaches using visual and verbal feedback to the ecological modification approach using increased load or distance to constrain movement patterns into an increased recruitment of muscular energy over a longer range of movement.

Ball Activity Patterns

This section discusses tasks pertaining to negotiation with static or moving objects, such as balls, that are used in physical education and sports. Movement patterns once used for combat such as throwing and striking are now used mostly for sport and recreation purposes.

Throwing

Throwing is functionally defined as using one or more arms to propel an object held in the hand(s) of the arm(s) being employed (Davis and Rizzo 1991). Throwing has two main outcomes: distance and precision. In throwing for distance, an increase in coupling of body segments is required to increase rotational energy. In throwing for precision, a decrease in joint degrees of freedom is required to limit errors in the control of movement coupling. The pattern of the throw is dependent on the performer's attributes and the object to be thrown. In petanque boules, for instance, a straight-arm, underhand pendulum throw is preferred in order to achieve both distance and precision.

Children with disability display a variety of self-selected throwing patterns. Analyzing the spontaneously selected patterns provides astonishing insights into their degree of efficiency. For example, an adolescent boy who has L_{3-4} complete spinal cord lesion due to spina bifida and lacks ankle and knee force and stability tries to increase the rotational forces of one arm and the trunk by stabilizing with his legs on the surface and one hand holding on to the wheelchair in a semiseated position. An adolescent girl with spinal motor atrophy who is lacking stability and strength of her back muscles, thus eliminating trunk rotational moments, attempts to gain momentum using both her arms in a chest throw.

On the basis of these examples, it appears that professionals should very carefully consider the patterns they would change. An attempt to modify these patterns toward the gold standard pattern might eventually impose greater functional limitation. If, however, the functional circumstances for a pattern are available but the typical learning process does not take place due to a lack of information input, constraint-induced teaching might help. For attaining the adult overarm throwing pattern (Ulrich 2000) in cases of decreased input, as in visually or proprioceptively impaired individuals, dynamic induction modalities could be applied. For example, smoothly pulling the throwing hand from behind with a rope or elastic band perpendicular to the shoulder line would induce a complete pattern shift from a primary push pattern into the mature pattern. The particular criteria changed include a controlled elbow hold during the trunk rotation and shoulder adduction preceding the extension of the underarm, with the elbow leading the rotational movement of the hand. An experimental paradigm using dynamic loading as well as scaled-up or scaled-down ball diameters, in contrast to conservative feedback-based instruction, is worth consideration.

Catching

Catching is defined as stopping and securing an object with one or more limbs (Davis and Rizzo 1991). In contrast to throwing, catching is a tracking activity requiring continuous control of the perceptual systems, primarily the visual system. Typical errors in catching are more perceptual than mechanical in origin and predominantly relate to impaired timing. Catching a rolling physiotherapy ball facilitates underarm and hand control due to the reduced difficulty in anticipating the angular approach of the ball. This practice appears to produce a pattern shift from the primary patterns of "hugging" the ball with the arms into the mature pattern of grasping and securing the ball with the hands. A research paradigm using rolling and catching versus catching-only trials is warranted to account for the anticipated effect of changing the dynamics of ball movement into a bidimensional rather than a three-dimensional space. Another option for inducing transitions in catching pattern is scaling ball size either up or down. This paradigm was used in the grasping experiment of Burton and colleagues (1993) and resulted in a transition from a one-handed to a two-handed grasp as ball diameter was scaled up. The likelihood of use of more mature catching criteria at ages 4 to 7 years as ball diameter is scaled up has been explored in preliminary case studies in our laboratories but not yet confirmed.

Striking

Striking is defined as using an arm-hand-implement to impart force to a stationary or moving object (adapted from Davis and Rizzo 1991). The tennis swing and golf swing are excellent examples of striking activities in a sport context. The striking pattern may include one or two hands and a variety of implements according to the distance and precision required. A set of golf clubs is a good example of the specificity that may be attempted in striking. The variety of implements and specific skills increase the likelihood of negative transfer. For example, during the tennis forehand strike, some beginners demonstrate a tucked elbow throughout the swing (e.g., Brown 1989). One example of the use of an ecological modification approach in correcting this inefficient pattern is increasing ball mass and size. This practice results in a spontaneous adaptation of the swing even in the unfamiliar conditions of striking from a wheelchair. The significant influence of different diameters and masses of table tennis balls on their velocity and speed has been demonstrated by Xiaopeng (1998), but the influence of this increased velocity on shifting patterns warrants further research. Another adaptation is holding the wrist with the other hand throughout the forehand swing, thus constraining the extension pattern of the dominant hand (Brown 1989).

Bouncing

Bouncing is defined as imparting force to an object continuously as it rebounds from a stationary surface (Davis and Rizzo 1991). Increasing ball diameter while keeping the same ball mass and density appears to facilitate a pattern shift from shoulder- to underarm- and particularly hand-controlled action (table 9.2). Task outcomes with this mature pattern are increased accuracy in controlling the position and height of ball bounce. While there is no empirical evidence for this modification as of now, it is being used clinically. However, the specific control parameters, such as the ratio of ball diameter to performer criteria or, more specifically, arm length and hand span, are not yet known. A paradigm similar to the one used by Burton and colleagues (1993) is recommended for detecting the appropriate ratio across age, gender, and limitations.

Swimming

Swimming is defined as locomoting in water (Davis and Rizzo 1991). It includes a number of strokes composed basically of a combination of propulsive and recovery movements. The aim is to increase propulsive momentum through arm pulls and leg kicks and decrease drag during the recovery movements. Among the most complex and difficult strokes to learn are the breaststroke and butterfly stroke. Both require a wave-like short-range body rotation around the waist. Wearing fins that increase the propulsive and buoyant forces (without kicking) has been encouraged as a means of overcoming the difficulty of acquiring the correct pattern (Gmünder 2003). In adapted aquatics, fins have also been shown to be beneficial for individuals with limitations in their plantarflexion strength, range of motion, or control. Hand pulleys are another device used in aquatics for dynamically constraining the proper pattern of sculling (outward and inward rotation of the hand) during the arm pull. Fins and hand pulleys are frequently employed in teaching the freestyle and backstroke to individuals with motor control disorders such as cerebral palsy. A 2 × 2 group design to examine the use of apparatus and the use of feedback in teaching the specific skill would be one way to account for the anticipated effect of constraining limb buoyancy and drag.

INSTRUCTIONAL STRATEGIES

- Facilitating and limiting conditions are found in individuals and the environment. Instructors should consider the impact of these conditions when suggesting the adaptations to be utilized.
- Using treadmills is recommended for initiating and maintaining stepping patterns across a variety of ages and disorders.
- Manipulating ball size and mass for constraining patterns used in fundamental ball skills such as bouncing, catching, and batting is recommended.
- Using a bi-dimensional space for rolling rather than a three-dimensional for throwing is expected to facilitate efficient catching patterns.
- Using fins and pulleys may facilitate acquisition of efficient pulling and kicking patterns in swimming.

Summary

This chapter presents a model for systematic modification of environmental factors across task learning conditions. The advantages of using systematic ecological modification as an extension of the ETA model can be summarized as follows: (a) increasing the effectiveness of adaptation, due to a more goal-directed analysis; (b) increasing the efficiency of adaptation, due to decreased experimentation time; and (c) decreasing unnecessary adaptations, which may inhibit players' self-efficacy and socialization. The examples described are expected to increase current intuitive use of ecological modification for constraining shifts between proficiency patterns within physical education instruction in general and APA in particular. It is proposed that the approach described in this chapter follows up on the paradigmatic concepts of Burton, Greer, and Wiese-Bjornstal (1993) to provide a well-established analysis of control parameters across fundamental and sport-specific skills.

Providing Decision-Making Opportunities for Learners With Disabilities

Jane Taylor, PhD, Donna L. Goodwin, PhD,
and Henriëtte Groeneveld, PhD

I n human society, independence, self-worth, and dignity are reflected in the ability and opportunity to make choices about our lives (Glausier, Whorton, and Knight 1995). In the past, opportunities to make decisions, exercise choice, and express preferences have been absent from many educational programs for persons with disabilities (Guess, Benson, and Siegel-Causey 1985), particularly programs designed to promote physical activity. Although there are many practical reasons given for not providing choice to people with disabilities (such as constraints of time, scheduling, knowledge), perhaps the most disturbing is the perception that they are incapable of making choices (Kishi et al. 1988) or that professionals know what is best for all (Szymanski and Trueba 1994). It was not until we attended a presentation at the International Federation of Adapted Physical Activity meeting in Miami and followed up by reading the first paper on Ecological Task Analysis (Davis and Burton 1991) that we became aware of a comprehensive model attempting to address this issue. More than a decade later we are continuing to struggle with the application of this model, although we remain stubbornly convinced of its utility. As educators who have spent much of our lives advocating for the independence of people with disabilities, the ETA model has provided us with an excellent framework, but one that has not been without its challenges.

Since its authors and proponents began the task of changing our minds about traditional instructional practices using task analysis in the domain of physical activity, they have promised the following. Ecological Task Analysis is equally applicable to instruction and assessment; it takes all of the relevant task, performer, and environmental factors into account;

it is learner centered and is functionally based (Balan and Davis 1993; Burton and Davis 1992, 1996; Davis and Burton 1991). As the model has evolved, the authors have placed more emphasis on its applicability to all learners, not just those with disabilities. In particular, the refusal to dictate movement form is, in its own way, a celebration of diversity. All persons can strive to achieve the same functional goal; therefore all persons can be successful. Requiring, rather than just allowing, the student to choose the goal, the skill, and the movement form may in turn enhance motivation, develop skills in decision making, and foster ownership of the learning environment (Burton and Davis 1996). All of these outcomes are desirable in and of themselves and are the gifts of ETA. But with respect to application of ETA in our own physical activity settings, two major barriers need to be addressed if we are to be successful in teaching others to embrace and implement this model.

The first obstacle is the instructor who is entrenched in the traditional, teacher-centered model of skill instruction. In this model the instructional setting is established and controlled by the instructor. Although we may see advantages to learner choice making, our entrenchment in the expert model gives privilege to the knowledge and authority of the instructor. We do not generally have a history or instructional tradition that recognizes choice making as an instructional goal. Although encouraging decision making and choice is intuitively and ethically pleasing, it is difficult to embrace without personal commitment, professional preparation that emphasizes self-determination as an outcome of student learning, and curricula in which choice and decision making are a foundation to their design and application.

The second impediment relates to our own knowledge and understanding of the interactions of task dimensions and participant characteristics and the necessary role they play in presenting an environment that encourages choice making from any and all participants. Typical physical activity skill instruction focuses on the completion of skills according to predetermined criteria of correctness that are often developmentally based (Herkowitz 1978b). Deviation from these criteria can be deemed an incorrect motor response or an underdeveloped skill form. Even Herkowitz herself acknowledged that users of her developmental General Task Analysis (GTA) model had to rely on intuition to select task and environment factors, as there has been little research to substantiate the environmental variables that best promote motor skill development. The present authors agree that this uncertainty is still a major impediment to the conceptual understanding and ease of applying ETA (Davis and Burton 1991). This uncertainty is complicated further when we must also be aware of the elements in the task and environment that need to be manipulated in order for a child with a disability to be successful.

Choice is defined by Brigham (1979) as "the opportunity to make an uncoerced selection from two or more alternative events, consequences, or responses" (p. 132). It has been further defined as "a process of selecting between alternatives based on individual preferences" (Wehmeyer et al. 1997). Some of the questions we have pondered over the years include (a) why choice making is an important instructional goal; (b) what reasonable conditions must exist in order for teachers or coaches to provide alternatives; (c) what variables within the environment, the task, and the person affect a learner's ability to make choices and act on the choices made; and (d) how the application of decision making can be facilitated in applied physical activity settings. The purpose of this chapter, therefore, is to discuss the challenge of applying the decision-making aspect of the ETA model within physical activity environments for learners with disabilities.

Rationale for Providing Choice

The importance of choice making becomes particularly palpable when we think about quality of life and persons with intellectual disabilities. Exercising choice and making decisions are life skills that are expected of those who live in the community (Bannerman et al. 1990; Harchik et al. 1993), and have been cited as among the main reasons why persons with intellectual disabilities struggle with the transition from school life to employment as young adults (Schloss, Alper, and Jayne 1993). Brown (1996) argues that self-determination is central to the education of students with disabilities and should receive educational emphasis through the school years. Choice making is a determinant of self-determination as it is fundamental to goal setting, decision making, and problem solving (Wehmeyer et al. 1997). Leisure contributes substantially to the quality of life we experience (Glausier, Whorton, and Knight 1995). As leisure, by definition, refers to time spent as one chooses, the need for skills at choice making becomes abundantly clear (Parsons et al. 1997).

Harchik and colleagues (1993) reviewed 100 research articles addressing the effects of providing people with intellectual disabilities increased opportunities for choice. Among other things, they concluded that individuals most frequently chose, participated in, and rated as more pleasant, those situations in which choice or control was available.

Another review article by Kern and colleagues (1998) looked at studies between 1975 and 1996 in which opportunity for choice making was purposefully implemented as an intervention to decrease problematic behavior and increase desirable behavior. They reviewed 14 papers, three of which were in the area of recreation and leisure, and concluded that "choice making was an effective procedure for both decreasing the occurrence of undesirable responding and increasing the quantity and quality of desired behaviors" (p. 165). A recent pilot study employing ETA illustrates this point (Taylor 2002). Although the instruction was implemented to increase swim skill behaviors of youths with developmental disabilities, the variability in skill levels dictated that for one participant, comfort in the water was the goal. Through an instructional period of 14 sessions the participant went from "not in the pool, in pool but upset and agitated" in sessions 1 and 2 to "very content, eager to play and move" by session 10. Similarly, Groeneveld (1999) reported that when viewing the "new-found" functional abilities of their children, parents in South Africa were shocked at the independence demonstrated in skills they presumed their children were incapable of performing. If we are convinced that choice is a desirable instructional goal, what is needed to make choice an embedded component of our instructional-leisure settings?

Knowledge and Skills Needed for Implementing Choice

Creating opportunities for choice making in instructional settings requires numerous instructor and learner conditions to be in place. The instructor must provide more than opportunities for choice. The choices offered must be meaningful, must be within the understanding and ability of the learner, and must reflect the abilities of the learner. Furthermore, in some instances, choice making may need to be taught in small incremental steps.

Teacher or Instructor Considerations

There is empirical evidence to suggest that children as young as 8 years old with severe intellectual disabilities and individuals with profound multiple disabilities can learn to make choices in a leisure setting (Dattilo and Rusch 1985; Realon, Favell, and Lowerre 1990). The ability of a person to make choices known to others is dependent on a number of interrelated variables. For instance, the person must be able to make choices and then act on the choice made. "[C]hoice is really only a choice when one is able to act on the decision" (Mobily 1985, p. 23). To provide an alternative that is beyond the understanding, ability, or interest of the student is pointless. Participants who do not respond to opportunities for choice that are presented verbally may need to be provided with visual representation. This representation may be either the actual object, a picture of an object or activity, or a physical demonstration to identify the options available. Moreover, for individuals who are nonverbal, a two-object choice, which in this instance may be more appropriately labeled preference, may need to be presented initially and their responses judged behaviorally (Dattilo and Rusch 1985; Parsons et al. 1997).

For there to be a true indication that a choice has been made based on saliency of the contexts offered, the options presented must be meaningful to the person. Offering an unattractive choice is equivalent to offering no choice at all (Harchik et al. 1993; Monty et al. 1979). The disadvantage to this form of choice making is that the alternatives are presented to the person by another and may develop into a standard repertoire of choices that may limit further opportunities to grow in choice making and thereby restrict participation options. To facilitate the experience of choice, the person must be engaged with the elements of the environment and feel that there is an element of control over the surroundings due to the choice made (Dattilo and Barnett 1985; Monty et al. 1979). To lack the opportunity to exhibit self-determined behavior can lead to feelings of helplessness. Individuals learn over time that their actions have no effect on the environment, and future attempts to exhibit choice may result in reaction based on habit rather than choice (Schloss, Alper, and Jayne 1993).

On the other hand, alternatives for choice may need to be offered along a continuum as the person's skills and interests expand. One method that has proven helpful in teacher training related to choice offering and selection is the creation of "ETA simulations" (Taylor 2002). Student teachers choose a task goal and then detail three choices that could be offered to the student. They arbitrarily select a response and then proceed to write environmental manipulations that might encourage the desired outcome. The ETA model is followed through to inevitable instruction or some success with achieving the goal until the student teachers think they have written a reasonable application of the model. These simulations are presented to teaching peers for critique and then prepared in a manual of ETA suggestions. Although use of the manual is optional, the process of preparing these simulations helps the student teachers learn the model and gives them a repertoire of ideas that is particularly helpful when they finally meet their pupils, who often have a wide range of abilities. Implementing this peer review process is an alternative to submitting plans to a master teacher, who acts as a sounding board and critical observer of student applications, as is the practice in Davis' teaching laboratory (Davis and Klingler 2001).

To make choices, the person must comprehend the consequences of each alternative (Mobily 1985). To assume that the performer would know not only what the alternatives may be, but also what the outcome of the choice selection is, within the realm of disability and physical activity, is erroneous. The same concern applies to the instructor. Determination of the alternatives from which a performer can choose given the interacting variables within the environment, the task, and the performer is an enormous task and responsibility. Thus, while freedom of choice may be available, knowing the alternatives from which to choose becomes perhaps the largest challenge of the learner and the instructor.

Knowing how to approach the analysis of and subsequent presentation of alternatives from which the learner can choose is somewhat easier if we return to the model and use it to complete a movement skill assessment prior to beginning the instruction process. In fact, Davis and Burton (1991) clearly indicated the interconnection and seamless transition between assessment and instruction in their ETA model. Furthermore, it does not seem logical or useful to try to create a choice paradigm in an instructional setting for students with disabilities if the skill repertoire and functional level have not been previously determined. The advantage of applying the entire model is that instruction follows naturally from the assessment process and is "set up" for success. On the other hand, the joy of discovering a successful movement form when an individual responds to a particular environmental manipulation cannot be overstated. Perhaps as instructors, we need to relinquish our roles as "movement experts" a bit and let the students take the lead in choosing and acquiring suitable movement forms.

However, an absence of instructor constraints to choice making as a valuable learning outcome may not be a sufficient condition for experiencing choice. Additional circumstances are required within an instructional setting. For example, asking a student to "figure it out" may be insufficient even in the face of numerous alternatives for participation. Positive and facilitative resources may be needed to encourage and teach choice making, particularly in first-time situations or as the difficulty of tasks increases across grade level. Giving a student enough time to explore the options or the consequences of various choices within a supportive environment is essential. Certainly, presenting alternate movement forms, making environmental modifications, and maximizing learner performance variables, and repeating these options until the student is able to actively make and act on his or her choices, are skills required by instructors who use ETA.

There may be clusters of alternatives or modifications that can be made across contexts and across many different students to enhance participation and learning (e.g., decrease or increase distance, decrease or increase time available to respond, decrease or increase size of projectile). Moreover, choice in participation as expressed through rule changes, equipment alternatives, and changes in skill demands may enhance participation of many students (Bulger, Townsend, and Carson 2001; Canadian Association for Health, Physical Education, Recreation and Dance [CAHPERD] 1994; Davis and Klingler 2001; Taylor 2001). Although the process of determination of alternatives should not become mechanical, it may on the other hand become more natural or automatic. "Choice making is highly complex and contingent on the individual's dynamic interaction with the environment" (Schloss, Alper, and Jayne 1993). The process by which these alternatives are generated and presented may be the greatest pedagogical challenge to the instructor toward the creation of a self-determined learning environment. A dynamic tension should exist in the process of providing opportunities for choice, the determination of alternatives, and the consequence of the choices made. The ability to make choices is dynamic and may increase as the person benefits from more opportunities to choose and to learn (Schloss, Alper, and Jayne 1993). Short- and long-term goals along a continuum of choice difficulty within a given context would recognize the individual's choice-making capabilities and build an ecological repertoire of choice-making strategies.

For students for whom the completion of a task goal through traditional movement forms is not viable or safe, achieving the outcome through alternate means becomes the instructional focus. The student plays an active choice- and decision-making role in determining the focus of the skill and movement forms that will best achieve the task goal (Davis and Burton 1991). The achievement of the desired task goal should not be interpreted, however, as the only outcome of the ETA process. Providing opportunities for students to make choices and be self-determined in their actions and to recognize their own agency is a concomitant benefit of the ETA approach that should not be lost to teachers and coaches of learners with disabilities. The opportunity to foster feelings of self-worth and self-efficacy through the choice-making process not only is meaningful to the learner, but also instills a sense of internal agency and responsibility for the learning. A self-determined learning environment is created when the students are provided with an opportunity to make deliberate choices from alternatives that are well understood, are goal directed, are meaningful, and have an achievable outcome. Without knowing what alternatives exist and their relationship to the goal, the learner is really not experiencing conscious and deliberate choice making.

Learner Considerations

The opportunity for choice may also be mediated by learner variables such as age, ability, personal history, and age of onset of disability. The implementation of ETA as it applies to the type and level of ability of students has not been explored in detail. The model is said to apply to all students, including students with and without disabilities (Davis and Burton 1991). However, if its application is to be consistent across students and settings, additional guidelines for adaptation are necessary. For example, the early work of Herkowitz (1978b) on developmental task analysis is essential in determining alternatives from which students may choose to alter the perceptual demands of a task. Herkowitz constructed these hierarchies, however, with the underlying assumption of normal development. If in a striking task, a particular student needs to eliminate the need to track a moving projectile by placing a ball on a T-ball stand, then this option needs to be built into the available task options (Robb 1972). Similarly, students in wheelchairs and their able-bodied partners would need a number of different adjustments in ball size, trajectory, and force absorption in learning a catching task if success is to be promoted. It appears that teachers need a protocol to follow in determining the nature of choice-making alternatives needed to enhance performance and thereby also encourage choice-making skills that are meaningful and success oriented (Parsons et al. 1997).

There may also be a psychological comfort that comes with having decisions made by others. The students are absolved of responsibility and there is no consequence, either positive or negative, for making an incorrect choice (Mobily 1985). For example, Neumayer and Bleasdale (1996) completed a study in which 30 adults (mean age 33) with intellectual disabilities were interviewed about their preferences regarding four major areas of their lives: home, work, leisure, and relationships. Forty-seven percent of the participants wanted more choices in their lives, while 43% felt it was not important or preferred fewer choices. Wanting fewer choices was related to "it gets too confusing, makes it overwhelming for me, I don't know what to do if there are too many choices, and a few choices make it easier" (p. 106). The need for choice opportunities and choice instruction was summed up by one of the participants in this study: "It depends on how hard the choice is, what the choice is, and if you are capable of making the choice" (p. 107).

Another complicating factor is whether a lack of expressed preference for presented alternatives should be respected as an active choice. In this situation it is always important to know if the person has had the opportunity to learn to make choices, or if history has resulted in the no-choice behavior. Not hearing complaints from students about the extent or nature of their participation should not be taken to mean that further alternatives and opportunities for choice are not required. The question arises whether acquiescing to the impact of the disability within a given setting is something that is valued within a physical activity setting. If active participation is valued, then the task of creating opportunities to express choice becomes not only desirable, but also essential to the participation of many students with disabilities. The impact of history is most apparent in the study of young South African children given the opportunity not only to use wheelchairs for the first time but also to play wheelchair basketball (Groeneveld 1999). Since many of the children had no experience in either context, independent decision making in the form of choosing how to get in and out of the chair, get into a van, or direct a basketball from A to B on the court took on a whole life of its own. In addition, these experiences were brand-new, as teachers had felt it was more efficient if they physically transferred the children from van to chair than allowing them to solve the problem themselves.

Providing opportunity for choice within a physical education setting is challenging. The pressures of curriculum implementation with large classes of diverse students, in teaching environments that can be cramped and underequipped, and while working within inflexible schedules, demand a great deal of teachers. Teachers must be creative in the interpretation of the curriculum, present alternatives in the completion of tasks, and address individual student needs. There is an inherent tension between the teaching of a prescribed curriculum that has been formulated on the principles of normal development and choice for students. This tension is exacerbated when the achievement of prescriptive educational objectives based on behaviorism is the focus of the program (Fredericks 1980).

In summary, utilizing ETA as an instructional model in the context of motor skill development requires a committed and highly knowledgeable instructor. The instructor must embrace a learner-centered approach to teaching that recognizes the significance of choice making in self-determined behavior. An initial understanding of the instructional curriculum is necessary, as the teacher is required to deconstruct the learning activities particularly in light of learners with disabilities. Thus there is less emphasis on the skill process or how closely the skills utilized emulate a normative standard of performance, and more focus on the task outcome. The instructor's role shifts to providing opportunities to explore and develop skills and movement forms that can be used to successfully achieve the task goal by encouraging the learner to choose between performance, task, and environmental variables. Variables pertaining to the learner cannot be overlooked in the implementation of ETA. Personal histories of learned helplessness may undermine the instructor's efforts to enhance choice making.

An ETA approach to instruction requires considerable skill on the part of instructors. The instructional setting should reflect pedagogical sensitivity to the subjective experience of the learner based on an interpretive understanding of how many forms of movement can achieve the same task goal (van Manen 1993). This sensitivity to the learning experience from the learner's perspective includes an appreciation of the physical, emotional, and social attributes the learner brings to the task. Within the context of ETA, pedagogical tactfulness means assisting learners to comprehend the possibility of multiple choices in skill and movement forms. As learners are provided with the time to explore these choices within the context of their own abilities, they will learn to interpret environmental supports or the support of others who can facilitate their participation.

We cannot expect or assume that practicing teachers have the inclination or the professional background to embrace, in essence, this new way of approaching skill instruction. Nor is it necessary for all students to use the ETA model of instruction to become successful performers. The blending of the traditional skill approach and the ETA approach may provide the most salient instructional climate for skill development in the context of diverse learners. Indeed, the challenge of implementation of ETA as an instructional model may have to lie with our future instructors. Those who are committed to the field of adapted physical activity have promoted and will continue to promote ETA as an instructional model through their university- and college-based programs. Getting the message to our colleagues who are directly involved in teacher education is the true challenge. We present no quick solutions to bridging this chasm. The departmental and attitudinal barriers to sharing our knowledge bases are immense. The preparation of an instructional unit that could be incorporated into existing courses, or the publication of an instructional manual that brings the tenets of ETA to bear, may be of some value. Certainly, personal contact with educationally based colleagues would go a long way to bring the ETA model to students who will ultimately be teaching in the school system.

Teaching Choice: Role of the Instructor

Whether the teacher's role involves prior arrangement of the movement environment for student self-discovery or timely manipulation of environmental prompts to encourage choice, the teacher's role is crucial in the application of ETA. It has been suggested that infants as young as 4 to 5 months can indicate preferences through eye gazing, cries, and smiles, and by 10 months through motor skill acts such as pointing and crawling toward a desired object (Wehmeyer et al. 1997). The advent of language increases the ease with which alternatives can be offered and children can signal their preferred choices. But for children who are nonverbal, the teacher's challenge of presenting choices iconically can become exceedingly difficult in terms of time, creativeness, and energy to persevere. For learners with developmental disabilities, it may be difficult to ascertain their ability to link the outcomes of the choices made to the ultimate goal that is to be achieved (Wehmeyer et al. 1997). The functional level of each child will determine in large part the role of the teacher and the progressive learning steps needed as the student becomes more experienced with making choices. Wehmeyer et al. (1997) provide suggestions for educational practice in the promotion of self-determination that have direct relevance here to the instruction of choice making given the embedded nature of choice in self-determination.

Teacher support may be needed to assist children to recognize alternatives and the relative contribution of each in facilitating the achieved outcome. This support may include the following:

- Restricting choices that are unsafe or are detrimental to the achievement of the goal
- Suggesting alternatives that complement the abilities of the student
- Reinforcing the identification of multiple alternatives and the match between the options selected, the task goal, and the student's ability
- Facilitating active engagement by encouraging students to revisit a decision and its effectiveness, particularly when the choice has not resulted in the desired outcome
- Promoting meaningful organization of choice making by asking students to identify alternatives and describe the consequence of acting on the different choice options

Although choice making and choice-making skill development through instruction have received considerable research attention over the past several decades (Harchik et al. 1993; Parsons et al. 1997), the focus of this research has been primarily persons with intellectual disabilities (Kern et al. 1998). Research attention has been given to decreasing problem behaviors by offering choices in activities (e.g., Dyer, Dunlap, and Winterling 1990; Dunlap et al. 1994; Kern et al. 1998; Munk and

Repp 1994), demonstrating that individuals with disabilities are capable of purposefully making choices (e.g., Parsons and Reid 1990; Stancliffe and Wehmeyer 1995), and enhancing quality of life by increasing access to preferred activities through the exercise of choice (e.g., Harchik et al. 1993; Kern et al. 1998; Neumayer and Bleasdale 1996).

In addition, a number of researchers have developed programs to teach choice making (e.g., Gothelf et al. 1994; Parsons, McCarn, and Reid 1993; Warren 1993). With the exception of ETA, none of the instructional frameworks have addressed choice making for students with disabilities within the physical activity setting (Davis and Burton 1991; Groeneveld 1999; Taylor 2002). Reid, Parsons, and Green (1991) identified the instruction of choice making as consisting of two components, the act of choosing and the identification of a preference. Other instructional frameworks have made use of teacher prompts (e.g., Schloss, Alper, and Jayne 1993; Zetlin and Gillmore 1983).

Schloss and colleagues (1993) illustrate the levels of prompted choice making along a continuum dependent on the potential for risk to the individual and the skill level of the person in question. Choice making is placed on the following continuum: total independence in making a choice; guidance that does not restrict the actual response of the individual; guidance that may partially restrict the actions of the individual; guidance that more fully restricts the actions of the individual; and full restriction of action on behalf of the student (p. 223). The levels of prompting used in conjunction with the continuum are (a) identifying the discrete choice situation; (b) providing a priori restrictions in the choice; (c) providing a reasonable period of time for the student to self-initiate with no input; (d) providing partial and then full restrictive guidance if no response is made; and (e) finally, making a choice on behalf of the learner. If at any time a high-risk choice is made (e.g., refusal to wear helmet for ice-skating), the choice is negated and restrictive guidance is provided. As Schloss and colleagues (1993) indicate, this approach is highly concrete and uses the natural cues available in the specific context.

These authors also point out that because inclusionary classrooms generally involve large numbers of students, the often lone teacher may not be available to provide input on a vast number of choice situations. The implication is that either smaller class settings are needed to allow the required input (self-contained classroom setting) or additional support personnel are needed (e.g., paraprofessionals). An alternative suggestion, however, that might help maximize the effectiveness of implementation is to be selective regarding where and when ETA is implemented. As both participants and instructors become familiar with the system, it can be implemented in other, less predictable environments. It may be of considerable merit to investigate further the sticky points in the curriculum for children with movement difficulties and ways in which ETA can be gradually introduced to both the instructors and the students. Curriculum modules (or lesson plans or worksheets) that provide templates for use by the teachers and students may be of immense support. These modules would also assist in bridging the instructional gap identified in preservice university education as well. Although we cannot overemphasize the importance of the role of the teacher in increasing students' awareness of affordances in physical education, it is equally important to relieve the teacher of "having all the answers." One of the joys of ETA is the assumption that there is always an answer to a movement question. It just needs to be discovered. This answer undoubtedly will not necessarily be the same for any two people, and that is probably the biggest challenge and yet the greatest benefit of implementing ETA. Preservice and practicing teachers need to be supported in learning how to identify environmental affordances within the physical activity context that can moderate the experiences of diverse students.

Shevin and Klein (1984) identified three component skill clusters requiring instruction within a choice-making curriculum—discriminative skills, affective skills, and generalization of skills to real settings. The discriminative skills cluster includes the ability to use visual, tactile, and auditory skills to identify and discriminate among alternatives. The affective skills component involves the identification of the students' interests, abilities, likes and dislikes, and wants and needs. The generalization of skills refers to the making of choices within authentic contexts and beyond the classroom. Choice making is embedded in the broader skill of decision making.

To make a decision requires a number of steps, including listing relevant alternatives, identifying the consequences of acting on the alternatives, assessing the probability of the consequence occurring, establishing the value or utility of each consequence, and identifying the most attractive course of action (Beyth-Maron et al. 1991; Bullock and Mahon 1992). It is only after alternatives have been identified and their consequences understood that choice making may occur. However, "choice making is often not taught" (Bannerman et al. 1990) but relegated to a permissible activity rather than a target of our teaching (Shevin and Klein 1984). Although curricula have been developed to teach students to make choices (see Harchik et al. 1993), they have been developed for segregated settings and have not been accessed by generalist teachers of physical education. Moreover, methods on how to instruct choice making are not often included in teacher preparation programs (Bannerman et al. 1990).

Meyer (1991) cautions us that a success-based paradigm can become a paradigm trap. As a result of the behavioral research paradigm, the lives of people with severe disabilities, autism, and multiple disabilities became less restrictive and more hopeful as expectations increased and intervention programs were implemented. On the negative side, the success of the applied behavior analysis approach meant that a diagnostic-prescriptive approach based on a deficit-remedial assumption was applied across many disabilities, contexts, and instructional settings without thought as to alternate approaches or the long-term implications of the efficacy of the approach in natural settings. Success was judged by how much the individual had moved toward that which was considered typical. This almost singular reliance on one instructional approach served to reinforce the need to "reduce the gap between disability and typical" (Meyer 1991, p. 634), a gap based on a developmental reference.

Ecological Task Analysis has shifted the curriculum focus away from a rigid developmental reference to one that is environmentally referenced and therefore far more flexible in its approach. Task goals can be completed using numerous solutions, reflecting the dynamic interaction of variables within the task, the environment, and the person (Davis and Burton 1991). With respect to choice making, the intent is not only to enhance performance, but also to teach choice-making skills. When the student does not possess the skills needed to make choices or to act on the choices made, the structure of ETA fills in the gaps. Facilitation of choice making with ETA is easily supplemented with a prompting continuum that ranges from physical support to environmental enticement (Taylor 2002; Watkinson and Wall 1982). As the learner displays more comfort with choice, the prompts become less supportive until they disappear entirely. Ecological Task Analysis departs from previous intervention strategies that were designed to change the person with a disability (Skrtic 1986) based on the assumption that the person with a disability was deficient and that the focus of instruction should be remediation directed at the individual (Meyer 1991). Ecological Task Analysis brings the teacher and the student into a closer relationship resulting in a closer balance of input and problem solving by both parties.

Practical Tools for Applying ETA

We remain convinced of the importance of choice making as an instructional goal for students with disabilities in physical activity settings. Although we have given some examples of relatively successful attempts to implement choice making, we also acknowledge that lack of experience is still a barrier for both instructor and student. The only way to overcome lack of experience or absence of history in choice making is to start implementing it as an instructional goal. However, a little skepticism may be a healthy perspective from which to further investigate the practical implementation of choice making within the context of ETA for both school and recreational settings.

Skepticism may cause us to wonder if choice making can be taught within the confines of school physical education programs as we know them. Again, part of the answer lies in the desire to value personal decision making as an instructional goal. If the desire is there, then teachers and students will find a way to make it work. We do not have all the answers, but it seems quite obvious that instructors must be equipped with the ability to identify or task analyze environmental and task variables that can influence motor skill performance. The GTA work of Herkowitz (1978b) provides a process and completed templates for many of the fundamental locomotor and object control skills on which our elementary school curricula are based. To this we would add that starting slowly, in a skill domain that is well known to the instructor or perhaps highly motivating to the learner, would help to relieve a lot of the pressure of "getting it right." The assumption is of course that once the methodology starts to work, there will be a concomitant desire to apply it to other skill domains. It might actually become contagious!

We might also wonder if students with physical disabilities perceive, attend to, or actively seek out affordances that are to their advantage in physical activity settings. If we consider the young wheelchair basketball players in South Africa who were challenged with devising ways of getting from A to B on the basketball court, when they had no experience with the skill, the answer is yes, a qualified yes (Groeneveld 1999). When the pairs of players were brought together to demonstrate their solutions, a critique of each solution ensued that eventually led to each player's choosing the method that was best for him. In this way, choice making was valued, affordances were demonstrated, and individuality was respected. Ecological Task Analysis takes time and requires careful observation and continual review.

Clearly students can be encouraged to seek and find strategies that would guide their own learning in physical education settings (Bulger, Townsend, and Carson 2001). Preparing students to take full advantage of affordances that contribute to positive experiences, while minimizing the constraining qualities of those that do not, would appear to be vital to the development of student self-determination. Fortunately, when ETA is working, it is usually fairly obvious to the student which choice has given the best result. But to solidify the development of effective strategic behavior, the instructor needs to follow up with intelligent practice of same-choice solutions. Positive practice is still an effective learning tool.

The complexity of recognizing and utilizing environmental affordance is illustrated by the example of a ramp. A ramp affords ascent or descent to horizontal surfaces that are on different planes for persons who use wheelchairs. Each person will perceive and experience the qualities of the ramp differently; however, successful negotiation of the ramp will occur only if the ramp is strong enough, at a low enough angle, and wide enough for the person using it. A ramp that does not have these characteristics affords the negative consequence of falling. Furthermore, the parameters of a safe and negotiable ramp for one person may be different from those for another. Similarly, other people within the environment are of particular interest, because students with disabilities are often put in the position of needing assistance due to environmental or attitudinal barriers.

Whether this assistance is direct or indirect, the role of the teacher or instructional assistant in the ETA model is essential. It is not only teachers who afford students an opportunity to learn; peers can also play a major role in the movement experiences of students with disabilities (Block, Oberweiser, and Bain 1995; Goodwin 2001; Tripp, French, and Sherrill 1995). If personal decision making is valued, then peers in turn afford enhanced participation by sensitively judging the force and effort needed to exchange a ball successfully in a partner activity. If not, peers can detract from the experience by overhelping and removing choice and opportunity for decision making. Although success is important, it is also necessary to allow students to fail, as these experiences provide the information that leads to better choice making and eventual success. Implementation of a "teaching audit trail" is one way of documenting the role of the teacher in this process (Taylor 2002). Although in some ways it merely fulfills the requirement of "observe and record" as outlined in the ETA model, there is an opportunity to trace the decision making of both student and teacher that is invaluable in the instruction process.

The largest challenge to teachers in the application of ETA may be the generation of alternatives to present to students as they choose among movement forms and environmental alternatives that will enhance performance. If instructors are to favorably alter and encourage their students to take advantage of what the environment offers, they must either intuitively perceive what will be supportive to particular pupils, teach the pupils to make this assessment themselves (Bulger, Townsend, and Carson 2001), or create and systematically test a menu of adaptations that extends the work of Herkowitz to participants with various functional abilities.

In the meantime, from our own experience, we can recommend the following ideas.

Always Include Assessment

It is essential to initiate the implementation of ETA with an assessment process. Sometimes instructors choose to leave out this process because they think it takes too much time and effort. However, assessment is an integral part of instruction in ETA and easily sets the stage for success and effectively minimizes instruction time. There is, however, no prescription for the process itself. That is, the entire process needs to fit the knowledge, skills, resources, and environment in which the instructor or coach abides. In large classes or groups it may work well to choose the task goals by setting the environment up in self-discovery stations. The performers can choose from a hierarchy of relevant task variables and then record their own success rate and their preferred combination of distance, ball, target size, and outcome, for example, in a target-shooting task. Whatever the result, we have a baseline performance from which to work.

Davis and Klingler (2001) offer a quantitative approach to assessment that involves awarding points for the outcome of each trial. In throwing for accuracy and distance, the participant is given four trials in which he or she chooses the skill, object, and movement pattern and is awarded 3 points for a center hit, 2 points for an intermediate circle, 1 point for an outer circle, and 0 for missing the target. If the performer is successful in 75% of the trials using a particular style and set of task variables, then a challenge is introduced via changing the task variables. The results are again recorded using the same scoring system. This method provides a good quantitative baseline to use in evaluating instructional success.

Document Customized Adaptations

A more hands-on approach, which may be necessary for some students who do not engage easily or who need customized adaptations, might involve the instructor's setting up the environment and then verbally offering the student a choice of task goal and movement form. Prompts might be just the equipment, verbal images, actual visuals or physical demonstrations, or physical assists. In this case the instructor records the choice made by the participant, the prompt used, and the success achieved in reaching the goal. This information still provides a baseline for instruction but also provides valuable information on successful and unsuccessful environmental manipulation, prompting, or enticement (Taylor 2002). For example, if the desired task goal in a swimming session is body submersion to promote breath control, task goal choices could be blowing bubbles under water, underwater races with a peer, or underwater treasure hunting. The movement form is up to the student, and the skill is exhaling air under water. In the actual instructional setting in Taylor's study, a student chose racing under water. On his initial attempts while his peer was swimming along the bottom of the pool, the student who had made this choice had his back exposed to the air as he raced along the surface. His peer encouraged him to submerge, then handed him a brick to make sinking easier. On the second try the student sunk to the bottom. He continued playing this "game" and by the end of the class had reached the 75% mark in exhaling under water.

Another adaptation of the ETA assessment model can be seen in an example of coaching young wheelchair basketball enthusiasts in South Africa (Groeneveld 1999). The task goal and rule limitations were provided to the players, and they would then explore ways in which they could achieve the goal. After 5 or 10 minutes, each group would be asked to demonstrate how they thought the skill would best be performed. Then each child would be given individual instruction to maximize the efficiency of his or her chosen movement form. Each individual's demonstrated movement form provided the baseline for skill development and visual guidance for other performers without requiring a movement form that was not yet possible.

Record the Perceptual-Motor Match

Compilation of successful adaptations, or what we see as extensions to the compilation of task and environmental influences on motor skill performance as outlined by Herkowitz's GTA, is also particularly useful when one is trying to provide meaningful choice to participants with disabilities. For instance, if students have functional implications for object manipulation, there are various ways to alter speed besides just physically slowing down the delivery of the moving object, including changing the throwing style, increasing the size of the ball, using balloons, decreasing the weight of the ball, decreasing the air pressure in the ball, rolling the ball, or bouncing the ball (CAHPERD 1994). There are many useful suggestions in a number of the *Moving to Inclusion* manuals. The success of any of these suggestions depends on how they accommodate for the specific abilities of the person—a type of perceptual-motor match. In the absence of systematic evaluation as was done by Burton, Greer, and Weise-Bjornstal (1993) on the impact of ball size on catching and throwing, we encourage instructors to continue testing the utility of these adaptations.

Implications for Research

We have attempted to identify some of the barriers to implementing ETA while at the same time giving some suggestions on how they might be overcome. More documentation is needed, however, "toward translating the ideology concerning an individual's right to choose into a workable technology for evaluating, facilitating, and training choice making skills" (Parsons et al. 1997, p. 125). For although the research suggests that choice making results in favorable outcomes in the areas of classrooms and vocational, recreation, and leisure settings, there is still little guidance as to the most effective and parsimonious way to proceed with choice-making strategies (Kern et al. 1998). Documentation of the implementation of ETA at multiple sites with different disabilities would definitely be a worthwhile step in providing this guidance.

To address instructor entrenchment in the traditional teacher-focused instruction of motor skills, there is a need for more research that documents student success in meeting task goals without passing through the motor skills sequences often found in the curriculum. Measures of student success, number of trials or amount of time needed to meet task goals, degree of instructor input, amount of decision making and choice, and student agency would be documented. The work of Gelinas and Reid (2000) provides an excellent base on which to expand.

The stereotypic belief that students with disabilities cannot decide for themselves, or that the choices they select will be made without due consideration of the consequences, needs to be reframed. There is a need for instructional activities that incorporate increasingly complex and risk-laden opportunities to make choices and enjoy the benefits of the outcomes. For teachers to find choice making a sufficiently useful strategy to teach and employ pedagogically, further explanation as to what is involved and how it can be implemented needs to be communicated by teachers who are using ETA.

The impact of environmental, performer, and task variables on task goal achievement is in need of further investigation. Instructors are often left to use their expert knowledge, or intuition, in determining variables that may positively influence affordance identification and choice alternatives. A systematic review of affordances that are most influential in goal attainment may be warranted. It is even more important that we gain a better understanding of how, within their learning environments, children identify (or fail to identify) variables that are open to manipulation to their benefit.

INSTRUCTIONAL STRATEGIES

- To maximize the effectiveness of ETA, be selective about the setting where it is implemented rather than resorting to making the choice for the participant. As both participants and instructors become familiar with the system it can be implemented in other, less predictable environments.

- Alternatives for choice may need to be offered along a continuum as the person's skills and interests expand. That is, you don't have to open up the whole curriculum to choice. Allow everyone time to get comfortable with the idea.

- Asking a student to "figure it out" may be insufficient even in the face of numerous alternatives for participation, but giving a student enough time to explore the options or the consequences of various choices within a supportive environment may create the right atmosphere. Be patient.

- A lack of expressed preference for presented alternatives can be interpreted *and should be accepted* as an active choice.

- Providing opportunity for choice within a physical education setting is desirable and challenging, but not impossible.

Summary

Providing decision-making opportunities for learners with disabilities in physical activity environments is the joy and the challenge of applying the Ecological Task Analysis model. Two obvious obstacles to successful application of this model are: teacher-centered as opposed to choice-driven or student-centered models of instruction and lack of teacher knowledge in manipulating task and environmental dimensions in a way that promotes both choice making and consequent skill development. As self-determination is a central goal of the education of students with disabilities, and exercising choice is fundamental to self-determination, implementing ETA can enhance the quality of life of people with disabilities.

Although there is ample evidence that people with disabilities can make choices, instructors may find it necessary to teach choice making. Setting up the environment and offering the choice may not be enough to facilitate the process. Instructors may find that it is helpful to place choice making on a continuum with decreasing levels of support. Start by implementing choice in an area of the curriculum that is well known to the instructor and highly motivating to the learner; respect the initial refusal of the learner to choose, as a conscious choice; and give the student time to process the consequences of each choice. We encourage full implementation of the model. Always begin with an assessment process, keep a record of successful adaptations particularly for students with functional constraints, and continue to test the utility of task and environmental manipulations on skill attainment. Conducting research as to the most effective way to proceed with choice-making strategies with different disabilities is recommended.

Using Ecological Task Analysis in Physiotherapy

Gerald Mullally, MSc, and Mary Mullally, DipPhysio

The learning of motor skills is particularly salient for young children. This is evident in the motor milestones (such as reaching, crawling, cruising, and walking), the fundamental movement skills (such as jumping, throwing, catching, and kicking), and the fine motor skills (such as buttoning trousers or tying a lace) that children learn and that skilled adults take for granted each day. Motor skills are particularly salient because their impact is multidimensional, affecting cognitive and social as well as subsequent motor skill development (Ulrich et al. 2001). For instance, Butler (1986, 1991) observed that when preschool-aged children with mobility problems learned to use powered wheelchairs, there was an immediate increase in their language, play, and exploration. Most interesting was the occurrence of the "movement domino effect," whereby the rewarding experience of being able to control their movement in one context inspired these children to engage in self-propelled locomotion when not in the wheelchair. The field of motor learning since its inception has sought to understand and facilitate the control of movement and the learning of movement skills in both children and adults. However, the principles uncovered within this field have had little impact on clinical applications in the field of pediatric physiotherapy. This is in spite of the fact that learning is central for rehabilitation. On the positive side, more functional approaches are emerging from the motor learning and control literature. In particular, the Ecological Task Analysis approach (Davis and Burton 1991) holds great promise for physiotherapists as described in this chapter. The four principles of ETA are described and illustrated using case studies from physiotherapy practice.

Special thanks to Professor Nancy McNevin for her valuable contributions to our thinking and helpful comments on an earlier version of this manuscript. Thanks also to Aoife O' Connor for proofreading the final version of this manuscript.

Across the Motor Learning– Physiotherapy Divide

The failure to apply motor learning concepts and principles to pediatric therapy cannot rest just with therapists. The use of simple laboratory-type tasks by motor learning researchers, tasks that lack the complexity of skills used in real-world situations, has certainly contributed to this failure. According to McNevin, Wulf, and Carlson (2000), these simple laboratory tasks have "little in common with types of functional skills patients learn as part of their rehabilitation" (p. 374). This situation is beginning to change, however. In recent years researchers have begun to examine complex skills, and although there is still a lack of clinical research from a motor learning perspective, much can be learned from this complex skill research.

The second reason for this failure lies on the other side of the motor learning–physiotherapy divide. The field of physiotherapy has been dominated in recent times by neurofacilitation approaches developed during the 1950s and early 1960s. Neurofacilitation approaches include the Bobath approach (Bobath and Bobath 1965), sensory integration therapy (Ayres 1972), proprioceptive neuromuscular facilitation (Voss, Ionata, and Meyers 1985), the Rood approach developed by Margaret Rood (Stockmeyer 1967), and the Brunnstrom approach (Brunnstrom 1966). Developed in response to clinicians' dissatisfaction with muscle reeducation approaches (Gordon 1987; Horak 1992), the neurofacilitation approaches were based on reflex and hierarchical theories of motor control (Shumway-Cook and Woollacott 2001). Two key assumptions of neurofacilitation approaches as outlined by Shumway-Cook and Woollacott (2001) go a long way toward explaining why motor learning principles have not influenced clinical applications. Assumption 1 is that functional skills will automatically return once abnormal movement patterns are inhibited and normal movement patterns facilitated; assumption 2 is that repetition of these normal movement patterns will automatically transfer to functional tasks (Shumway-Cook and Woollacott 2001). Consequently, motor learning principles that can aid in the achievement of functional tasks are not required, as functional tasks will be accomplished if normal movement patterns are facilitated and then repeated.

According to recent motor control theories (Kelso et al. 1980; Kugler, Kelso, and Turvey 1980; Schöner and Kelso 1988a), however, it is not correct to assume that functional skills will automatically return once normal movement patterns are facilitated and then repeated. According to the dynamic systems approach to motor control, movement emerges from a confluence of constraints (Newell 1986). A constraint is simultaneously an enablement and a limitation on movement (Kugler and Turvey 1987). Constraints arise from three sources and thus are of three kinds: individual, environmental, and task. A motor cortex lesion, for instance, acts as an individual constraint, and the movements observed may be adaptive solutions to a particular task and environmental context. This means that what is observed is not the result of just the lesion itself but also of the efforts of the remaining systems to compensate for the loss and still be functional. However, the compensatory strategies developed by the child may not always be optimal. Thus, a goal of intervention according to Shumway-Cook and Woollacott (2001) is "to improve the efficiency of compensatory strategies" (p. 25). However, a practical example indicates that this goal is not tenable in all cases. A child with a right hemiplegia will decrease weight bearing on the affected side; thus, to accomplish the goal of standing from floor sitting, the child will invariably weight bear on the unaffected side. Obviously the goal of treatment is not just to improve the efficiency of this strategy but rather to aid in the emergence of a coordination pattern that utilizes the affected side and accomplishes the task of standing from floor sitting. In essence the goal of pediatric physiotherapy is to improve the efficiency of compensatory strategies *and* to aid in the emergence of coordination patterns that enable the child to engage in more adaptable solutions to a given task in a given context and across a variety of tasks in many different contexts.

Therapeutic intervention, as Badke and DiFabio (1990) argue, should focus on limb movement patterns "as they fit into a full functional pattern because individual muscle action may be insignificant to the biomechanics involved in a total integrated motor response" (p. 78). This approach, termed the systems approach (Woollacott and Shumway-Cook 1990) or a motor control or motor learning approach (Carr and Shepherd 1987) to therapeutic intervention (see Perry 1998; Corcos 1991), is beginning to be incorporated into the traditional neurofacilitation approaches as motor control and motor learning chapters appear in neurofacilitation texts (see Roley, Blanche, and Schaaf 2001). A discernable blurring of boundaries is occurring as each approach integrates dynamic systems principles into its theoretical base and moves toward a functional task-oriented approach to therapy (Shumway-Cook and Woollacott 2001).

Ecological Task Analysis Applied to Physiotherapy

Although a task-oriented approach to pediatric physiotherapy has been implicated by neurofacilitation theorists, a coherent framework that incorporates recent theories of motor control and motor learning has not been provided. Ecological Task Analysis, originally presented by Davis and Burton (1991) and expanded in numerous papers by Davis and colleagues (Balan and Davis 1993; Burton and Davis 1992, 1996; Davis and Van Emmerik 1995a, 1995b), may provide such a framework. The four tenets of ETA (Davis and Burton 1991) are these:

1. Establishing task goals by structuring the physical and social environment
2. Allowing choices of movement solutions
3. Manipulating performer, environmental, or task variables
4. Providing instruction

Structuring the Physical and Social Environment

The first step of ETA elucidates its child-centered approach to therapy. Establishing task goals by structuring the physical and social environment is one of the features distinguishing ETA from traditional approaches in all therapeutic disciplines. In these traditional therapist-centered models, the therapist plays the gatekeeping role in which he or she controls, circumscribes, and legitimizes the task goal (e.g., applied behavioral analysis [ABA]) (Lovaas 1987, 1993). In contrast, ETA positions the therapist inside the learning system as a learning facilitator and moves toward a participatory-based model in which the child in collaboration with the therapist is involved in the problem-solving process. The role of the physiotherapist in pediatrics is to structure the physical and social environment to invite meaningful activity. This can easily be accomplished through play situations that facilitate the intrinsic motivation of the child. Such structured play situations facilitate the emergence and evolution of the task goal(s). These intrinsically motivating play situations add meaning and enhance commitment to the task goal.

An inherent weakness of strict behavioral approaches to learning and skill acquisition is the separation of the task goal from its meaningful context. Such polarization inevitably leads to the production of an impoverished task goal (an inert task goal)—a task goal that the child can realize when explicitly requested to do so, but not something that can be readily applied to relevant real-world situations. In general, there appears to be a relationship between the practices involved in an intervention approach and the type of gains that one observes. It is perhaps to be expected that a child will develop the skills or capacities that are practiced. As Stanley Greenspan, an internationally renowned clinical professor of Psychiatry and Pediatrics at George Washington University Medical School, states:

> . . . more structured approaches have tended to be associated with being able to perform under structured conditions, while relationship-based, developmental models have tended to be associated with more spontaneous social interactions and meaningful language and communication. (Greenspan, unpublished paper, p. 3)

CASE STUDY 1:
Fireman Sam and the Elderly Woman

We recently created a play situation in which a child with difficulties planning and organizing fine motor sequences, together with body control issues, was facilitated in his learning of the task of buttoning. The importance of the buttoning skill cannot be overestimated in relation to self-dressing and self-toileting, particularly in a school context. The child was 5 years of age and two months from commencing his first year of formal schooling. We created a play situation whereby the child chose to dress up and play the role of his favorite cartoon character, Fireman Sam. The therapist played the role of a distressed elderly woman who couldn't get out of her jacket and needed to go to bed. Fireman Sam saved the day numerous times, using his own movement solutions to varying task difficulties. The task constraints were varied (i.e., button size, buttonhole size, shirt, trousers, levels of stress such as in an emergency and a nonemergency), and the conditions were established in which Sam could always, sometimes, and never accomplish the task of buttoning garments that he wore and garments that the elderly woman wore. The whole process was videoed to analyze the coordination tendencies under varying task and environmental constraints. Particular difficulties in relation to the task included the following:

- Poor positioning of the button in relation to the buttonhole
- Frequent use of only one hand during attempts at the task
- Application of force to pull the buttonhole over the button at a suboptimal position high over the buttonhole

By the following visit, an evil frog puppet had put a spell on the elderly woman and she had to relearn buttoning, a task she had learned as a young girl. A creative instructional technique was created whereby a sticker depicting Fireman Sam's head was placed on every button of Fireman Sam's jacket. A red sticker cut to resemble a small jumper was placed around the buttonhole (i.e., the buttonhole represented the hole for the head). Within a collaborative learning environment, the elderly woman and the child learned to button together. The elderly woman, like a good nanny, gently nudged the child forward at critical points, creating and sustaining an environment in which the child's curiosities about his own movement solutions flourished. By the end of the session, Fireman Sam, with help from the elderly woman, had created the following instructions:

1. Turn Sam's head to face the ground so he won't hurt his head when he puts on his jumper
2. Hold Sam's head and pull the jumper over Sam's head

It is important to understand that what is being proffered here is not the instructional solution but rather the process by which the task goal of buttoning was made meaningful for the child as the child identified with the buttoning task through his favorite cartoon character. As we shall see in the following section, one can encourage this identification with the task goal by allowing the child to choose his or her own solutions to the movement problem, that is, implementing the second step of ETA.

Allowing Choices of Movement Solutions

The goal of pediatric physiotherapy, as we have defined it, involves facilitation of the emergence of coordination patterns that allow the child more adaptable solutions to a given task and across a variety of tasks in many different situations. In accordance with Davis and Strand (this volume), we emphasize the fact that the more movement skills one possesses, the more choices one has. Thus the goal of therapy is to facilitate the child's ability to make choices. There are two main reasons for allowing children choices with regard to their movement solutions.

Firstly, encouraging children to choose their own movement solutions may provide the therapist with important clues about the child's "preferred behavioral mode," that is, interests, attributes, or characteristics that may constrain the child's movement options (Burton and Davis 1996). Establishing the child's preferred behavioral mode, "intrinsic dynamics" (Zanone and Kelso 1992, p. 565), or "unique developmental profile" (Greenspan and Wieder 1998, p. 22), under given task and environmental conditions that are not overly constrained by the therapist, will likely provide the therapist with important insights about the anatomical, physiological, psychological, and social constraints on the child's behavior that may then be used in designing therapy (Burton and Davis 1996). In traditional therapeutic approaches, specified movement patterns of the child are contrasted with age-related developmental norms, the foundation of the majority of neurofacilitation approaches. The idea that by a particular age an infant or toddler "should" have achieved a particular motor milestone has not only become a standard developmental diagnosis, but has also become completely entrenched in our cultural beliefs about child raising (Thelen 2000). Perhaps it is important to remember that many of these descriptive data sets were collected more than 60 years ago when the experimental work was driven in many instances by prescriptive theorizing of a genetically motivated maturational perspective (e.g., Gesell 1933; McGraw 1943; Shirley 1931), elevating the "typical child," who of course was no child, into a biological reality (Thelen and Adolph 1992).

However, many of these ideas of developmental timetables can now be recast in different terms. Instead of a phylogenetically determined sequence of stages, development is better conceptualized as a changing landscape of patterns whose stability depends not only on the organic status of the child but also on his or her experiential history and how these interact with the particular task at hand (Thelen 2000). Thus, a proviso can be added to the "normal" developmental sequence, namely that alternate or nonnormative forms may offer optimal solutions for some children under certain task and environmental conditions.

The second reason for allowing choices with regard to children's therapy sessions relates to the well-established fact that increasing one's perception of self-control enhances learning and motivation (Bandura 1993; Chen and Singer 1992; McCombs 1989). The positive effect of perceived self-control on learning has also been demonstrated for those with disabilities (Berk 1976; Lovitt and Curtis 1969). For instance, Berk (1976) found that persons with disabilities were more self-confident and self-directed when given choices. Children, particularly those deemed incapable of making good decisions for and by themselves, are at particular risk of having their choices limited by others. Simple strategies for enhancing the child's perception of self-control over therapy situations may include facilitating choice with respect to therapy equipment, that is the use of objects representing therapy equipment, photographs and PECS (Picture Exchange Communication System) pictures of therapy equipment; sending videos of fun segments from the therapy session; writing and addressing some therapy recommendation letters to the child rather than to the parent; and talking on the phone to the child about his or her likes and dislikes in relation to different tasks, different toys, and therapy activities.

In the motor learning literature, self-control has been found to be beneficial in three areas: in the provision of feedback (when and how much feedback is provided), when or how often an assistive device is introduced, and in the scheduling of the practiced tasks themselves (McNevin, Wulf, and Carlson 2000). Studies by Janelle and colleagues (Janelle et al. 1997; Janelle, Kim, and Singer 1995) have shown that participants who self-select their feedback schedule outperform matched participants who have no control over the provision of feedback, as indicated by retention performance in throwing tasks. Wulf and Toole (1999) found that the effectiveness of learning was enhanced when individuals were given the choice of when they wanted to use an assistive device relative to those who had no control over the use of an assistive device. Interestingly, the self-control and yoked (no control) group demonstrated very similar performances during practice; it was only in the retention test that the effectiveness of self-control was clearly seen. Titzer, Shea, and Romack (1993) found that learners who could self-select the order in which they practiced different versions of a barrier knockdown task performed better than the blocked and random practice groups as demonstrated by each group's ability to repeat their performance after some interval of time had elapsed and without the benefit of feedback.

Allowing the child choice in the therapy session may also facilitate the child's intrinsic motivation. Intrinsically motivated behaviors are performed out of interest and require no "separable" consequence, no external prod, promise, or threat (Deci 1975). When intrinsically motivated, a child is motivated simply to perform the activity—or perhaps, to perform it well—and to have the spontaneous experiences of interest, enjoyment, excitement, and satisfaction that accompany the behavior. Csikszentmihalyi (1975) used the term *autotelic* to describe such behaviors for which the purpose of the activity is, in a sense, the activity itself. In contrast to intrinsic motivation, being extrinsically motivated involves performing an activity with the intention of attaining some separable consequence such as receiving a reward, avoiding guilt, or gaining approval. Behaviors that are extrinsically motivated would generally not occur spontaneously, so their occurrence must typically be prompted by some type of instrumentality. It is clearly evident that behavioral approaches facilitate extrinsically rather then intrinsically motivated behavior, with behavior controlled by demands or contingencies external to the child.

Although behavioral approaches such as the prominent ABA approach to disorders like autism have been found to work relatively well (Lovaas

1987, 1993; McEachin, Smith, and Lovaas 1993), serious methodological problems have been noted in regard to these studies (see Gresham and MacMillan 1998; Gresham, Beebe, and MacMillan 1999). And in a recent and unbiased investigation of this approach, Smith, Groen, and Wynn (2000) reported results showing only modest educational gains and little to no emotional or social gains. In spite of this, the ABA approach remains excessively popular. In light of our discussion about the importance of choice for the child and the importance of facilitating intrinsic motivation, serious concerns can also be raised with respect to the ABA approach itself. Inherently, the ABA approach or any strict behavioral approach to therapy or education is the antinomy of choice, in which the use of rewards and punishments amounts to a manipulation for compliance. As Kohn (1993, p. 27) states, "the point to be emphasized is that all rewards, by virtue of being rewards, are not attempts to influence or persuade or solve problems together, but simply to control." Davis and Strand (this volume), in a beautifully written account of the importance of choice, state:

> Rewards may be successful at changing our actions, but they also may change our reasons for the actions and our attitude toward those actions and ourselves. The question then is not whether rewards are effective in changing actions, but what changes and why. (p. 73)

Rewards and punishments are attractive for those working with children with autistic disorder. In many respects their use is much easier than good teaching and management practices of a poorly understood disorder. Anything that makes the task easier, regardless of the consequences, is tempting (Davis and Strand, this volume). In contrast, we recommend a child-centered, choice-centered model such as the ETA approach, Sensory Integration (see Bundy, Lane, and Murray 2002), or Greenspan's Developmental, Individual-Difference, Relationship (DIR) model (see Greenspan and Wieder 1998), whereby the focus shifts from changing surface behaviors and symptoms to the underlying individual differences or the missing basic foundations of relating and thinking.

CASE STUDY 2:
Self-Control in a Therapy Session

A 7 1/2-year-old child with Asberger's syndrome and severe motor planning problems, of which he was highly aware, provides a good example of the application of self-control in a therapy setting. During initial sessions, the boy was avoidant of any of the sensory integration play equipment offered to him. His choices of play situations were frequently erratic and disorganized; for example, he wished to sit on a peanut roll while swinging on a platform swing! When the therapist tried to enter his game and encourage adaptive responses, he became overly aroused and survival behaviors emerged, such as flight and fight. Because he was acutely aware of his motor planning problems, he attempted to exert control on the play session and frequently became avoidant and deregulated. Although the child had explicit control over the content of the play session, that is, what play equipment, if any, was used, he still frequently became overwhelmed and deregulated. The solution to this problem emerged when the child was given control over the organization of the play session (i.e., the order in which the play equipment was used) rather than the content of the play session. His developmental profile indicated particularly high reading and an acceptable level of written ability. Thus, at the beginning of each therapy session, the child in collaboration with the therapist wrote and structured the entire session. Each task was carefully and thoughtfully laid out to regulate his arousal and provide the "just-right challenge." As he had explicit control over what came next, his arousal level dropped and he then became willing to engage with the therapist and adapt to changing demands during movement activities. Through the facilitation of choice, regulation with adaptive responses was facilitated.

Although it seems evident that allowing children choices and self-control in learning increases their feeling of responsibility for and their involvement in the learning process, it is important to point out (and this will already be easily apparent to those working in the field of special needs) that the motor learning principles advocated earlier (i.e., when and how much feedback is provided, when and how often an assistive device is introduced into the practice session, and the organization of practice) are case dependent. In other words, these principles will have little relevance to cases in which the child has severe compromises in the basic foundations of relating, communicating, and thinking, as in the child with autistic spectrum disorder and in the lower range of intellectual functioning. However, this certainly does not imply that choice should be limited to higher-functioning children. As previously stated, a potentially damaging aspect of behavioral approaches is the distinct lack of choice provided to the child. As the next case study illustrates, choice can be provided to any child regardless of his or her range of intellectual functioning.

CASE STUDY 3:

Choice at Any Level of Functioning

Children with autistic spectrum disorder typically have challenges at two levels. At one level, as already indicated, they have compromises in the basic foundations of relating, communicating, and thinking, such as a difficulty with exchanging emotional and social signals as part of a relationship. At a second level, they frequently evidence symptoms such as repetitive behavior, self-stimulation, and self-absorption. A 4 1/2-year-old child with autistic spectrum disorder at the lower range of intellectual functioning presented with many of these symptoms. His play involved throwing objects, particularly throwing balls to the ground in an excessive, repetitive manner. Speech therapy reports indicated severe problems with expressive and receptive language. His parents' key concern was his lack of interaction and engagement and the frustrating repetitive ball-throwing activity. The goal of therapy in this case was to regulate this child and to have him engage while in play activity.

From assessment, the therapy environment was structured to invite floor play. The boy initiated play by throwing a ball repetitively to the ground. Importantly, this play activity, instead of being something to modify, was used to regulate, engage, relate, and problem solve in many sequences of interaction in ways that the boy perceived as fun. For instance, a frog puppet would collect the ball so that the child could continue his play activity. The frog created novelty and surprise by sometimes throwing the ball into a crawling tunnel or a roly barrel. Rather than continuing with his repetitive behavior, the child began to problem solve by searching for the ball, which involved heavy body-regulatory intake and handing the ball back to the frog in many sequences of interaction.

The frog then handed the ball to the child's father. The father took the frog puppet and continued the play with his son. The task evolved into rough-and-tumble floor play when the frog went under a soft mattress with the ball. The child went under the mattress to retrieve the ball, thus facilitating deep touch pressure and working his muscles and joints against resistance. He began to throw the balls to the floor from the roly barrel. His father, coached by the therapist, placed a cardboard box at a strategic point to catch the ball. The child, intrigued by this, collected all the balls and began to throw them into the cardboard box. When the child bent down to pick up a ball in the roly barrel, the child's father would move himself and the cardboard box to introduce novelty and surprise. This play sequence eventually led to father and son engaging and relating in throwing and catching activities. Thus the right sensory motor pattern was found to pull the child in and engage him. The frustrating repetitive behavior that his parents perceived as worthless was transformed into a warm and loving interaction. The beginnings of two-way communication were initiated by following the child's lead (i.e., by allowing the child choice and self-control).

Manipulating Performer, Environmental, and Task Variables

We believe that the theory and research surrounding and underpinning the step of manipulating variables have the potential to transform the way therapists conceptualize and conduct their clinical work. Although a small portion of the dynamic systems approach to motor control was sketched in the first section of this chapter, further elaboration is required. As previously stated, movement arises due to a confluence of constraints: individual constraints, both physical (e.g., muscular, skeletal, endocrine) and psychological (e.g., memory, attention); environmental constraints such as gravity, ambient light, support surface, and the sociocultural milieu; and finally task constraints such as object speed, size, weight, task duration, target size, and distance. As Thelen and Smith (1994, 1998) indicate, the key feature of dynamic systems is that the many heterogeneous parts of the system are free to combine in a virtually infinite number of ways. Theoretically at least, there is no limit to the actual number of combinations that might occur, yet movement is a coherent, coordinated event. The resolution to this problem offered by Russian physiologist Nikolai A. Bernstein led to a revolution in the way movement was conceptualized (Bernstein 1967). Bernstein's seminal insight was that the individual variables are organized into larger groupings called linkages or synergies. During a movement, the internal degrees of freedom are not controlled directly but are constrained to relate among themselves in a relatively fixed and autonomous fashion. The second, absolutely crucial aspect of the synergy concept is that it was hypothesized to be function or task specific. Indeed, Bernstein showed that movement was function specific and not muscle specific. His classic example was that a person can write his or her name using a pen on paper or using a broomstick on a blackboard, but the signature remains the same (Bernstein 1967).

Drawing on this concept of synergy and in complete opposition to the then-popular information-processing ideas of the early to mid-1970s (e.g., Keele 1973; Marteniuk 1976; Schmidt 1975), Kugler and colleagues introduced the concept of coordinative structures, which they defined as "a group of muscles often spanning a number of joints that is constrained to act as a single functional unit" (Kugler et al. 1980, p. 17). It was suggested that *self-organization* (Prigogine and Stengers 1984) was the mechanism or principle underlying the formation of coordinative structures (Kugler et al. 1980; Kelso and Schöner 1988). Self-organization denotes a conceptual framework for looking at the *spontaneous emergence of order* in physical, chemical, and biological systems. Here was a brilliant solution to Bernstein's degrees of freedom problem. Rather than the degrees of freedom being a curse, a computational load to be overcome, they became the very source of organization and, indeed, of change. Self-organizing systems have several properties (Clark 1997) that have consequences for therapists:

1. Self-organizing systems exhibit multiple stable states.
2. These states change when a constraint or subsystem (referred to as a *control parameter* in this instance) is scaled to some critical level.
3. As the control parameter is being scaled, the system passes through a region of instability. At that time, the system is particularly sensitive to perturbations or changes in constraints.

To understand the crucial control parameter concept, we wish you, the reader, to try the following—a replication of what has become known affectionately as the "finger twiddling" experiments. Hold your two hands up in front of you and begin to flex and extend the index fingers of both hands simultaneously or "in-phase" (similar muscles in each hand contracting simultaneously). Increase the pace or frequency of the motion and you will see that you are able to maintain a stable pattern for quite high frequencies. Now begin the sequence again, but this time flex and extend your index fingers "out of phase"—that is, flex one while extending the other. Now gently but continually increase the frequency of the motion and see what happens. What is remarkable about this paradigm is that when subjects begin their movements in an anti-phase pattern, they spontaneously switch to an in-phase mode at particular, individually reproducible pacing frequencies. The two patterns are stable at low frequencies, but the neuromotor system produces only one stable "attractor" at higher movement frequencies (Kelso 1995).

Experimentally Kelso (1984) used a metronome to increase the frequency and then plotted the phase relationship between the two fingers.

As you may have seen for yourself, this variable is constant for a wide range of oscillation frequencies but is subject to a dramatic shift at a critical value—the moment of the anti-phase to in-phase shift. Plotting the unfolding of the relative phase variable is plotting the values of a collective variable, since relative phase is determined by a relation between the behaviors of more basic system components (finger motions). The collective variable captures the intrinsic order of the system; it is the integrative variable that emerges within an open system to reduce its dispersion and increase its organization, or pattern. The emergence of such collective variables not only reduces the theoretically infinite number of combinations within a dynamic (open) system to some much smaller actual subset (two in this case, in-phase and anti-phase); but, as this occurs, the integration reflected by the collective variable provides continuity and stability within the system. In terms of dynamic systems, stability is defined as the persistence of behavioral or neural states in the face of systematic or random perturbations. All observable behavioral or neural states possess stability to some extent, as loss of stability leads to a change of state (Kelso and Schöner 1988). In dynamic terminology, this behavioral or neural mode is an attractor state, as the system—under certain conditions—has an affinity for that state; that is, the system prefers a certain topology in its state space. In the simplest case, the physics of the body itself can provide stability; that is, the elastic and viscous properties of the muscles can keep joints stable against perturbing forces. Often, however, the nervous system generates stability by, for instance, constantly monitoring and updating movements using sensory feedback.

A change of a system that leads a particular state to become unstable is referred to as an instability. Returning to the finger experiment, what caused the phase shift from one stable state (anti-phase) to another stable state (in-phase)? In other words, what caused the system to go through an instability? It was of course the pace or frequency of the motion, known in dynamic systems terms as a *control parameter*. More formally, the control parameter is the parameter that induces a phase transition from one stable state of the system to another. This phenomenon is called a bifurcation or nonequilibrium phase transition. For instance, using locomotion as an example, quadrupeds perform different gaits depending on the velocities of their movements; that is, velocity is the control parameter that causes a transition from one stable state to another. The gaits performed are those that are the most energy efficient for the particular speed. For patterns to change, the system must lose stability: Internal or external elements must disrupt the coherence so that the components can reorganize into a new and more stable state.

For example, a person can walk up hills of various inclines, but when the steepness of the hill reaches some critical value, the person must shift his or her locomotion to some type of quadrupedal gait—climbing on all fours. The slope change acts as a control parameter on the gait style. The control parameter does not really "control" the system in traditional terms. Rather, it is a parameter that the collective behavior of the system is sensitive to and that moves the system through collective states.

A wide range of variables could in principle act as control parameters in the reorganization of the system's state space. For instance, Thelen and Ulrich (1991) noted that the "disappearance" of the newborn stepping response (i.e., stepping movements made by the newborn when he or she is held upright), which occurs after a few months of life, occurs in relation to the dramatic increase in leg weight, primarily from fat, during the first two months of life. With the great increase in leg weight without a corresponding increase in muscle strength, the stepping reflex disappears, not because of neuronal suppression of the reflex as supposed by nativist theories, but because the infant has insufficient strength to lift the now-heavier legs. It is also important to note that the control parameter, that is, body fat deposition, is a growth change that is not specific to leg movements, yet it affects the system such that a qualitative shift in behavior results.

These data demonstrate that relevant control parameters and the resultant instabilities are central to behavioral switches from one pattern to another. Instabilities also occur when a new pattern is learned. For instance, Zanone and Kelso (1992) studied the learning of 90° of relative phase in "finger twiddling." Many participants in this study had difficulty learning the new pattern because of the persistent influence of intrinsic coordination tendencies of the in-phase (0° relative phase) and anti-phase (180° relative phase) pattern. However, the bias toward the in-phase and anti-phase pattern diminishes as learning proceeds; that is, a new attractor is established close to the requirement. This is an effect indicating that the different contributions to the pattern dynamics change in weight, with the learned pattern progressively overwhelming the intrinsic coordination tendencies.

Thus, the entire attractor layout changes with learning, not simply the coordination pattern being learned; that is, learning has stabilized the new pattern, but also destabilized previously stable states. In summary, skill acquisition involves matching one's own intrinsic dynamics or preferred coordination tendencies to the dynamics of the task. If the intrinsic dynamic is matched with the task dynamic, the pattern will be stable. As indicated earlier, instability will arise if there is not a match, but may then result in a new stable pattern of movement that matches the task dynamic. Such instabilities can be brought about not only by continuous change of relevant control parameters and by learning (Schöner and Kelso 1988a; Schöner, Zanone, and Kelso 1992) but also by perceptual information (Schöner and Kelso 1988c) and by an intention to change pattern (Schöner and Kelso 1988b; Kelso 1995).

The identification and manipulation of control parameters may provide the therapist with important information regarding at least four aspects of movement performance, according to Burton and Davis (1996):

1. The critical value marking a transition to a new movement form
2. The range of values within which the movement forms are stable or unstable
3. The optimal value at which the movement outcome is achieved most effectively and efficiently
4. Boundary conditions in which the task goal is not achievable and new patterns do not yet emerge

How do you find the relevant control parameter? Control parameters can be hypothesized based on (1) theory and research in the field of movement science and (2) past experience. These control parameters can then be manipulated and subsequently verified or rejected (Burton and Davis 1996). Control parameters include such things as object speed, object size and weight, and task duration criteria. Changing the energy requirements of the task, as in changing the speed or force requirements (i.e., increase or decrease movement speed, project objects to greater or lesser distances), can also result in a change in the movement pattern if a critical value is reached. For instance, Wagenaar and Van Emmerik in two separate studies have found that scaling walking speed can have positive effects on disordered gait patterns (Wagenaar and Van Emmerik 1994) and can influence rigidity and pathological tremor in patients with Parkinson's disease (Wagenaar and Van Emmerik 1996).

Burton and Davis (1996) suggest that a transition from a down-ward to an upward backswing in a child's throwing motion may occur when the ball diameter/hand width ratio exceeds 1.0. This is known as a performer-scaled value or dimensionless intrinsic measure. Environmental and actor properties are measured in the same units and thus allow the computation of a dimensionless number or ratio (Davis and Van Emmerik 1995b). The use of intrinsic measures has distinct advantages over the dominant extrinsic measures in clinical settings. Performer-scaled measures can establish direct links between task goals and the constraints of the performer and the environment (see Burton and Davis 1996 for an extensive discussion on this theme). The use of performer-scaled measures is in stark contrast to the pervasive use of assessment tools that are constant or invariant, for example the standard Halversonian 1 inch (2.5 centimeter) cube or the standard 2.25 inch (5.7 centimeter) diameter tennis ball. As Newell, McDonald, and Baillargeon (1993) suggest, the normative sequence of movement forms may be due more to these externally imposed or extrinsic constraints, which affect each individual differently, than to the actual limitations of the individual performers.

Corbetta and Vereijken (1999) suggest that whole-body coordination and force production can be modified and implemented if one loads the system with new perturbing forces to deal with, for example, by giving a heavier object to throw or by adding weights to the ankles of a jumper. These movement perturbations during the process of skill learning have the potential to break the initial coordination tendencies of the system, destabilize preferred patterns of coordination, and affect coordination by forcing the system to adopt a new and more efficient way of functioning. Corbetta and Vereijken describe the following thought experiment: Imagine a young child trying to produce an overarm throw with a slightly heavier object. This will raise the center of gravity. This situation can be compared to an inverse pendulum, which is by definition generating instability in the system (Kugler and Turvey 1987). When this instability is introduced into the system, the system is forced to develop a new solution to reach stability again, most likely by strengthening the base of support of the whole system. Eventually, the child will adopt a new posture with a wider stance by using his or her legs in conjunction with the throwing motion. This is a significant step forward in the process of gaining whole-body coordination. In addition, by throwing heavier objects, children have to build more strength in conjunction with adopting new forms of behavior, which ultimately should help improve force production with performance timing. If the weight of the ball is then progressively decreased, it is likely that the child will hold on to the new movement form. The reason is that abrupt changes in movement form (at a critical point) is dependent on the direction of the scaling of the control parameters, a phenomenon known as hysteresis (Kelso 1984).

Loading the limbs with appropriate weights in jumping and hopping will similarly modify the position of the center of mass and force children to enhance the use of their arms to propel their body forward or upward. Weighting is not the only strategy provided by Corbetta and Vereijken (1999) to enhance whole-body coordination. Exercises in a pool, where gravitational forces act differently on the body, or placing a blindfold on some children (case dependent) to encourage them to pay more attention to their body rather than external visual cues, may also be effective ways to break habitual (and possibly pathological) patterns and promote development and learning. Encouraging the system to explore variations of a movement pattern will destabilize the preferred or pathological modes of functioning and promote the emergence of new and adapted forms of behavior. Manipulating performer, task, and environmental variables may have a distinct advantage over didactic teaching methods for children with language or cognitive difficulties, as there is no heavy emphasis on specific cognitive processes. In addition, some children may have difficulties with traditional observational learning techniques, since observational learning requires children to be able to translate observed information to their own body parts. As Corbetta and Vereijken (1999) suggest, reproduction tasks may pose significant problems for young children due to their egocentric view (Piaget 1952), difficulty perceiving and assuming another person's perspective (Selman 1980), and the fact that young children do not have a good perception of their own body or fully developed spatial and temporal awareness (Gallahue and Ozmun 2002). This may be especially true of severely learning-disabled children; thus the third step of ETA may provide a wonderful means of evoking change without a reliance on higher cognitive functioning and reasoning.

Currently, in many instances it is not feasible to implement the manipulation of relevant control parameters because the therapy equipment that is sold is of a generic nature. For instance, balls of the same size but different weights, balls of the same weight but different sizes, or a required combination of both weight and size are not sold by equipment manufacturers. However, as knowledge of the importance and effectiveness of the manipulation of relevant control parameters diffuses throughout the therapy community, demand for such products will increase, and supply will no doubt follow suit.

CASE STUDY 4:
Scaling the Control Parameter

Scholz (1990) suggests that the degree of weight shift to the weight-bearing hip and its degree of extension may be important control parameters in facilitating the emergence of a reciprocal pattern in children with cerebral palsy who normally display a quadrupedal pattern of interlimb coordination in which limbs at the same girdle (pelvis and shoulder) move in-phase and limbs at different girdles move out of phase (i.e., a bunny-hop pattern). We recently applied this hypothesis in a clinical setting as a 3-year-old child with cerebral palsy wore yellow knee pads with two small teddies tucked halfway into each knee pad, encouraging an external focus of attention (discussed later). At first, strips of tape were placed on the ground in front of each knee, which the child could not touch. In our game the strips of tape represented the magic gate into dinosaur land, through which the child had to safely negotiate the Barney dinosaurs. Only one Barney could go at a time or the gate would not open and Barney would not meet his friends Baby Bop and BJ. This simple game facilitated weight bearing and extension of the hip as the child successfully negotiated the Barneys through dinosaur land. In subsequent games the Barneys negotiated slightly harder obstacles than tape, such as small pieces of foam, which caused more weight bearing and extension. Through gradual scaling of the relevant control parameters the child achieved a diagonal crawling pattern.

Providing Instruction

The last step of the ecological task-oriented approach to therapy utilizes applied research in the field of motor learning. The therapist can, through experiential knowledge, assist the child in discovering other solutions to the movement problem (i.e., "the range of possible new solutions") (Kamm, Thelen, and Jensen 1990, p. 774). However, the manner in which this discovery learning (Newell and McDonald 1992) is achieved is vitally important. We feel that when one is dealing with children, the direct solution to the problem should not be provided even after the child has been given his or her own choice of movement solutions. Instead we subscribe to a much more subtle approach, built on the foundations of dyadic training. Recent studies in the motor learning literature have provided evidence for the notion that having people practice in dyads not only can be more efficient than individual sessions but also can be as effective as, or even more effective than, individual training (Shebilske et al. 1992). There may be feasibility issues or parental restrictions in regard to working with two or more children at the same time, but this does not mean that the principles of dyad training cannot be employed. Rather we suggest that the therapist partner or collaborate with the child in the learning process. For instance, in the buttoning task we described earlier, one of the authors, when welcoming the child into her clinic, opened the clinic door wearing an improperly buttoned pajama top. Immediately the child laughed and engaged with the therapist as they entered into the task of buttoning together.

We have utilized this technique with great success in numerous tasks. Throughout each task, roles are alternated frequently in accordance with Shea, Wulf, and Whitacre's (1999) finding that alternate practice with a partner was more effective than individual practice or dyad practice in which partners did not alternate roles from trial to trial. The therapist can make explicit mistakes, sometimes exaggerations of the child's errors, and allow the child to correct these mistakes. The child may then be asked to demonstrate for the therapist and instruct the therapist regarding what to do. As a therapist, listen to the way the child instructs you to perform the task (i.e., what the child emphasizes and perhaps hence perceives as important in the completion of the task). This may provide an important window into the understanding that the child has of the task and what components the child feels (either correctly or incorrectly) are the most important. We believe that the success of this method is founded on three principles (McNevin, Wulf, and Carlson 2000). To list these in order of importance, (1) the child is facilitated to become an active participant in the learning process, thus gaining an increased feeling of responsibility for and involvement in the learning process; (2) dyad training adds a competitive element to the learning process, encouraging the child to set higher and more difficult goals; and (3) dyad training may be a successful form of observational learning (Shea et al. 2000). We have also found that our frog puppet is an extremely fun partner for the child in the dyadic training process. He gently nudges the child forward with subtle suggestions and always manages, no matter what the task, to fall flat on his face.

Motor learning research has also got something to say about what form these suggestions take. Instructions should always direct the child's attention away from his or her own movements. In other words, an external focus of attention versus an internal focus of attention is prescribed. Wulf and colleagues (Shea and Wulf 1999; Wulf, Hoss and Prinz 1998; Wulf, Lauterbach, and Toole 1999) have provided robust and general support for this phenomenon. In a study by Wulf and colleagues (1998), one group (internal focus group) was instructed to focus on their feet during a ski simulator task, specifically to exert force with the right foot when the platform moved to the right. A second group (external focus group) was instructed to focus on the wheels of the platform that were located directly under their feet and to exert force on the right or left pair of wheels when the platform moved to the right or left, respectively. The external focus of attention group was much more effective in the production of large movement amplitudes, in both practice and retention, than the internal focus group, which was not different from a control group that received no special instructions (Wulf, Hoss, and Prinz 1998). Similar results were obtained for a stabilometer task (Wulf, Hoss, and Prinz 1998) and generalized to a sport skill (Wulf, Lauterbach, and Toole 1999) under fieldlike conditions (i.e., golf).

Interestingly, Shea and Wulf (1999) found that an external focus of attention not only is relevant for the formulation of instructions, but also has implications for the feedback given to the learner. In a wonderfully designed experiment, two groups were presented the *same* concurrent visual feedback, with the platform movements displayed on a computer screen. One group of learners was informed that the feedback represented their own movements (internal focus), whereas the other group was told that the feedback represented lines marked on the platform in front of each of the performer's feet (external focus). Even though the feedback display was identical for the two feedback groups, the feedback group that adopted an external focus of attention performed better than the one that adopted an internal focus of attention.

CASE STUDY 5:
Fairies Doin' Some Stair Climbing

An 8-year-old child with developmental coordination disorder who had difficulty climbing stairs provides a nice example of external focus of attention instructions and feedback. Her parents had offered information that she continually stubbed her feet while climbing stairs. A play activity was initiated in which the child wore pink socks with pictures of fairies on them. She named the fairies Tinkerbell (left foot) and Marinda (right foot). A strip of red tape was placed at the front of each step on the stairs. This red strip represented hot fire that Tinkerbell and Marinda needed to avoid in order to rescue the young princesses (i.e., dolls) at the top of the stairs. An alternative approach (internal focus of attention) would have instructed the child to lift her feet over the step. Although the differences between the two approaches may seem insignificant, research indicates that the former method may be more beneficial.

Organization of Therapeutic Play: Emphasis on Fluidity

As tasks emerge and dissolve during play activity, choices are first allowed, variables are then manipulated, and dyadic instruction follows before the emergence of a new task goal. The fluidity of the play situation is constrained by an overall therapeutic goal. In other words, play revolves around this overall goal and returns to this specific goal many times during the therapy session. For instance, in a recent clinical case, the overall therapeutic goal was to improve a 6-year-old boy's writing ability from the perspective of a physiotherapist. The results of assessment of sensory integrative functioning indicated that this child had difficulties processing vestibular and proprioceptive sensation, which affected tonic postural control, stability, position sense, orientation from a center, and pencil control. The play activity incorporated Ecological Task Analysis with principles from sensory integration.

The child, as a veterinarian, received a phone call and wrote down the name and address of the caller and the problem with the animal (structured at the child's level of performance). He then got into his four-wheel jeep (platform swing) and drove out to the farm (i.e., pumping the swing and pushing hard with his arms as he went over bumpy terrain, caused by therapy balls, which encouraged supine flexion and body control). The farmer (therapist) was there to greet him. The cow needed an injection (i.e., the fine motor sequence of drawing water through a syringe). The farmer had a wall chart on which he wanted the vet to write the instructions (i.e., experiencing the movement of the letters with his whole body, gravity assisting, and also facilitating wrist extension). The vet, along with the farmer, made tablets out of therapeutic putty (i.e., facilitating thumb and index pincer grasp). On a subsequent call, the vet used a quad bike (i.e., a scooter board to enhance prone extension) and since he was far out in a field, he was constrained to write while on all fours (i.e., assisting shoulder stability). The vet then rescued a donkey using a rope tied around his waist, pulling the donkey out of a deep drain (i.e., facilitating sense of his hands and sequences of movement). He then had to swing to safety using a trapeze bar. He returned to his office on numerous occasions to take down calls using various writing implements (i.e., pencils, crayons, paintbrushes) and at times writing in sand. This structure contrasts with the task objective example cited by Bundy and Murray (2002, p. 27), which adheres to the underlying assumptions of sensory integration (see above). The task objective of stair climbing was not included as an activity in the therapy sessions. Instead, the goal of therapy from assessment was to improve vestibular proprioceptive processing under the assumption that it would transfer to achievement of the task of stair climbing.

Interspersing the specific therapeutic goal with other tasks that revolve around this task goal takes advantage of an established principle in the motor learning research literature (i.e., random or variable practice). In the laboratory, it has been found that "variable" or "random" practice is detrimental to performance during acquisition of a skill but leads to better performance during transfer tasks under novel conditions. Conversely, a blocked practice regime for the example just described would involve writing at the start of the therapy session for assessment purposes and at the end of the therapy session for evaluation purposes (i.e., in blocks). Many therapists incorporate blocked practice into their therapy or home programs to enhance performance. It has been found that blocked practice is beneficial for performance during acquisition but leads to decrements during transfer (Gentile 2000; Schmidt 1988). A classic explanation for the difference between blocked and variable or random practice is that the former leads to repeating a particular solution over and over on successive trials whereas the latter leads to a process of continually generating new solutions or generating old solutions anew (Gentile 2000; Schmidt 1988). The change in context during variable or random practice may actually prevent the child from merely repeating solutions by causing interference so that the current solution exits working memory and the child is required to construct or reconstruct a solution on successive attempts (Lee and Magill 1985). Put simply, variety of experience promotes "learning to learn" rather than learning particular solutions (Bernstein 1967, 1996; Harlow 1959). Such variety of experience might be exactly the kind of practice children need in order to achieve adaptive responding when challenged with novel contexts.

Self-Regulation of Arousal

Self-regulation is the ability to attain, maintain, and change arousal states appropriately for a task or an interpersonal situation (Williams and Shellenberger 1996). It is an inherent feature of biological systems that maintains internal order and underlies the ability to adapt to new situations (Porges 1996; Schore 1997). Facilitating the child's self-regulation should underlie every other therapeutic and educational goal. In other words, paramount to sharing attention, engaging, and performing all tasks in play and learning is the regulation of arousal. This underlying goal of all therapeutic intervention has been implicit in each of the clinical examples cited in this chapter and is a central tenet of sensory integration theory. A task-based approach that neglects the importance of self-regulation, particularly an approach that wishes to deal with children who have special educational needs, remains incomplete and is destined to fail. The appropriate interventions were based on the "right match" between each child's internal dimensions (based on sensory profiles and assessments) and the external dimensions of tasks, environments, relationships, and culture (Miller et al. 2001). There is much evidence throughout the neuroscience literature to support the use of active sensory experiences to enhance self-regulation as a basis for learning, brain maturation, and neural organization (Davidson 1994; Derryberry and Reed 1996; Ryan, Kuhl, and Deci 1997; Schore 1996, 1997).

Providing opportunities in all environments for self-regulation is critical for a child with issues of sensory, motor, or emotional modulation. Too often, opportunities for self-regulation are not provided in the task or the environment. For instance, the opportunities for movement or sensory input in the current school setting are not conducive to self-regulation and adaptive functioning in all children, particularly those with special educational needs. Consequently, children with behaviors that are seen as maladaptive in the classroom, such as excessive movement, fidgeting, making noise while working, chewing on things, rubbing or exploring objects with their skin, and wrapping their body around furniture or people, are in some cases using regulatory strategies as they attempt to meet their sensory needs. These sensation-seeking children are demonstrating what they need; thus the therapist, teacher, or caregiver must first provide what is needed in order to enable learning, rather than make it contingent (Dunn 1999).

In addition to sensory-seeking children such as those just described, children with a variety of sensory thresholds have been identified and characterized (see Dunn 1999). These include the child with poor registration, the child with sensitivity to stimuli, and the child who avoids sensation (Dunn 1999). Children with underlying emotional deficits such as separation, loss, abuse, or neglect may also have problems with everyday events that stem from an emotional attachment, a sensory base (sensory attachment intervention, Bhreathnach and Gogarty 2000), or both. These diverse individual constraints require alternative tasks and environments at the "just-right challenge" in order to facilitate self-regulation, a provision not usually given or understood in the current educational curriculum. As with an elite athlete who can attain his or her Individualized Zone of Optimal Functioning (Hanin 1989; Raglin and Hanin 2000) through simple sensory and cognitive techniques, the ultimate goal of regulation is self-monitoring and modification on the part of the child. But since this is not possible for all children, careful monitoring is required on the part of well-educated parents, caregivers, teachers, and professionals to enable provision of regulatory inputs and intake when required.

A poignant example of understanding regulation is as follows. A child with sensitivity to stimuli (tactile and auditory) did not participate in circle time (group time) or make friends. He was highly distractible and hyperactive, which made him unavailable for learning and behaving in class. The therapist, working with the child's parents, teacher, and special needs assistant, structured the environments and tasks based on the child's sensory profile and assessment to offer regulatory, discriminatory inputs and intake that supported organized information without additional arousal. For example, the boy had a water bottle on his desk, fidgets to squeeze, a piece of Velcro discretely hidden under his desk to rub at circle time, a piece of tubing on his pencil to chew, and a quiet corner in the classroom to retreat to fitted with heavy cushions, covers, and rolls, which he often used at reading time. His work desk was devoid of distracting visual inputs, and auditory cues were predicable. Movement breaks offered linear movement against resistance, for example pulling himself on his scooter board. His specific task goals offered working his muscles against resistance, for example making his shapes with therapeutic putty and performing coloring tasks on the floor using bumpy wallpaper. All of these offered deep touch pressure, using his muscles against resistance in linear patterns of movement. Utilizing these simple techniques of regulation has allowed this child to become available for learning, interaction, and participation in group work.

Ecological Task Analysis in Assessment Procedures

Although we have made reference to the use of ETA in the assessment of children with learning disabilities, an elaboration and clarification of our position is required. The sequential order (although not rigid) in the form outlined earlier is recommended for assessment. Thus, structuring the physical and social environment and allowing choices of movement solutions should precede formal assessment procedures. Therefore the four-step approach for assessment may be as follows: (a) establish the task goal by structuring the physical and social environment, in other words, invite play activity; (b) allow choices of movement solutions to help identify the intrinsic dynamics of the system; (c) manipulate performer, environment, and task variables to assess the stability of the system and to hypothesize about what control parameters are affecting this stability; and (d) undertake formal assessment procedures (e.g., tests) to help verify or call into question the hypothesis generated in the preceding step (these may be performed on another day).

This differs from the general therapy procedure, in which in many instances formal tests are administered first and then play is examined. However, two important questions must be asked. First, are the current movement tests assessing the intrinsic dynamics of the system? Secondly, are they assessing the stability and flexibility of these dynamics? We feel that the answers to these questions are most definitely in the negative. At best, the tests add credibility to the therapist's observations. At worst, they are rigid and inflexible, assessing deviations from "normative" movement patterns that may in fact be adaptive solutions to the current task and environmental constraints (see Holt, Obusek, and Fonseca 1996). As a therapist, you may learn a lot more from a natural play environment where task goals emerge and dissolve, where the child pulls you into her world to have a look around. Then you may see the preferred behavioral mode of the child. Then you may see, in the words of Stanley Greenspan, "how the child is cooking." And when you're there, add a few ingredients, change a few things, and see what happens. In so doing, you may get to see the stability and adaptability of the child's coordination dynamics.

Implications for the Therapist's Role

The effectiveness of therapy is significantly limited by the current trends of (1) localizing intervention by providing a block of therapeutic input, restricted in many instances mainly to the clinical setting, and (2) offering general cookbook intervention plans that are not tailored to the specific needs of each child. Both of these trends have emerged in response to the therapist's time limitations (i.e., the amount of time that can be spent with each child as waiting lists continue to grow). However, it is from this limitation that a solution can emerge once the therapist recognizes his or her limitations with regard to the time spent with the child relative to the amount of time the child spends outside of therapy (i.e., with family, friends, or in school).

Thus, intervention, rather than being bestowed solely by the therapist, is distributed or dispersed throughout the community of the child. Consequently, the therapist's role must shift to one of coach and consultant (Rush, Shelden, and Hanft 2003), modeling, supporting, and informing those within the child's community of the rationale behind the therapeutic techniques, the therapeutic techniques themselves, and ways in which these therapeutic techniques can be incorporated into the child's daily life, including the child's Individualized Educational Plan at home and in school. In many instances, this also moves the therapist out of the clinical setting and into the natural environment of the child, for example the classroom and the home, so that the therapist is immersed within the learning system as a learning facilitator and his or her contributions have to do with establishing an appropriate climate for learning. We have named this type of intervention *distributed intervention,* as it occurs when intervention and treatment are dispersed throughout the child's personal as well as professional community. As laid out in this chapter, the intervention itself utilizes the principles of ETA. We feel that this task-based intervention procedure, coupled with recognition of the importance of self-regulation and distributed throughout the community of the child, has the potential to transform the way therapists conduct their clinical work by helping them become more efficient, effective, and affective in meeting each child's unique therapeutic and special educational needs.

INSTRUCTIONAL STRATEGIES

- Provide a context for learning functional tasks through play and relationships rather than emphasizing solely the neurophysiological aspect.
- By understanding the child's unique sensory-motor profile, you can actively facilitate choice to make the therapeutic goal meaningful for the child and to stimulate the child's motivation.
- Understanding the dynamic systems theory may fundamentally change your "mental model" of therapeutic practice and your practices within it.
- Use motor learning principles such as dyadic practice, external focus of attention, and random/variable practice, as they are particularly valuable for learning functional skills.
- Become aware of the importance of the child's regulation of arousal, which is inherent in all tasks, environments, and relationships.
- *Have fun!*

Summary

This chapter indicates the usefulness of Ecological Task Analysis for physiotherapists. The four principles of ETA (i.e., structure the physical and social environment; allow choice of movement solutions; manipulate the task, environment, or the individual; and provide instruction) are illustrated with reference to actual case examples in pediatric physiotherapy. As outlined in the text, ETA provides not only a structured process for a single task or therapy session but also general principles that physiotherapists may find valuable in their clinical work. For instance, this chapter discusses the implications of ETA for other therapeutic approaches, for the organization of the therapy session, for assessment procedures, and for the role of the therapist.

CHAPTER 12

Ecological Approach to the Care of Persons With Neurological Disabilities

Adri Vermeer, PhD

Traditional therapy for persons with disabilities focuses on the identification of individually determined developmental tasks and skills to be learned by these persons for coping with the demands of their daily life. This approach aims at changes in cognitive, motor, or social structures of the individual. However, the determinants of behavioral performance are less likely to be individual structures than they are to be the immediacy of the situation and the task at hand (Thelen and Smith 1994). This "alternative" approach with respect to behavioral development is based on ecological psychology, dynamic systems theory, and related theories of human development and action as described in Davis and Burton's (1991) Ecological Task Analysis model. The ETA model implies that performance and behavior are

> determined by the mutual constraints (both limitations and enablements) of the task goal, environmental conditions (physical and social) and the performer's intent and attributes. Thus, performance is not based upon a normal model per se, as are most traditional approaches of understanding disorders. We make no apriori assumptions about an optimal performance, instead, we take a functional, exploratory, discovery approach to perception and action. (Davis and Van Emmerik 1995b, p. 34)

This chapter utilizes the ETA model to examine the practice of caring for individuals with neurologically determined disorders, such as persons with cerebral palsy, brain injuries, and intellectual disabilities. In particular, the behavioral patterns and outcomes for these individuals were considered to be the result of the mutual interaction between the task goal, which has its specific significance according to the perception of action possibilities of the person involved; the performer constraints; and the affordances of the environment. Both dynamic systems theory and ecological psychology stress the role of the environment in developmental change. For example, Thelen and Smith (1994) write:

> Of course, there is order, direction and structure just as there is in development. But there is no design written anywhere in a cloud or a program in the genes or a homunculus in the brain of any particular species that determines the final community structure or behavioral performance. (p. xix)

Thelen and Smith (1994) further state, "In particular we invoke Gibson's (1988) beliefs that the world contains information and that the goal of development is to discover relevant information in order to make a functional match between what the environment affords and what the actor can and wants to do" (p. xxi).

Context is the environment in which a human being perceives possibilities for action, while provision for action is afforded by information present in the environment. We act when there is information available that corresponds to our possibilities of action and our desire to act. Without such information we do nothing. Normally, the process is automatic; but if the individual is severely limited in his or her capacity for information pickup, the process may need conscious assistance, referred to as tuning. In general, tuning seems so simple as to be self-evident. We execute thousands of actions daily, many of them without conscious reflection.

However, for many individuals, tuning the system is not as self-evident as it seems. For some, every action costs considerable effort, time, and patience. For a child with disabilities and for his or her parents, every day means adapting, exercise, and support. Gerda and Siegfried (Mentz and Mentz 1982), who received an important presidential award in Germany for their work on the integration of persons with intellectual disabilities by means of sport, gave a vivid account of their daily efforts with their son Andreas, a boy with Down syndrome:

> Day after day we lay with him on the floor, we show him every movement, how we roll over, crawl, come to sit and to stand up. Andreas shows no attempt to undertake any action. We try everything, but without success. Finally, after 18 months, it happens: Andreas can crawl. We celebrate this as the first step of a normally developing child. (p. 3)

Andreas' parents came to wonder whether he achieved this and other milestones as a result of or despite their efforts. They felt that there were many moments when they observed no progress, but that from time to time there were sudden breakthroughs. The question is what to expect when the biological basis of human development is disturbed, as is the case with many persons with disabilities.

Brain and Behavior

Our brains are part of what makes it possible for us to be who we are and to do what we do. Our brains are flexible. They change and reorganize themselves continuously according to the pattern of stimulation (Mulder 1996). Less flexible brains or impaired brains are less capable of coping with an ever-changing environment. If a person receives information from the environment that the central systems cannot organize, the person cannot react adequately and will withdraw, exhibit unsuccessful behavior, or fail to act. Koot's (1992) concept of "goodness of fit" explains the fact that some persons react with behavior labeled as "handicapped" while others with the same impairments and disabilities do not. In other words, adaptive behavior and a feeling of well-being depend on the extent to which the expectations or demands and facilities of the environment fit with the biological and psychological capabilities of the person.

On the basis of studies of persons with an impaired cortex, Mulder (1996) states that "central and peripheral structures, in other words brain and environment, the biological system and its surroundings are a unity" (p. 459). The way these elements attune to each other is a very rapid process, and a fascinating one, in which conscious regulation is usually unnecessary. Indeed, we are looking at a fundamental characteristic of the neurological system: It's a self-organizing system. Cicchetti and Tucker (1994) describe the organic coherence within the dynamic differentiation of neuronal networks of the human cortex: "The self-organizing structures of the human mind are the most important stabilizing forces within the chaotic play of psychological and neurological development" (p. 547).

Approaches to Persons With Disabilities

In the history of the care for persons with disabilities, two paradigmatic shifts are discerned. The first shift concerns the change from an individually oriented approach to persons with disabilities toward a societal approach. The individual approach focuses on the impairments or disabilities of the individual, with care aimed at the curing of the disorders or compensation of the disabilities of the person. This paradigm is based on a medical model or a developmental model. Both models focus on changes "in" the person. However, evaluations of health care based on this approach show unsatisfactory results. The progress evident in the person's development seems more associated with casual environmental factors, in relation to the actual development of that person, than with any specific aspects of the health care itself (Becher and Douwes Dekker 1997).

This conclusion is also reached from an evaluation of individually oriented educational programs for children with cerebral palsy or for children with intellectual disabilities. Even when these children are still young and parents have high expectations about their developmental growth, the results of early intervention are disappointing (Van Gennep et al. 1997; Zijlstra 1997). Sipma (1996) concludes, from her research on the effects of the Portage Program for young children with developmental disabilities and their parents, that the development status of the children is more influenced by the education within the family and the physical and social environment of the child than by the Portage Program.

The societal model is widely known as "normalization" and implies that persons with disabilities have the right to live within the normal societal systems. The supposition is that normalization of living circumstances, education, work, and so on will have positive effects on the well-being of persons with disabilities. This places a heavy burden of responsibility on society to provide individuals with disabilities the possibilities for social participation. The first consequence of this model was attempts to change social attitudes toward persons with disabilities. The results, however, have not been very convincing. Secondly, considerable research on the effects of this paradigm on social integration has shown that although physical integration has been attained, social integration is more difficult (Van Gennep 1997). The main problem is that the environment is not usually fitted to the personal needs and social capabilities of individuals with disabilities. "Normalization alone is not sufficient, a personal kind of support is also necessary to avoid being normalized as incompetent" (Van Gennep 1997, p. 16).

Van Gennep therefore introduced a new paradigm, which he called "support." The person with the disability does not have to be "ready" for admission to all kinds of living, work, and leisure-time facilities. On the contrary, the aim is that the person can live and experience in the situation that he or she chooses (Van Gennep 1997, p. 26). In this situation, support is provided according to the person's capacities. Hereafter, this paradigm is referred to in this chapter as a functional model.

Personal Experience Related to the Functional Model

For an initial explanation of this view, some examples of personal experiences with individuals with disabilities are offered.

Functional Support at an Airport

A few years ago I accompanied a group of 25 young men and women with intellectual disabilities, as a researcher, on a trip to the United States for the Special Olympics Summer Games. During the journey we changed planes in Atlanta, one of the biggest airports in the country. So that they could take care of each other in this busy airport, the group was divided into smaller groups. I was responsible for four young men, with their passports in my pocket (why not in their own pockets?) and the firm look of a leader in my eyes. After less than a couple of hundred meters, the group was running 10 to 20 meters ahead, showing me the way to the other terminal. They had quickly figured out the system of colored pictograms in the airport that guided their way. How to operate the fully automatic shuttle train also was immediately understood by each person in my group. These young men with disabilities started experimenting with the distance to the door of the shuttle to find out when the speech chip warned that somebody was standing too close to the door for it to shut. In short, the group proved to be more than capable, governed by the rules of the airport systems that were suitable to almost everybody.

However, this changed once we arrived at customs. First, there was a sign saying that only couples could approach together and that others should wait behind the yellow line. I observed as the first young man, a person with Down syndrome, went alone to the customs official, who observed his passport and asked, "What is your purpose for this visit?" Fear and confusion appeared in the young man's eyes. He looked at me helplessly. The customs official also seemed not to understand the situation, or was not willing to understand. In short, the behavioral rules here did not fit at least some of the visitors who daily arrive at this airport.

My experiences during this trip suggest that given the appropriate attention from the customs official, this young man would have quickly learned to cope with the situation. For example, after a week's stay with a host family with an English-speaking father and a Dutch-speaking mother, this same young man answered a local journalist's question about what he had to do during the games. "I shall swim the breaststroke," he responded. This is social integration as a result of an adequate context, suitable to the capabilities of a person, and a suitable stimulation.

External Compensation During Walking

The second example concerns a situation observed in a rehabilitation center for persons with physical disabilities. A young woman who had suffered brain damage as a result of a road accident was attempting to maintain a straight line while crossing an inner court. However, the woman was unable to follow a line drawn on the pavement by the physical therapist. Her movement pattern was so erratic that she had to stop after a couple of meters. When the physical therapist walked beside her across the court, however, she could walk in a straight line to the opposite side. When the therapist next asked her to clap her hands in accompaniment to the rhythm of her steps, she walked straight to the other side unassisted.

I believe this is explained by the fact that normal brains are flexible and adaptive. They organize themselves according to the situation at hand. The gathered information remains available for subsequent use. In case of brain damage, however, the central system does not always respond to the relevant environmental information. It also might be that the detection is adequate, but that there is a failure in the control needed to act according to this perception. External compensation is then needed to execute the desired behavior (Mulder 1996; Hochstenbach 1997; Mulder, Nienhuis, and Pauwels 1996). The two examples just presented show that the loss of central capabilities to control can be compensated by means of peripheral or environmental control. Much research has been carried out to discover whether this kind of peripheral reorganization of lost coordination and control could be used for therapeutic purposes (e.g., Wagenaar and Meijer 1998).

Verbal Guidance in Gymnastics

The final example of experience-based knowledge involves my observations during a Special Olympics event. In gymnastics, the coach or the trainer is allowed to guide the performance of an athlete verbally if the athlete has difficulties executing a sequence of exercises because of intellectual disability. We know from both practical experience and research that many people with intellectual disabilities have difficulty with the transition from one situation to another and in coupling one exercise with another. Through the provision of verbal guidance, such a person can participate in these types of events and enjoy and experience a task successfully executed. Such involvement enhances feelings of competence, which in turn increase the motivation to continue. Increased motivation after a successfully performed task may also help provide motivation to act in other situations. However, a person is motivated to act only if there is something in the present environment that will give significance to that action.

Behavior and Development as Self-Organization

Fogel (1990), who has investigated early development, claims that the functionality of developmental processes is lost, whether in education or treatment, when the person is separated from his or her environment. Fogel (1990) sees communication and social interaction as the construction of a common communication frame and social frame in which the two partners—person and environment—play equal roles. In terms of well-being and social integration, this means that there is no external motor or motive; the mutual adaptation and cohesion between person and environment result in a dynamic and self-changing health-social system. "Self-organization takes place when a large number of components of a system interact. This interaction is determined by a small number of rather simple rules. These are sufficient to result into complex patterns" (Fogel 1990, p. 122).

For example, rather normal walking patterns arise in patients with Parkinson's disease when the velocity of the gait is enhanced (Van Emmerik and Wagenaar 1996a). Guess and Sailor (1993) discussed the complex interaction between psychological, biological, and environmental factors in children with conduct disorders. They described the occurrence of periods of aggressive behavior in a child who had severe emotional disorders. It was established that the aggressive behavior of the child coincided with the monthly visit of his father. The upcoming visit of the father also resulted in sleep problems and shortage of sleep and accompanying tiredness. In and of itself, a small event in the child's context disturbed the entire (i.e., biological, psychological, and social) functioning of the child. The interaction of these variables results in a dynamic change of behavior, which may be triggered by a significant environmental parameter. The implication for school and family education is that much more attention should be given to the immediate environmental conditions, both social and physical.

Implications for the Development of Physical and Social Well-Being

The implications of the preceding examples and the explanation for the occurrence of certain behaviors lead to the conclusion that behavior and development can be understood only from the viewpoint that the individual and environment are inextricably connected. Our biological makeup enables us to do what we do in context. In the case of disorders of biological capabilities, a person is less likely to cope because the environment does not contain suitable information and therefore no action possibilities. It is, then, the task of educators, coaches, and trainers to create a context in which the person can perceive action possibilities. Although this sounds simple, this approach requires the careful observation of the interaction between individuals with disabilities and their surroundings. Too often we are inclined to provide our "normalized" models of interaction to "not-normalized" people. Whether there are action possibilities or not depends on the landscape offered. It is the task of caretakers to create openings into such a landscape.

The person also has to be motivated to enter a new landscape. "Recent studies from psychology and neurosciences suggest that motivational processes play a central organizing role. First, the motivational system operates at the behavioral level and enables a communicative response or an avoidance response. Second, the motivational system operates at the attentional level and directs one toward the most important sources of information" (Derryberry and Reed 1994, p. 656).

The organization and reorganization of the brain depend on use and activity, implying a functional approach to education. A research project was conducted to test the efficacy of this approach (Ketelaar et al. 2001). A functional (disability oriented) treatment program for children with cerebral palsy was compared with a traditional (impairment oriented) therapy regime. The outcomes showed a significant increase of mobility and self-care skills in the daily life of the functional group in comparison with the reference group. Although no significant differences were found between the two groups with respect to the level of performance of the skills, the functional group accomplished more with the skills learned. They were more independent in daily life with the same skill level compared to the control group.

Outline of Context-Oriented Care

Care facilities for individuals with disabilities have to differ from facilities for healthy individuals in the way the environment plays a role in affecting the well-being and the behavior of the residents. There must be sufficient movement space that is not overly structured. The environment must be one in which individuals can find their own way and can perceive affordances according to their action possibilities. This means a diversity of spaces, of landscapes, trees, animals, and objects. Providing care means that caretakers are creating landscapes wherein individuals with disabilities can act.

Living and working in such environments result in feelings of competence of the persons involved. If individuals feel accepted within their environment, their motivation will be positively affected and they will continue to be active and to master new tasks. We define "development" as an increasing level of mastery of being effective in one's environment (White 1959). The expectation is not that individuals with disabilities must adapt to their environment; rather the expectation is that there will be a goodness of fit between the capabilities of the individual and the possibilities of that environment—a coupling of affordances and effectivities.

"Taking care" means guiding and supporting people as they learn to perceive these affordances, to act and to perform according to these affordances, and to experience the emotional effects of action and performance. Every individual with a disability has his or her own possibilities, and accordingly, his or her individually determined affordances. Not every individual is capable of clearly expressing his or her desires and preferences; therefore, it is necessary that caretakers be creative and flexible in providing learning and care environments. Interaction with individuals with disabilities is a continuous experiment. An important skill needed by caretakers is observing before doing. This implies an open view regarding the specific development of the people they are responsible for. Based on these principles, a set of instructions has been formulated for the care of individuals with disabilities (Vermeer 2005).

- *Taking time.* Allow time to discover the capabilities of the person and the aspects of the environment that best fits that person. Also take into account the previous care, whether in an institutional, home, school, residential, or other setting. It will take time to change any established behavioral patterns.

- *Recognition.* Recognize the uniqueness of persons with a disability and do not necessarily try to change them from "being different." Accept them as equal in value to all other persons. Acknowledge successes and help make these the focus of the individual's attention as well.

- *Role of the environment.* Living, working, and leisure-time environments become an important focus for those responsible for supporting people with disabilities—parents, teachers, therapists, and so on. Both the physical and the social environments are important and are the basis for the choices and challenges given to people. The caregiver looks for the point of contact that each individual has with the environment.

• *Interaction.* The attitude of the caregiver is extremely important and is part of the social environment. Respect, spontaneity, and high positive energy should all be part of the demeanor of the caregiver. Physical contact is important, but it should not be controlling. Establishing a good rapport is essential and requires mutual trust and confidence brought about by clear communication.

• *Open settings.* Parents and caretakers have the right to know what will happen in learning and instruction processes. Any therapeutic or residential setting should be open to all those with a legitimate concern for the person with disabilities. Parents and caregivers should have some say in the services afforded their children and should provide their consent. On the other hand, parents and others should not be controlling of either their children or the service providers. Everyone concerned must take equal responsibility and accountability.

PRACTICAL APPLICATIONS

• Training, education, and therapy do not have to focus on changing the characteristics of the person, but on changing the characteristics of the environment.

• Because of their disorders, persons with chronic disabilities do not always perceive the action possibilities in their environment. It is then the task of the caregiver to restructure the environment so that the person is afforded action possibilities.

• Motivation has a controlling and organizing function for a person's attention. It facilitates the perception of action possibilities.

• Training, education, and therapy have to use task- and context-specific exercises. Training of discrete functions is not effective.

Summary

In this chapter an ecological approach to behavioral development is applied to the care for persons with neurological disabilities. This approach emphasizes the role of the environment in carrying out and changing behavior. The environment contains information that determines the behavior of an individual. If the information perceived fits with capabilities of a person, this will result in effective behavior. If not, this will result in inadequate behavior. It's the task of a trainer, educator, or therapist to structure the environment in such a way that the person can observe action possibilities. This approach is based on concepts from ecological psychology, dynamic systems theory, and the Ecological Task Analysis model.

CHAPTER 13

Interface of the KB
and ETA Approaches

A.E. Wall, PhD, Greg Reid, PhD,
and William J. Harvey, PhD

The Knowledge-Based (KB) and Ecological Task Analysis models are both heuristic, but they differ significantly in underlying assumptions, theoretical explanation, and points of emphasis. Notwithstanding these differences, both have provided guidance for assessment and instruction in physical activity for over a decade that, at the level of application, are often similar or complementary. The purpose of this chapter is to outline the KB model and to describe how it interfaces with ETA with respect to assessment and instruction.

Before beginning the chapter, it is important to acknowledge that there are some fundamental differences that distinguish the cognitive approach, which supports our KB model, from the ecological perspective, which supports the ETA model (see Fodor and Pylyshyn 1981). As Gardner (1987) observed over 15 years ago, those who adhere to the ecological approach reflect "a belief in the real world as it is, with all the information there, and the organism simply attuned to it;" in contrast, those who adhere to a cognitive approach reflect "a belief in the constructive powers of the mind, with the external world simply a trigger for activities and operations that are largely built into the organism" (p. 317). Although there are significant differences between the two approaches, there are some important areas of agreement. For example, cognitive psychologists have gained very important insights about the nature of perception from those who have taken a Gibsonian stance; moreover, their emphasis on the role of the environment has prompted many cognitive psychologists to place much greater emphasis on the ecologically validity of their research efforts (Neisser 1976, 1984). However, as Gardner (1987) wisely noted, the fundamental issue of "whether the study of organisms and environments can suffice or whether an additional layer of analysis is necessary still separates the two approaches and only future research will be able to resolve which approach is correct" (p. 287).

Knowledge-Based Approach

In 1985, Wall and colleagues described a cognitive approach to motor development that stressed the importance of knowledge about action with special reference to the developmental problem of physical awkwardness. In a subsequent paper published the next year, Wall (1986) described the role that different types of knowledge about action play in the skill acquisition process. Essentially, the KB model contends that increases in relevant knowledge directly influence the quality of cognitive functioning as a person learns and develops physical skills (Bruner 1986; Gardner 1987; Piaget 1956). A review of some of the major observations that were made in those initial papers may be of help as we try to understand the interface between the KB approach and ETA.

Figure 13.1 presents a model of the KB approach to motor development. As the figure shows, in the KB approach a fundamental distinction is made between structural capacity and acquired knowledge. Structural capacity refers to the anatomical and physiological potential inherited by a person that supports performance, learning, and development. Recent research has shown that genetic endowment as well as environmental stimulation plays an influential role in the developmental process (Bouchard, Malina, and Perusse 1997; Howe, Davidson, and Sloboda 1998; Plomin and DeFries 1998). Thus, structural capacity is placed at the base of the figure to acknowledge the vital role that genetic endowment, as well as physiological and neurophysiological structures, plays in the development of skilled action.

Skeletal, circulorespiratory, digestive, endocrine, neuromuscular, and sensory systems of the body support the development of skilled action. In addition, the human brain with its billions of neurons and countless nerve pathways plays a critical role in supporting the developmental process. In fact, recent advances in neuroscience document the dynamic role that neural networks play in the acquisition of skill. Based on such research, it is clear that the human brain and its associated nervous system are extremely adaptable and are, in fact, structurally modified by learning and experience (Calvin 1990, 1996; Damasio 1999; Edelman and Tononi 2000; Gazzaniga 1999).

The other major component of the KB model is acquired knowledge. This is defined as knowledge that is learned through experience and is stored in long-term memory, which increases with development. Given its central importance in motor development, acquired knowledge is divided into several major categories. Specifically, the KB model contends

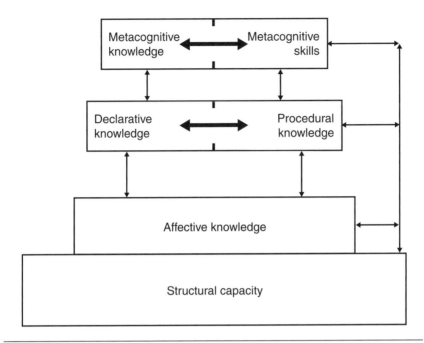

Figure 13.1   A knowledge-based model of motor development. The arrows in the model reflect the interactive nature of the components of a person's knowledge base. The bold arrows emphasize the interaction between declarative and procedural knowledge as well as between metacognitive knowledge and metacognitive skills. An essential aspect of the model is the impact that increases in one's developmental knowledge base have on the processes underlying learning and performance.

that individuals acquire five types of knowledge about action, namely, declarative, procedural, and affective knowledge, as well as metacognitive knowledge and metacognitive skills that are also referred to as self-awareness and self-regulation.

These five types of acquired knowledge about action are presented in figure 13.1 in such a way as to highlight the ongoing interaction among them during learning and performance. While it would be difficult to distinctly identify the exact role of any one form of knowledge in any given physical performance, it is helpful to differentiate among these forms for analysis and discussion purposes. Let us briefly describe each of the types of knowledge about action that are illustrated in figure 13.1.

Affective Knowledge

The KB approach defines affective knowledge about action as the subjective feelings that people store in memory about themselves in various action situations. By including affective knowledge, the model highlights the critical role that affective and motivational influences play in the development of skilled action. Moreover, affective knowledge about action is placed directly above the structural capacity base in figure 13.1 to underscore the close relationship between affective reactions to task demands and the physiological responses they invoke within the person. Take, for example, a novice golfer who must tee off on the first hole in front of a group of seasoned players. It is very likely that in this situation the person will experience increases in resting heart rate and galvanic skin responses due to the anxiety linked to such a performance environment. As the bidirectional arrows from the affective knowledge box show, affective factors are purported to interact with all of the other components in the model (Bandura 1997; Damasio 1999).

In recent years, the role that one's physical proficiency and motor competence play in the development of a positive physical self-concept has become widely recognized. Studies of physical self-efficacy and sport confidence have broadened the notion of affective knowledge and heightened interest in the role of affective factors in the acquisition and development of motor skills. Physical self-efficacy and sport confidence are extremely important components of the knowledge base of athletes. In competitive, tension-filled game situations, competent athletes are able to focus their attention and execute key skills in a calm, almost relaxed, manner. In contrast to their less skilled peers, competent athletes are often able to perform at their peak in such stressful, competitive situations. Most importantly, physical self-efficacy beliefs have been shown to positively or negatively affect a person's ability to learn and perform in a variety of sport settings (Bandura 1982, 1986, 1997; Vealey 1986; Vealey et al. 1998).

Declarative Knowledge

As figure 13.1 shows, declarative and procedural knowledge are given a prominent place just above the affective knowledge base in the model. Declarative knowledge about action is defined as conceptual information stored in memory that can influence the development and execution of skilled action. Declarative or conceptual knowledge about action is acquired through experience, and its development is facilitated through the use of language. During their preschool years, children have been shown to learn verbal labels for objects and actions that eventually become integrated into their physical activity vocabulary (Bruner 1983). For example, a person must know what a "softball" actually looks like in order to pick out this distinct type of ball from a variety of balls. The term *softball* can be misleading, as the object is actually hard and not soft as the label suggests. The term is related to the sport and not to the characteristics of the ball. Hence, the person must be aware of this difference in order to pick out the correct object and not a Nerf ball or foam ball. Similar logic can also be applied to verbal labels for actions. For example, different names can be used for the skill of throwing because there are many ways in which a person can throw a ball (underhand, overhand, sidearm, etc.), at various heights (high, low, etc.), with differing amounts of force (fast, hard, strong, slow, soft, light, etc.), to a variety of locations (at a target, to a friend's hands, etc.).

In addition to developing a declarative knowledge base about one's actions, the action of others, and the effects of one's actions on objects and people in the environment, individuals develop specific information related to the culturally normative games that they play (French and Thomas 1987; Grehaigne, Godbout, and Bouthier 1997; McPherson 1993; McPherson and Thomas 1989). For instance, in Canada, hockey is a game that is watched or played by a high percentage of the population from early childhood. Thus, it is not surprising that many Canadians develop a rather well-structured knowledge base about the sport of hockey, including the rules of the game and specific contextual cues that are stored in the form of declarative knowledge. However, in addition to this basic declarative knowledge, competent athletes acquire an even more extensive and coherent conceptual knowledge base about their sport; that is, they develop true "knowledge of the game"—an understanding of the rules, the equipment, and the environment in which they play, as well as of the contextual strategies related to personal and team tactics needed to play successfully. Research has documented the importance of such conceptual knowledge in the acquisition and performance of skilled action (Paull and Glencross 1997; Williams and Davids 1995).

A number of observations can be made regarding the nature of declarative knowledge. In the KB approach, schemas are viewed as packets of knowledge that store information in a highly interconnected, yet accessible, manner. Moreover, these declarative schemas are purported to play a major role in the storage, organization, access, and retrieval of information within specific domains, that is, circumscribed areas of knowledge. Thus, sport-specific knowledge is developed as a person acquires expertise in a given sport. Such conceptual knowledge is stored and organized in networks that facilitate categorization, pattern recognition, and the chunking of information into meaningful units (Chiesi, Spilich, and Voss 1979; Rumelhart 1980; Schacter 1995; Tulving 1972). The size and organization of a person's declarative knowledge base play a major role in contextual understanding, problem solving, and the development of the procedural knowledge that underlies skilled action (Sternberg et al. 2000). It is important to appreciate that in addition to differences in the quantity of conceptual knowledge a person may acquire, there are differences in the depth of such knowledge. In fact, it has been shown that depth of knowledge may range on a continuum from superficial understanding of tasks to meaningful, deep, structured task knowledge. For example, consider the idea of an offside in the sport of ice hockey: novice players may know superficially that they cannot pass a puck to a teammate if he or she is inside the opponent's blue line. A more experienced defensive player may be able to use a deeper understanding of the concept of an offside to force an opponent into an offside situation so that the offensive action is strategically halted.

To stress the close connection between declarative and procedural knowledge, these two types of knowledge about action are represented in figure 13.1 within one box, along with a bidirectional arrow that emphasizes the ongoing interaction that takes place between them. It has also been shown that there are wide interindividual differences in declarative knowledge. For example, the "Great One," Wayne Gretzky, possesses a much more extensive declarative knowledge base about playing hockey than any of the authors, if not more than all of their declarative knowledge combined.

More importantly, we now know that declarative knowledge is organized in a coherent fashion so that it can be accessed quickly at the appropriate time from memory. For example, as just noted, it is essential that hockey players understand the notion of an offside so that when they are executing a pass they appreciate the personal and environmental constraints under which the pass must be made. In order to become highly proficient movers, they must develop a deep understanding of the factors affecting the task and the situation, as well as construct personal knowledge related to the skills, tendencies, and attitudes of their teammates and opponents. On the basis of their conceptual knowledge, competent athletes understand the situations facing them, the key players in those situations, and the important factors in the game that may change, often very quickly, as play unfolds. The close association between procedural and declarative knowledge in the model underscores this fact (Williams and Davids 1995).

Procedural Knowledge

In the KB approach, procedural knowledge is purported to underlie all aspects of an action sequence, including the anticipation and prediction, decision-making, response selection, and response execution aspects of information processing. With respect to the performance of any sport skill, procedural knowledge represents the neurophysiological processes in the information-processing system that facilitate the execution of that skill. For example, in a situation in which a person is attempting to catch a ball, the sensory information in the flight of the ball, that is, its trajectory, speed, and size, as well as the actions of the thrower in relation to the environment, will be processed based on the perceptual knowledge that the person has acquired related to the act of catching a ball. Moreover, it is assumed that the goal of the performer provides a framework that limits the number and type of relevant cues within a given situational display. Thus, the more expert person is able to identify and encode relevant cues relatively early for perceptual processing (Abernethy 1988, 1990; Abernethy and Russell 1987).

Once the key features in the environmental display have been perceptually processed, it is assumed that relevant information is processed to facilitate the making of a decision regarding when and how to catch the ball. Once again, it is the quality of the sport-specific knowledge base of the learner that facilitates making these decisions effectively and efficiently. Once a decision is made to try to catch the ball, then the most appropriate response that is available is activated and relevant information is processed so as to initiate the execution of a response action. At this point, the model assumes that ongoing feedback, from intrinsic and extrinsic feedback loops, controls the actual execution of the action. Throughout the entire process, these intrinsic and extrinsic feedback loops provide pertinent information by which the system can update and modify itself. Of course, much of this knowledge will be procedural and will be mainly tacit in form, which makes it difficult or impossible to describe verbally. The physical process of riding a bike is often described as tacit knowledge, as it is difficult to explain exactly what we do in the situation once we have learned the skill (Logan 1985; Norman and Shallice 1980; Sternberg et al. 2000).

Procedural knowledge can also be viewed from a developmental perspective in terms of the repertoire of skills that a person has acquired. Viewed from this perspective, procedural knowledge reflects the accuracy, consistency, and automaticity with which a person can perform the various physical skills he or she has acquired. In fact, measuring the degree to which a person attains culturally normative skill expectations in relation to the performance of his or her peer group can provide a basic assessment of the developmental level of a person in a given sport. For example, hockey players acquire a number of fundamental skills, such as skating, stick handling, shooting, and passing, in order to play effectively in competitive game situations. Moreover, with considerable practice, competent hockey players develop their skills so well that they can use these skills almost automatically in fast-paced hockey situations, that is, perform them without having to think very much about how or when to do so. In fact, recent research has shown that as expertise increases, knowledge base differences affect information processing from initial anticipatory and perceptual components to the selection and execution of responses (Allard and Burnett 1985; French, Spurgeon, and Nevett 1995; Smith and Chamberlin 1992).

Two Meta-Level Knowledge Bases

As important as structural capacity and the three basic types of acquired knowledge are in the motor developmental process, perhaps the two most important components of the model are those represented by the top box, labeled metacognitive knowledge and metacognitive skills. Before describing them let us consider the meaning of the word "metacogni-tion." The prefix "meta-" refers to higher level or above. Thus, when used with the word "knowledge," it refers to a higher-level understanding of a particular form of knowledge; that is, metacognitive knowledge is a higher form of declarative knowledge about one's knowledge base. In figure 13.1, metacognitive knowledge has been placed above the declarative knowledge base and metacognitive skills are represented above the procedural knowledge base in order to underscore their conceptual and procedural nature, respectively.

Metacognitive Knowledge

Metacognitive knowledge refers to conceptual awareness of one's knowl-edge base; that is, it is purported to be a higher-level form of declarative knowledge that allows one to understand and appreciate the knowledge and processes that have been developed (Anderson 1990; Brown 1984; Flavell 1979). In swimming, realizing that one's kicking action in the front crawl is effective but that one's arm motion is hampering move-ment through the water and needs refinement is an example of the use of metacognitive knowledge about action. Understanding that one can perform the front and back crawl relatively well and the breaststroke quite proficiently, but that one cannot perform the butterfly very well, is another example of the use of metacognitive knowledge in action situ-ations. Such metacognitive knowledge is based on the use of specific declarative terms that the learner has acquired within a given sport. For example, it is important to understand such concepts as streamlined body position and an effective flutter kick. The use of such declarative knowledge terms facilitates teacher–learner discussions of the specific procedural knowledge that the learner has developed in relation to each of the swimming strokes he or she is acquiring.

The KB approach also contends that with development, a person's metacognitive knowledge base becomes more organized, coherent, and accessible. Self-awareness, that is, knowing one's strengths and weaknesses, has long been recognized as an important aspect of human behavior, and the KB approach underscores that fact. For example, metacognitive knowledge about action in a specific sport refers to an awareness of one's strengths and weaknesses in relation to the situations faced in that particular sport. Competent hockey players understand their strengths and weaknesses in relation to the demands that they face. They are aware of how quickly they can skate, how accurately they can shoot the puck, and how precisely they can pass the puck to their teammates. Such metacognitive knowledge is very important, as it allows them to select an appropriate skill required at a given time based on their metacognitive knowledge of their own performance capabilities and their conceptual knowledge of the perceived demands of the task. More importantly, in performance situations, this knowledge may prevent them from choosing a skill or set of skills that they cannot effectively execute and might lead only to poor execution and an advantage for their opponents. From another perspective, metacognitive knowledge of their affective knowledge base allows them to assess how confident or unconfident they might be in a given situation. Such feelings of sport confidence will depend on a variety of factors. However, the metacognitive awareness of one's emotional and attitudinal state is an important aspect of motor development that has often been overlooked (Bandura 1997; Deci and Ryan 1985).

Metacognitive Skills

Metacognitive skills are viewed as a higher-level form of procedural knowledge as they represent the executive processes involved in the monitoring, planning, and evaluating of skilled action. Metacognitive skills are especially important in the selection and planning of goal-directed behaviors; as such, they concern the allocation of attentional resources and personal effort that are so important in the learning and development process. With sufficient practice, in many time-constrained sport situations, procedural knowledge, whether it is at the response execution level or at the metacognitive skill level of planning and predicting, often becomes so well learned that it can be used relatively automatically. Hence, it is often no longer possible to access and describe such knowledge in declarative terms; that is, it becomes tacit. Nevertheless, there are many occasions in physical activity and sport settings when self-regulatory processes are verbally accessible, and they are of fundamental importance in the learning and performance of motor skills (Bouffard and Dunn 1993; Downey, Neil, and Rapagna 1996; Ferrari 1996; Glaser 1996).

As athletes become more competent, they use highly adaptive problem-solving and planning strategies to monitor and control their own performance, learning, and development. For instance, to use a swimming example, elite swimmers may choose to hold their breath while finishing the last few meters of a close race. In fact, many coaches believe that the effective and efficient use of metacognitive skills may well be the most important feature that distinguishes elite athletes from their less skilled peers. The bidirectional arrow between metacognitive knowledge and metacognitive skills in figure 13.1 emphasizes the close relationship between these two elements and the interaction that is assumed to take place between them. In other words, the model contends that knowing and doing are different but intricately connected. Knowing may lead to doing, and doing leads to knowing at a basic level. Yet at the meta-level, it is the individual's flexibility in linking performance with the different types of knowledge in the appropriate context(s) that is vital to the development and refinement of highly proficient fundamental movement skills, specialized skills, and sport expertise.

Combining the KB and ETA Approaches

With this information in hand, our purpose in this section is to describe similarities and differences between the KB approach and ETA from the perspectives of assessment and instruction. The two approaches have quite different theoretical orientations, but the models are similar in practice since the importance of person, task, and environment factors is embedded in each framework. Assessment and instruction are theorized to function in an iterative fashion rather than a simple "assessment precedes learning" model. Moreover, both approaches and respective interventions focus on the specific needs of each individual learner. There is a common emphasis on problem solving in context, since physical activities are considered to be goal directed. Thus, the self-regulation of learning and performance are important end products shared by the two schools of thought. In general, the two approaches share a number of instructional similarities. Yet at a deeper level of understanding, there are substantial differences regarding how each framework portrays the development of expertise, with definite practical implications. For example, while ETA places considerable importance on individual structural constraints to explain development, knowledge-based viewpoints emphasize acquisition and refinement of various types of knowledge about action. Moreover, KB also emphasizes the importance of developmentally appropriate experience and practice; hence, three increasingly more demanding environments are described, namely, instructional, practice, and competitive. Perhaps the addition of these three environments to ETA might further enhance the guidance it provides to instructors.

In 1986, Wall examined the influence of knowledge differences on the skill acquisition process. That article noted the effect of expert–novice differences on the learning of different types of tasks while stressing a central principle, that "task difficulty must always be viewed from the perspective of the individual learner" (p. 43). In addition, it was suggested that special attention be paid to how learners view the chances of success or failure before attempting to perform a given task. If learners feel that a task is within their capabilities, they will usually view it as a skill task that, by definition, is to some extent subject to their control. However, if learners' subjective expectancies for success in a task are low, they will probably view the task as a chance task, that is, one they can have little control over. In this regard, Smith (1978) noted the important role that instructors play by adjusting the difficulty of a task; as he aptly put it, "[By] simplifying the skill-to-be-learned we not only make it more understandable but we may redefine it as a skill task that is subject to learner control, rather than a chance task in which the learner feels relatively helpless" (p. 11). On the basis of these observations, Wall (1986) called for a careful analysis of the task to be learned in relation to the developmental level of the learner and recommended that during the skill learning process the following types of questions be posed: Does the task require mainly perceptual, cognitive, or response-loaded processing? Is it to be learned in a closed or open environment? Where will it ultimately be used, in a competitive, stressful, or cooperative environment? (p. 44)

Context

Given the importance of practice in the developmental skill learning process, it is not surprising that the KB approach, like ETA, places considerable emphasis on the nature of the learning environment and its effect on the learner. Thus, inherent in KB assessment and instruction is the recognition that environments can differ enormously in social pressure and performance expectations. For example, consider the increasing performance demands that would be placed on the learner in three progressively more challenging environments: instructional, practice, and competitive.

Instructional environments are defined as relatively closed, supportive environments in which developmentally appropriate instruction and feedback are provided. Such instructional learning environments are typically found in physical education class settings where ample practice opportunities are provided with progressively more difficult tasks and environmental conditions. For example, in these settings, novice learners can practice basic skills with peers or with a small group under minimal social pressure, with sufficient time to organize their initial attempts at performing the new skills. In less demanding environments, the less physically skilled learner has the opportunity to practice and acquire sufficient skill proficiency to participate in more demanding settings and may do so with considerable enjoyment, but this same person may become overwhelmed when asked to participate in a 5-on-5 lead-up game in a practice environment during a physical education class at school.

A practice setting is a more demanding learning environment; by definition it is a controlled environment that emphasizes proper execution of specific skills under increasingly more demanding spatial and temporal constraints as established by the instructor or leader of the practice session. Typically, the performance demands within a given practice setting are controlled through determination of the number of players involved, the roles they must play, the equipment used, and the space provided for them. Lead-up games and practice drills are examples of this more demanding learning environment. Even in this relatively controlled practice setting there is greater emphasis on successful individual performance than in an instructional environment, because the team has some interest in winning, and the required skills must be executed with speed in an ever-changing environment.

The performance expectations in competitive environments, that is, age-appropriate or recreational settings in which individuals or teams compete against each other, can range from relatively simple to very demanding if the participants are at the elite level for a particular age group. In competitive environments, there may be the additional stress of watchful and evaluative fans and of outcomes, which may have implications for social prestige and peer acceptance. The instructional, practice, and competitive environments can be viewed as a continuum; seeing them in this way underscores the need to recognize and assess the performance capabilities of learners in different performance environments.

Task Goal

An instructor using ETA may suggest that skilled human movement emerges from the complex interaction between an individual's multiple dynamic systems, the task, and the environment. As such, the end product of successful goal-directed activity is more important than the movement skill(s) chosen to complete the goal itself. In the first two steps of the ETA applied model, a movement goal is established, followed by observation of how the individual attempts to achieve the goal. Instructor challenges or intentional cues enter the learning equation only after observation of the individual attempting to solve the task goal. An instructor from the KB approach would be inclined to suggest that human movement develops with increases in specific knowledge and experience. As noted earlier, instruction would focus on the development and refinement of specialized skills that are relevant in a given environmental context. Hence, the instructor would assume that certain specific movement patterns would be more suitable for a person to learn given the goals of the movement context. For example, one of the main sport-specific goals in hockey is to shoot the puck and score into your opponent's net so that your team may win the game. A variety of shots may be used (e.g., slap shot, wrist shot, backhand), and the instructor would focus teaching and learning on these specific skills. As already noted, relevant declarative and procedural knowledge is initially taught in a closed instructional learning environment.

Thus, instructional environments can involve activities ranging from deliberate practice of selected skills in a noncompetitive atmosphere to the incorporation of these skills in more open, competitive contexts. In other words, with time and increases in developmental skill level, the learner is introduced to increasingly challenging situations including practice and competitive environments. Moreover, in these increasingly difficult contexts, the learner is challenged not only to perform the skills to be learned but also to evaluate their effectiveness in relation to the goals of each situation. The KB approach is therefore quite comfortable with identifying typical movement patterns for learners and providing a host of challenging tasks that promote domain-specific practice and experience. As the learner practices and is encouraged to problem solve, unique movement solutions for that individual, influenced by personal constraints and the environment, will become apparent and accepted.

Individual

From a KB perspective, it is assumed that highly proficient movers will most likely have acquired better specialized skills and more extensive knowledge structures than their less proficient counterparts. A basic premise of the KB approach is that people are assumed to be more proficient in some skills than in others, depending on the activities in which they have been participating. Quite simply, depending on his or her developmental history, someone can be an excellent swimmer but not be very competent in ice hockey. Since theories of expertise underlie the KB approach, it is assumed that highly proficient movers will most likely have acquired better specialized skills and more extensive knowledge structures than their less proficient counterparts. It is important to underscore that as proficiency and knowledge of specific skills within a sport develop, this does not mean that performers are limited only to the use of those specific skills. Rather, they have access to a variety of skilled responses that can be used to meet the task demands in a given situation. Put simply, increases in expertise result in greater flexibility of relevant responses from which to choose.

Expert–novice research shows that achieving excellence in a sport usually requires approximately 10,000 hours or 10 years of sustained practice (Ericsson 1996, 2003). While the process of developing expertise has not been fully explored, we suggest that skill proficiency progresses from initial, or novice, performance levels to mature, or expert, performance levels over time and with experience. Therefore, the process of skill proficiency can be observed as a continuum from novice to expert performance levels. For example, less proficiently skilled individuals are expected to possess superficial knowledge about the performance environment and its constraints. In fact, there can be considerable differences in the quality and quantity of knowledge that is related to the various aspects of skilled action.

For example, a person may have minimal knowledge of particular task constraints and related goals. These performers would be assumed to have less extensive knowledge about their own physical constraints in relation to the types of movement strategies that might be useful when they are solving different physical activity problems. Given their lack of experience and knowledge, we would not expect less skilled performers to be aware of their strengths and weaknesses. Also, these novice movers would not be expected to effectively self-regulate actions in relation to the constraints of the task and performance environment. Given that the performers are not highly competent movers, they may well experience some difficulties in the control of their emotions when attempting to complete goal-directed activities.

Therefore, the essence of assessment from a KB viewpoint would be to identify specific strengths and weaknesses of each learner. From a more general perspective, a domain, that is, a circumscribed area of knowledge or action, may be viewed from a variety of perspectives. For example, knowledge can be acquired related to fundamental skills such as object control and locomotor skills, or sport-specific skills such as golf or basketball skills. Most norm-referenced and criterion-referenced tests are not comprehensive enough to capture the depth of required knowledge and skill within a domain and the manner in which the specific individual interacts with it. The strengths and weaknesses of an individual go much beyond physical proficiency and include movement confidence, knowledge of task constraints, self-regulation, and so on.

Even if we restrict our focus to physical proficiency of a youngster in the skill of catching, assessment guided by the KB view would insist that catching with balls of different sizes, from varying distances, and with different speeds is necessary; this is similar indeed to what would occur with ETA. But again, expertise is much more complex than simple physical proficiency. Hence, a comprehensive assessment of catching might include a checklist of questions to ascertain declarative knowledge of task constraints that influence catching (e.g., impact of trajectories, ball size), movement confidence (e.g., how successful will you be in catching a ball when the teacher throws it, when a peer throws it?), or knowledge of personal constraints (e.g., I have to get into the open to catch a ball in a game in particular because I am shorter than my peers). Instruments of this type should be developed, as they could be of value to many instructors. Most importantly, effective instructors know that they should approach learners who have rather negative feelings of physical self-efficacy in a more careful and considerate manner than with those who demonstrate high levels of confidence due to acquired physical proficiency. Similarly, athletes who have developed a strong initial conceptual understanding of the rules, strategies, and tactics of a given sport along with enhanced physical proficiency can be taught the finer aspects of a sport much more easily than those who have a more limited declarative and procedural knowledge base.

Individualizing Evaluation

Given the preceding observations, it is clear that the instructor can evaluate and instruct individual movers based on each learner's strengths and weaknesses in both skill proficiency and knowledge. Inasmuch as individuals may choose different methods of solving movement problems, the teacher can help guide individuals to refine their skills and knowledge about action in context. Instructors can also help each person to recognize the task, environment, and physical constraints that are unique to that person. For example, in baseball, an overhand throw would seem to be the most logical skill for a second baseman to use to throw a runner out at first base. However, the infielder may be more comfortable throwing sidearm and may adopt that particular movement pattern for the majority of baseballs hit in her or his direction. The learner would be encouraged to spend more time in deliberate skill practice to fine-tune the automaticity of the action.

Moreover, the instructor is able to observe many skill performances and provide specific individual feedback to increase the efficiency of the skill being performed in either practice or performance environments. Also, the learner is taught to continually evaluate the effectiveness of the skill in relation to contextual and environmental demands. For example, a performer with low physical skill proficiency might be encouraged to understand where his or her solution to a movement situation fell short (e.g., did not apply enough force on an overhand throw and did not throw the runner out at first base). On the other hand, a highly skilled performer might be encouraged to preplan for certain hitters by changing his or her position on the field in relation to the hitter (e.g., closer or farther away) at certain times in the game (e.g., no one on base, no outs in the top of the first inning; or bases loaded, two outs in the bottom of the ninth inning). Thus, evaluation is individualized, dependent on skill level, and domain specific knowledge.

We could also apply the notion of specificity to each physical activity instructor who teaches physical activity and sport, as each would be expected to possess different levels of teaching skill and knowledge. Instructional strategies and program effectiveness would be dependent on the strengths and weaknesses of each teacher and his or her unique relationship with each student. Thus, the process of developing movement skill expertise can be quite complex, as it is influenced by a host of factors. The KB model takes a holistic approach to understanding how movement expertise develops for each person and how each instructor teaches it. Therefore, we suggest that a reflective instructor will attempt to understand his or her strengths and weaknesses in teaching physical activity while at the same time trying to recognize and plan for the specific strengths and weaknesses of each and every learner.

Self-Regulation and Personal Empowerment

Finally, and perhaps most importantly, if one of the major aims of physical educators is to empower our students and encourage them to make wise decisions regarding their involvement in physical activity, then it surely follows that learners should be encouraged to develop their metacognitive knowledge and skills. Quite simply, being aware of one's strengths and weaknesses so that one is able to recognize when instructional support is needed, as well as choose activities that are within one's capabilities, seems very important, especially if we wish to encourage our students to pursue a lifetime of active living. Thus, during the learning process, the learner or performer is guided by the instructor to find creative and innovative ways to solve movement problems in context.

Encouraging students to take increasing control over their own learning and performance, and ultimately their own motor development, requires that we place increasing emphasis on the use of self-regulatory skills so that our students can manage their own learning and performance in an effective and efficient manner. Therefore, students should be encouraged to establish realistic learning goals, monitor their progress, and engage in self-evaluation as they move toward the goal. The ultimate instructional outcome is the creation of self-regulated learners and proficient performers. Thus, the relationship between a performer and a physical education teacher or coach is expected to develop and change over time. For example, it is assumed that the novice performer may require specific feedback and encouragement when faced with specific learning challenges. With time and experience, performance variability decreases, but the learner will still benefit from the external assistance of teachers and coaches. However, with further increases in expertise, the performer is expected to become a more proficient mover who is personally aware of and increasingly self-regulates his or her own learning and performance.

By combining the KB model with the ETA model, we may come to the best of both worlds. An increased appreciation of the importance of the knowledge base acquired with development may be of interest to those who take an ecological perspective, especially those who are interested in the manipulation of task and environmental variables to enhance instruction and learning. Given the clarity with which the ETA describes and explains the role of tasks and different learning and performance environments, it may be useful for those employing ETA principles to consider how the learner thinks about the challenges he or she faces in different environments. By recognizing these developmental differences in the person, professionals employing ETA may well be able to structure even more appropriate learning experiences.

At the same time, those who have adopted a KB approach will surely benefit from the insights into task and situational variables generated from research based on an ecological perspective. One has unique opportunities to gain important knowledge about learning and development by noting the assessment and instructional similarities and differences inherent in the ETA and KB models. In turn, professionals from both perspectives may better serve their students given a comprehensive understanding of the complex relationships between the variables of the person, task, and environment.

INSTRUCTIONAL STRATEGIES

- Physical activity instructors should develop a thorough understanding of each learner and their specific knowledge bases.
- Instructional settings and teaching–learning strategies should be designed on the KB needs of the learner.
- Physical activity instructors should promote an understanding of the activity's goal in relation to the task goals.
- The role of emotion in physical activity should be recognized, especially when providing student feedback.
- Physical activity teachers should use language carefully, and delivery of feedback is essential for mastery learning experiences.

Summary

This chapter began with a consideration of the differences in basic assumptions underlying the ETA and KB approaches and the guidance that an understanding of them might provide with regard to instruction and assessment in physical activity. The KB approach was then described, along with evidence from a variety of studies that support the importance of the development of affective, declarative, and procedural knowledge as well as of metacognitive knowledge and metacognitive skills, including self-awareness and self-regulation in movement development.

The next section examined the interface between the ETA and KB approaches. The fact that both models include the importance of the person–task–environment interaction is highlighted. Most importantly, each model places great emphasis on meeting the individual needs of the learner. At the same time, it is also recognized that both approaches underscore the important role played by problem solving in the acquisition of physical proficiency. While there is a considerable amount of agreement between the two approaches to instruction and assessment, the KB approach places greater emphasis on the developmental level of the learner and especially the role that affective and metacognitive factors play in the learning process.

To highlight the interface between the two approaches, the three major ETA variables of context, task goal, and the individual were addressed. The discussion of context dealt with the effects of learning in instructional, practice, and competitive environments by individuals who are at different developmental levels. Viewing performance environments from instructional, practice, and competitive perspectives may well lead to a deeper understanding of the person–task–environment interaction that is so central to the ETA model. Nevertheless, the clear conclusion of this discussion is that the learning and performance context must be appropriate to the developmental level of the learner as both approaches so clearly advise.

The discussion of task goal factors noted the emphasis placed on goal-directed activity by the ETA model and the role in the learning process played by the interaction between the individual and changes in the environment. In contrast, in the KB approach the instructor plays a more directive role, especially in the initial phases of learning, in terms of the selection of the skills to be learned and the application of relevant skill cues during practice within a closed instructional environment.

With regard to the individual, the KB approach underscores a developmental continuum that ranges from novice to expert performance that is accompanied by increases in all five types of knowledge about action. A key point within the KB approach is that physical proficiency is not related simply to the physical skills or procedural aspects of performance; rather, as expertise increases, knowledge related to affective, declarative, and metacognitive factors is also developed. Being aware of the increases in such knowledge might well be important to an instructor whether he or she is using an ETA or KB approach. It is especially important for instructors to recognize the influences of affective factors on the willingness of an individual to participate in a given physical activity environment or maintain an interest in practicing a set of skills.

The chapter ended with a discussion of self-regulation and personal empowerment. The KB approach places significant emphasis on the role of personal agency and the importance of encouraging learners to take control of their learning and performance. It is perhaps this emphasis on the growth of self-awareness in relation to the different types of knowledge about action that might be of most interest to instructors who are using ETA with their students. In a sense, as individuals become more proficient in certain contexts while performing goal-related tasks, they are acquiring relevant knowledge about the context, task goals, and themselves, which is at the heart of the approaches that have been considered in this chapter.

EPILOGUE

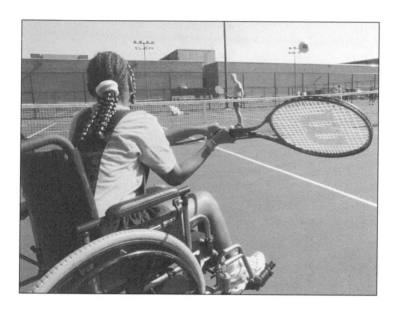

The question of where we might go from here is the challenge we put to the readers, because we believe that the significance of the book lies not only in the individual chapters that provide advancements to the ETA model, but also in the overall message delivered by the book. The ETA model embraces and promotes the revolutionary spirit of James Gibson (Reed and Jones 1979), the belief that transformations are required within each level—philosophy, theory, and research and practice—and in every setting from leisure and sport to education and work. The transformation visualized is from authoritarian models to empowerment models. Therefore choice, as one of the central components of the ETA applied model, is viewed not simply as a teaching strategy. Rather, choice is seen in its broadest ramifications whose importance has become considerably magnified in a society that on the one hand believes itself to be a democracy and on the other hand accepts with little question its largely authoritarian nature. From this perspective, empowering students in learning settings and participants in research settings, as well as students and scientists in universities, becomes part of a broader effort to bring about real democracy. This is the broader challenge we hope readers will accept.

Advances in Theory and Research

Theoretical challenges will always arise, as the nature of science is such that when one puzzle or conflict is solved, several more are posed. As Newell and Jordan (chapter 1) rightly point out, one of the important theoretical questions to be addressed is the status of task in the constraints model relative to the general ecological approach initiated by James J. Gibson and advanced by Michael T. Turvey and many of his colleagues. While acknowledging the goal directedness of human behavior, ecological theorists have been content with the duality of the individual and environment or context. Newell added task to the actor and context in his constraints model and thus aligned more with the theorizing of the cognitive symbolic approaches to action. Burton and Davis provided a variation to Newell's view of task by singling out and emphasizing the goal aspect of task.

How do goals, beliefs, and knowledge fit with the actor and environment? Are they to be given the same ontological status? Theorizing in ecological psychology can no longer avoid a confrontation with the issue of consciousness—the ultimate observer of the human drama. Recent theorizing in quantum physics may hold some of the keys to answering these important theoretical questions while simultaneously presenting new challenges to some of ecological psychology's currently held philosophical assumptions (e.g., Laszlo 2004). Most notable is the quantum physics challenge to Turvey's (1992) materialist ontology. For example, radical theorizing in quantum physics suggests that consciousness rather than matter may be the driving force in the universe and beyond (e.g., Goswami 2000). Thus, a belief in the constructive powers of the mind as advocated in cognitive psychology should not be dismissed by theorists of the ecological psychology persuasion.

Likewise, research is a never-ending endeavor if knowledge, understanding, and applications are to be advanced. We believe that the ETA model provides a solid foundation for efficacious methods of research. Research paradigms consistent with the ETA approach are discussed by Davis and Van Emmerik (1995b), but that book has not received wide circulation, especially in the United States. These paradigms were described in the Prologue as the study of how various subjects choose affordances; the use of intrinsic measures to identify the optimal and critical (phase transitions) points in performance; identification and measurement of higher-order variables; and the study of changes in movement coordination, stability, and variability in various populations. These paradigms are briefly described in this book, and examples are presented (chapters 4 and 5). We believe that it is largely a matter of promoting these paradigms to researchers, and we hold out the hope that this book contributes in this way. Research within the ETA framework includes both basic and applied emphases. Of course ETA philosophy stresses the functionality and application of science in general.

Advances in Application

The majority of chapters in this book are decidedly applied in their focus. As in research, we believe that the foundation for practice has been laid but not taken up by many persons in the field of movement. The issue of why this is the current status is addressed by some chapters. Nevertheless, numerous issues present themselves as challenges. It is far more exciting and beneficial to deal with questions and with what is unknown than to rest on any kind of certainty, false or otherwise. Taking context seriously puts one squarely into the social world where politics resides. Of course scientists as well as teachers must face the challenge of creating more democratic conditions in which decision-making responsibilities involve everyone. We hope that notions of empowerment and responsibility are taken to a deeper and more meaningful level within education and society. Expected outcomes are more inclusive settings and greater cooperation between groups and between individuals within groups. Likewise we would like to see the infusion of knowledge and information about people with disabilities into the educational curricula as a natural part of what everyone, not just specialists, learns. We want ETA to promote connection and unity rather than separation.

One important area for applied researchers and practitioners to explore is the categorization and description of skills, sports, and games. Burton and Davis began the processes with their general (functional) task categories. Davis and Strand add a modified version of the classification of games used in the Tactical Games model. Numerous games, sports, and other activities including cooperative games remain unanalyzed from this functional approach. Wall and his colleagues (chapter 13) add learning environments to the discussion.

Included in this classification should be a strong move away from terminology such as the "proper" or "correct" movement forms, which are value judgments. We suggest that functional descriptions of the movement form and the outcomes are more useful and more accurate. This is in keeping with the ETA belief that there is no one best way; movement form and outcomes are determined by goals, context, and individual constraints that are continually changing. We believe that this change in language is more than discarding what seems like innocuous terminology. Rather, it is a change in beliefs, attitudes, and perspectives leading to different actions. Functional and more precise descriptive language helps decrease the separation between scientists and practitioners as well as between labeled populations and their teachers, therapists, and coaches.

We believe this book will make a very significant contribution to spreading the practice of empowerment teaching, coaching, and treatment. To fully develop and realize empowerment models and practices, we believe that it is necessary to challenge the systems of rank ordering and credentialing and licensing. These are to be challenged in both education and society at large. We stress the intrinsic value of discovering, practicing, learning, and teaching and we challenge readers to join our revolutionary and evolutionary efforts. Methods and strategies for replacing authoritarian practices with empowerment models such as ETA will emerge as more people become convinced of the benefits to be realized.

Thus, we hope this book becomes a valuable resource for those who visualize, or desire to visualize, human movement in the broadest of contexts. We look forward to hearing and reading the reactions of those who examine this book, just as we look forward to the ETA model being used in a variety of ways in philosophy, theory, research, and practice. We anticipate with great relish the chance that the ETA theoretical and applied models can be agents for change. If this collection of papers validates, inspires, or challenges readers in some way, then we have achieved our purpose of honoring Allen W. Burton, who validated, inspired, and challenged us.

Walter E. Davis, PhD

Geoffrey D. Broadhead, PhD

REFERENCES

The numbers in square brackets following each reference indicate the chapters in which the reference is cited.

Abernethy, B. 1988. The effects of age and expertise upon perceptual skill development in a racket sport. *Research Quarterly for Exercise and Sport* 59: 210-221. [13]

Abernethy, B. 1990. Anticipation in squash: Differences in advance cue utilization between expert and novice players. *Journal of Sport Sciences* 8: 17-34. [13]

Abernethy, B., and D.G. Russell. 1987. Expert-novice differences in an applied selective attention task. *Journal of Sport Psychology* 9: 326-345. [13]

Abraham, R.H., and C.D. Shaw. 1982. *Dynamics: The geometry of behavior (part 1).* Santa Cruz, CA: Aerial Press. [1, 5]

Adams, J.A. 1971. A closed-loop theory of motor learning. *Journal of Motor Behavior* 3: 111-150. [1, 9]

Adolph, K.E., M.A. Eppler, and E.J. Gibson. 1993. Crawling versus walking infants' perception of affordances for locomotion over sloping surfaces. *Child Development* 64: 1158-1174. [4]

Alexander, R.M. 1984. Walking and running. *American Scientist* 72: 348-354. [9]

Alexander, R.M. 1992. *Exploring biomechanics: Animals in locomotion.* New York: Scientific American Library. [9]

Allard, F., and N. Burnett. 1985. Skill in sport. *Canadian Journal of Psychology* 39: 294-312. [13]

Almond, L. 1986. Reflecting on themes: A games classification. In: R. Thorpe, D. Bunker, and L. Almond (Eds.), *Rethinking games teaching* (pp. 71-72). Loughborough, England: University of Technology. [8]

Anderson, J.R. 1990. *Cognitive psychology and its implications* (3rd ed.). New York: Freeman. [13]

Angulo-Kinzler, R.M., B. Ulrich, and E. Thelen. 2002. Three-month old infants can select specific motor solutions. *Motor Control* 6: 52-68. [1]

Arai, S.M. 1997. Empowerment: From the theoretical to the personal. *Journal of Leisurability* 24(1): 3-11. [6]

Arnold, J.C. 2000. *Why forgive?* Farmington, PA: Plough. [3]

Arnold, P.J. 1997. *Sport, ethics and education.* London: Cassell. [3]

Auerbach, J.S. 1983. *Justice without law?* New York: Oxford University Press. [3]

Australian Sports Commission. 1997. *Games sense: Developing thinking players: A presenter's guide and workbook.* Canberra: Australian Sports Commission. [6]

Ayres, J. 1972. *Sensory integration and learning disorders.* Los Angeles: Western Psychological Services. [11]

Badke, M.B., and R.P. DiFabio. 1990. Facilitation: New theoretical perspective and clinical approach. In: J.V. Basmajian and S.L. Wolfe (Eds.), *Therapeutic exercise* (5th ed., pp. 77-91). Baltimore: Williams & Wilkins. [11]

Balan, C.M., and W.E. Davis. 1993. Ecological task analysis approach to instruction in physical education. *Journal of Physical Education, Recreation and Dance* 64(9): 54-61. [3, 7, 10, 11]

Bandura, A. 1982. Self-efficacy mechanism in human agency. *American Psychologist* 37: 122-147. [13]

Bandura, A. 1986. *Social foundations of thought and action: A social cognitive theory.* Englewood Cliffs, NJ: Prentice-Hall. [13]

Bandura, A. 1993. Perceived self-efficacy in cognitive development and functioning. *Educational Psychologist* 28: 117-148. [11]

Bandura, A. 1997. *Self-efficacy: The exercise of control.* New York: Freeman. [13]

Bannerman, D.J., J.B. Sheldon, J.A. Sherman, and A.E. Harchik. 1990. Balancing the right to habilitation with the right to personal liberties: The rights of people with developmental disabilities to eat too many doughnuts and take a nap. *Journal of Applied Behavior Analysis* 23: 79-89. [10]

Barrow, C.W. 1990. *Universities and the capitalist state: Corporate liberalism and the reconstruction of American higher education, 1894-1928.* Madison, WI: University of Wisconsin Press. [3]

Beak, S., K. Davids, and S. Bennett. 2002. Children's sensitivity to haptic information in perceiving affordances of tennis rackets for striking a ball. *Motor Development: Research and Reviews* 2: 120-141. [4]

Becher, J., and L.F. Douwes Dekker. 1997. Interventie onderzoek bij kinderen met cerebrale parese [Intervention research in children with cerebral palsy]. In: A. Vermeer and G.J. Lankhorst (Eds.), *Kinderen met cerebrale parese: Motorische ontwikkeling en behandeling* [Children with cerebral palsy: Their motor development and treatment] (pp. 171-180). Bussum: Coutinho. [12]

Beek, P.J., and M.T. Turvey. 1992. Temporal patterning in cascade juggling. *Journal of Experimental Psychology: Human Perception and Performance* 18: 934-947. [3]

Benello, C.G. 1981. Technology and power: Technique as a mode of understanding modernity. In: C.G. Christians and J.M. Van Hook (Eds.), *Jacques Ellul: Interpretive essays* (pp. 91-107). Urbana, IL: University of Illinois Press. [3]

Berk, R.A. 1976. Effects of choice of instructional methods on verbal learning tasks. *Psychological Reports* 38: 867-870. [3, 11]

Berkowitz, R.J. 1996. A practitioner's journey from skill to tactics. *Journal of Physical Education, Recreation and Dance* 67(4): 44-45. [8]

Bernstein, N. 1967. *The co-ordination and regulation of movements.* New York: Pergamon. [1, 2, 11]

Bernstein, N.A. 1996. On dexterity and its development. In: M.L. Latash and M.T. Turvey (Eds.), *Dexterity and its development* (pp. 3-244). Mahwah, NJ: Erlbaum. [2, 11]

Beyth-Maron, R., B. Fischhoff, J. Quadrel, and L. Furby. 1991. Teaching decision-making to adolescents: A critical review. In: J. Baron and R.V. Brown (Eds.), *Teaching decision making to adolescents* (pp. 19-59). Hillsdale, NJ: Erlbaum. [10]

Bhaskar, R. 1980. Scientific explanation and human emancipation. *Radical Philosophy* 26: 17-28. [3]

Bhaskar, R. 1989. *Reclaiming reality: A critical introduction to contemporary philosophy.* New York: Verso. [3]

Bhaskar, R. 1993. *Dialectic: The pulse of freedom.* Cambridge, MA: Blackwell. [3]

Bhreathnach, E., and H. Gogarty. 2000. The hero's journey, bridging the inner and outer world of the child. *Book of Proceedings IFCO European Foster Care Conference Ireland* 40-54. [11]

Block, M.E. 1993. Can children with mild mental retardation perceive affordances for action? *Adapted Physical Activity* 10: 137-145. [4]

Block, M.E. 2000. *A teacher's guide to including children with disabilities into general physical education* (2nd ed.). Baltimore: Brookes. [9]

Block, M.E. 2002. Developmental trends in perceiving affordances: A preliminary investigation of jumping distances. *Motor Development: Research and Reviews* 2: 142-161. [4]

Block, M., B. Oberweiser, and M. Bain. 1995. Using classwide peer tutoring to facilitate inclusion of students with disabilities in regular physical education. *Physical Educator* 52: 47-56. [10]

Block, M.E., S. Provis, and E. Nelson. 1994. Accommodating students with severe disabilities in regular physical education: Extending traditional skill stations. *Palaestra* 10(1): 32-35. [9]

Bloom, S.L., and M. Reichert. 1998. *Bearing witness: Violence and collective responsibility.* New York: Haworth Press. [3]

Blum, W. 1995. *Killing hope: U.S. military and CIA interventions since World War II.* Monroe, MI: Common Courage Press. [3]

Blum, W. 2000. *Rogue state: A guide to the world's only superpower.* Monroe, MI: Common Courage Press. [3]

Blumenfield, P.C., and R.W. Marx. 1997. Motivation and cognition. In: H.J. Walberg and G.D. Haertel (Eds.), *Psychology and educational practice* (pp. 79-106). Berkeley, CA: McCutchan. [7]

Bobath, K., and B. Bobath. 1965. *Abnormal postural reflex activity caused by brain lesions.* London: Heinemann. [11]

Booth, K. 1983. An introduction to netball. *Bulletin of Physical Education* 19 (1): 27-31. [8]

Bouchard, C., R. Malina, and L. Perusse. 1997. *Genetics of fitness and physical performance.* Champaign, IL: Human Kinetics. [13]

Bouffard, M., and J.G.H. Dunn. 1993. Children's self-regulated learning of movement sequences. *Research Quarterly for Exercise and Sport* 64(4): 393-403. [13]

Bouffard, M., W.B. Strean, and W.E. Davis. 1998. Questioning our philosophical and methodological research assumptions: Psychological perspectives. *Adapted Physical Activity Quarterly* 15: 250-268. [7]

Bouffard, M., and A.E. Wall. 1991. Knowledge, decision making, and performance in table tennis by educable mentally handicapped adolescents. *Adapted Physical Activity Quarterly* 8: 57-90. [3]

Boxill, J. 2003. Introduction: The moral significance of sport. In: J. Boxill (Ed.), *Sport ethics: An anthology* (pp. 1-12). Malden, MA: Blackwell. [6]

Breggin, P.R., and D. Cohen. 1999. *Your drug may be your problem: How and why to stop taking psychiatric medications.* Cambridge, MA: Perseus. [3]

Brigham, T.A. 1979. Some effects of choice on academic performance. In: L.C. Perlmutter and R.A. Monty (Eds.), *Choice and perceived control* (pp. 131-142). Hillsdale, NJ: Erlbaum. [10]

Brooks, J., and M. Brooks. 1993. *In search of understanding: The case for constructivist classrooms.* Arlington, VA: ASCD. [7]

Brophy, J. 1981. Teacher praise: A functional analysis. *Review of Educational Research* 51: 5-32. [3]

Brophy, J.E., and T.L. Good. 1986. Teacher behavior and student achievement. In: M.C. Wittrock (Ed.), *Handbook of research on teaching* (3rd ed., pp. 328-375). New York: Macmillan. [7]

Brown, A.L. 1984. Metacognition, executive control, self-regulation, and other even more mysterious mechanisms. In: F.E. Weinert and R.H. Kluwe (Eds.), *Metacognition, motivation, and learning* (pp. 60-108). Stuttgart, West Germany: Kuhlhammer. [13]

Brown, F. 1996. Self-determination and young children. *Journal of the Association for Persons With Severe Disabilities* 21: 22-30. [10]

Brown, J. 1989. *Teaching tennis: Steps to success.* Champaign, IL: Leisure Press. [9]

Bruininks, R.H. 1978. *Bruininks-Oseretsky test of motor proficiency.* Circle Pines, MN: American Guidance Service. [4]

Bruner, J.S. 1973. Organization of early skilled action. *Child Development* 44: 1-11. [1]

Bruner, J. 1983. *Child's talk.* New York: Norton. [13]

Bruner, J. 1986. *Actual minds, possible worlds.* Cambridge, MA: Harvard University Press. [13]

Brunnstrom, S. 1966. Motor testing procedures in hemiplegia: Based on sequential recovery stages. *Physical Therapy* 46: 357-375. [11]

Bulger, S., J.S. Townsend, and L.M. Carson. 2001. Promoting responsible student decision-making in elementary physical education. *Journal of Physical Education, Recreation and Dance* 7: 18-23. [7, 10]

Bull, R., and R.S. Johnston. 1997. Children's arithmetical difficulties: Contributions from processing speed, item identification, and short-term memory. *Journal of Experimental Child Psychology* 65: 1-24. [4]

Bullock, C., and M. Mahon. 1992. Decision making in leisure empowerment for people with mental retardation. *Journal of Physical Education, Recreation and Dance,* October: 12-16. [10]

Bundy, A.C., S.J. Lane, and E.A. Murray. 2002. *Sensory integration, theory and practice* (2nd ed.). Philadelphia: Davis. [11]

Bundy, A.C., and E.A. Murray. 2002. Sensory integration: A. Jean Ayres' theory revisited. In: A.C. Bundy, S.J. Lane, and E.A. Murray, (Eds.), *Sensory integration, theory and practice* (2nd ed., pp. 3-33). Philadelphia: Davis. [11]

Bunker, D., and R. Thorpe. 1982. A model for the teaching of games in secondary schools. *Bulletin of Physical Education* 18: 5-8. [8]

Burrows, L. 1986. A teacher's reactions. In: R. Thorpe, D. Bunker, and L. Almond (Eds.), *Rethinking games teaching* (pp. 45-52). Loughborough: University of Technology. [8]

Burton, A.W. 1990. Assessing the perceptual-motor interaction in developmentally disabled and nonhandicapped children. *Adapted Physical Activity Quarterly* 7: 325-337. [4]

Burton, A.W., and W.E. Davis. 1992. Optimizing the involvement and performance of children with physical impairments in movement activities. *Pediatric Exercise Science* 4: 236-248. [Prologue, 1, 3, 10, 11]

Burton, A.W., and W.E. Davis. 1996. Ecological task analysis utilizing intrinsic measures in research and practice. *Human Movement Science* 15: 285-314. [Prologue, Intro Part I, 1, 4-7, 9-11]

Burton, A.W., N.L. Greer, and D.M. Wiese-Bjornstal. 1993. Variations in grasping and throwing patterns as a function of ball size. *Pediatric Exercise Science* 5: 25-41. [9, 10]

Butler, C. 1986. Effects of powered mobility on self-initiated behaviors of very young children with locomotor disabilities. *Developmental Medical Child Neurology* 28: 325-332. [11]

Butler, C. 1991. Pediatric rehabilitation. In: K.M. Jaffe (Ed.), *Physical medicine and rehabilitation clinics of North America* (pp. 801-816). Philadelphia: Saunders. [11]

Butler, J. 1997. How would Socrates teach games? A constructivist approach. *Journal of Physical Education* 68(8): 42-47. [6]

Calvin, W.H. 1990. *The cerebral symphony.* New York: Basic Books. [13]

Calvin, W.H. 1996. *The cerebral code.* Cambridge, MA: MIT Press. [13]

Canadian Association for Health, Physical Education, Recreation and Dance (CAHPERD). 1994. *Active living through physical education: Maximizing opportunities for students with multiple disabilities* (pp. 1-146). Ottawa: Health Canada. [10]

Capra, F. 1998. Evolution: The old view and the new view. In: D. Loye (Ed.), *The evolutionary outrider: The impact of the human agent on evolution: Essays honouring Ervin Laszlo* (pp. 39-47). Westport, CT: Praeger. [3]

Carello, C., A. Grosofsky, F.D. Reichel, H.W. Solomon, et al. 1989. Visually perceiving what is reachable. *Ecological Psychology* 1: 27-54. [4]

Carr, J.H., and R.B. Shepherd. 1987. A motor learning model for rehabilitation. In: J.H. Carr, R.B. Shepherd, J. Gordon, A.M. Gentile, and J.M. Held (Eds.), *Movement science: Foundation for physical therapy in rehabilitation* (pp. 31-91). Rockville, MD: Aspen. [11]

Carron, A.V., and P.W. Dennis. 1998. The sport team as an effective group. In: J.M. Williams (Ed.), *Applied sport psychology: Personal growth to peak performance.* Mountain View, CA: Mayfield. [6]

Center for Active Learning and Empowerment. 2004. Adaptip: The support service for Adapted Physical Activity. Retrieved on August 30, 2004 from www.adaptip .com. [9]

Cesari, P., and K.M. Newell. 1999. The scaling of human grip configurations. *Journal of Experimental Psychology: Human Perception and Performance* 25: 927-935. [1]

Chen, D., and R.N. Singer. 1992. Self-regulation and cognitive strategies in sport participation. *International Journal of Sport Psychology* 23: 277-300. [11]

Chiesi, H.L., G.J. Spilich, and J.F. Voss. 1979. Acquisition of domain-related information in relation to high and low domain knowledge. *Journal of Verbal Learning and Behavior* 18: 257-274. [13]

Chorover, S.L. 1979. *From genesis to genocide: The meaning of human nature and the power of behavior control.* Cambridge, MA: MIT Press. [3]

Cicchetti, D., and D. Tucker. 1994. Development and self-regulation structures of the mind. *Development and Psychopathology* 6: 533-549. [12]

Clark, J.E. 1995. On becoming skillful: Patterns and constraints. *Research Quarterly for Exercise and Sport* 66(3): 173-184. [9]

Clark, J.E. 1997. A dynamical systems perspective on the development of complex adaptive skill. In: C. Dent-Read and P. Zukow-Goldring (Eds.), *Evolving explanations of development: Ecological approaches to organism-environment systems* (pp. 383-406). Washington, DC: APA. [11]

Clark, J.E., and S.J. Phillips. 1993. A longitudinal study of inter-limb coordination in the first year of independent walking. *Child Development* 64: 1143-1157. [9]

Collins, J.J., and C.J. De Luca. 1995. Upright, correlated random walks: A statistical-biomechanics approach to the human postural control system. *Chaos* 5: 57-63. [2]

Collins, J.J., C.J. De Luca, A. Burrows, and L.A. Lipsitz. 1995. Age-related changes in open-loop and closed-loop postural control mechanisms. *Experimental Brain Research* 104: 480-492. [2]

Collins, J.J., T.T. Imhoff, and P. Grigg. 1996. Noise-enhanced tactile sensation. *Nature* 383: 770. [2]

Condon, R., and C. Collier. 2002. Student choice makes a difference in physical education. *Journal of Health, Physical Education, Recreation, and Dance* 73(2): 26-30. [7]

Cook, F.J. 1962. *The warfare state.* New York: Macmillan. [3]

Corbetta, D., and B. Vereijken. 1999. Understanding development and learning of motor coordination in sport: The contribution of Dynamic Systems Theory. *International Journal of Sport Psychology* 30: 507-530. [11]

Corbin, C.B. 1994. The fitness curriculum: Climbing the stairway to lifetime fitness. In: R.R. Pate and R.C. Hohn (Eds.), *Health and fitness through physical education* (pp. 59-66). Champaign, IL: Human Kinetics. [7]

Corcos, D.M. 1991. Strategies underlying the control of disordered movement. *Physical Therapy* 71: 25-38. [11]

Cross, N., and J. Lyle. 1999. *The coaching process: Principles and practice for sport.* London: Butterworth Heineman. [6]

Crossley, R., and A. McDonald. 1980. *Annie's coming out.* New York: Penguin. [3]

Crutchfield, J.P., J.D. Farmer, N.H. Packard, and R.S. Shaw. 1987. Chaos. *Scientific American* 254(2): 46-57. [5]

Csikszentmihalyi, M. 1975. *Beyond boredom and anxiety.* San Francisco: Jossey-Bass. [11]

Damasio, A. 1999. *The feeling of what happens.* New York: Harcourt. [13]

Dattilo, J., and L.A. Barnett. 1985. Therapeutic recreation for individuals with severe handicaps: An analysis of the relationship between choice and pleasure. *Therapeutic Recreation Journal* 19(3): 79-91. [10]

Dattilo, J., and F.R. Rusch. 1985. Effects of choice on leisure participation for persons with severe handicaps. *Journal of the Association for Persons with Severe Handicaps* 10: 194-199. [3, 10]

Davidson, R.J. 1994. Asymmetric brain function, affective style, and psychopathology: The role of early experience and plasticity. *Development and Psychopathology* 6: 741-758. [11]

Davis, W.E., and A.W. Burton. 1991. Ecological task analysis: Translating movement theory into practice. *Adapted Physical Activity Quarterly* 8: 154-177. [Prologue, 1-12]

Davis, W.E., and T. Chandler. 1998. Beyond Boyer's scholarship reconsidered: Fundamental change in university and socioeconomic systems. *Journal of Higher Education* 69: 23-64. [3]

Davis, W.E., and J. Klingler. 2001/2004. Movement and leisure skills program: On-campus teaching lab manual. Kent State University. [Unpublished]. [Prologue, 10]

Davis, W.E., and T.L. Rizzo. 1991. Issues in classification of motor disorders. *Adapted Physical Activity Quarterly* 8: 280-304. [9]

Davis, W.E., and R.E.A. Van Emmerik. 1995a. An ecological task analysis approach for understanding motor development in mental retardation: Philosophical and theoretical underpinnings. In: A. Vermeer and W.E. Davis (Eds.), *Physical and motor development in persons with mental retardation.* Medicine and Sport Science Series (pp. 1-32). Basel: Karger. [3, 11]

Davis, W.E., and R.E.A. Van Emmerik. 1995b. An ecological task analysis approach for understanding motor development in mental retardation: Research questions and strategies. In: A. Vermeer and W.E. Davis (Eds.), *Physical and motor development in persons with mental retardation.* Medicine and Sport Science Series (pp. 33-63). Basel: Karger. [Prologue, 5, 11, 12, Epilogue]

Deci, E.L. 1975. *Intrinsic motivation.* New York: Plenum Press. [11]

Deci, E.L. 1980. *The psychology of self-determination.* Toronto: Lexington Books. [3]

Deci, E.L., and R.M. Ryan. 1985. *Intrinsic motivation and self-determination in human behavior.* New York: Plenum Press. [3, 13]

Deci, E.L., and R.M. Ryan. 1991. A motivational approach to self: Integration in personality. In: R. Diensbier (Ed.), *Nebraska symposium on motivation:* Vol. 38. *Perspectives on motivation* (pp. 237-288). New York: Plenum Press. [3]

Deci, E.L., R.J. Vallerand, L.G. Pelletier, and R.M. Ryan. 1991. Motivation and education: The self-determination perspective. *Educational Psychologist* 26: 325-346. [3]

Delin, C.R., and R.F. Baumeister. 1994. Praise: More than just social reinforcement. *Journal for the Theory of Social Behaviour* 24: 219-241. [3]

Derryberry, D., and M.A. Reed. 1994. Temperament and self-organization of personality. *Development and Psychopathology* 6: 653-676. [12]

Derryberry, D., and M.A. Reed. 1996. Regulatory processes and the development of cognitive representations. *Development and Psychopathology* 8: 215-234. [11]

Diedrich, F.J., and W.H. Warren. 1995. Why change gaits? Dynamics of the walk to run transition. *Journal of Experimental Psychology: Human Perception and Performance* 21: 183-201. [2, 4]

Dingwell, J.B., J.P. Cusumano, P.R. Cavanagh, and D. Sternad. 2001. Local dynamic stability versus kinematic variability of continuous overground and treadmill walking. *Journal of Biomechanical Engineering* 123: 27-32. [2]

Downey, P.J., G. Neil, and S. Rapagna. 1996. Evaluating modeling effects in dance. *Impulse* 4: 48-64. [13]

Drinnon, R. 1997. *Facing west: The metaphysics of Indian-hating and empire-building.* Norman, OK: University of Oklahoma Press. [3]

Dromeric, A.W., D.F. Edwards, and M. Hahn. 2000. Does the application of constraint-induced movement therapy during acute rehabilitation reduce arm impairment after ischemic stroke? *Stroke* 31: 2984-2988. [9]

Duff, A. 1996. Punishment, citizenship and responsibility. In: H. Tam (Ed.), *Punishment, excuses and moral development* (pp. 17-34). Aldershot, England: Avebury. [3]

Dunlap, G., M. dePerczel, S. Clarke, D. Wilson, S. Wright, R. White, and A. Gomez. 1994. Choice making to promote adaptive behavior for students with emotional and behavioral challenges. *Journal of Applied Behavior Analysis* 27: 505-518. [10]

Dunn, W. 1999. *Sensory profile: User's manual.* San Antonio, TX: Psychological Corporation. [11]

Dyer, K., G. Dunlap, and V. Winterling. 1990. Effects of choice making on the serious problem behaviors of students with severe handicaps. *Journal of Applied Behavioral Analysis* 23: 515-524. [3, 10]

Eckhardt, R.B. 2000. *Human paleobiology.* Cambridge: Cambridge University Press. [1]

Edelman, G.M., and G. Tononi. 2000. *A universe of consciousness.* New York: Basic Books. [13]

Edwards, P.N. 1996. *The closed world: Computers and politics of discourse in Cold War America.* Cambridge, MA: MIT Press. [3]

Eisler, R. 1987. *The chalice and the blade: Our history, our future.* San Francisco: Harper & Row. [3]

Ellul, J. 1967. *The technological society* (trans. J. Wilkinson). New York: Knopf. [3]

Epstein, S. 1994. Integration of the cognitive and the psychodynamic. *American Psychologist* 49: 709-724. [3]

Ericsson, K.A. 1996. *The road to excellence: The acquisition of expert performance in the arts and sciences, sports, and games.* Mahwah, NJ: Erlbaum. [13]

Ericsson, K.A. 2003. Development of elite performance and deliberate practice: An update from the perspective of the expert performance approach. In: J.L. Starkes and K.A. Ericsson (Eds.), *Expert performance in sports* (pp. 49-83). Champaign, IL: Human Kinetics. [13]

Erlhagen, W., and G. Schöner. 2002. Dynamic field theory of movement preparation. *Psychological Review* 109: 545-572. [1]

Eskes, T.B., M.C. Duncan, and E.M. Miller. 1998. The discourse of empowerment: Foucault, Marcuse and the women's fitness texts. *Journal of Sport and Social Issues* 23(3): 317-344. [6]

Facoetti, A., M.L. Lorusso, P. Paganoni, C. Cattaneo, R. Galli, C. Umilta, and G.G. Mascetti. 2003. Auditory and visual automatic attention deficits in developmental dyslexia. *Brain Research* 16: 185-191. [4]

Ferrari, M. 1996. Observing the observer: Self-regulation in the observational learning of motor skills. *Developmental Review* 16: 203-240. [13]

Ferrel-Chapus, C., L. Hay, I. Olivier, C. Bard, and M. Fleury. 2002. Visuomanual coordination in childhood: Adaptation to visual distortion. *Experimental Brain Research* 144: 506-517. [4]

Fetz, F., and B. Jaeger. 1995. Development of throwing accuracy. *Sportonomics* 1(1): 17-26. [5]

Fitch, H.L., and M.T. Turvey. 1977. On the control of activity: Some remarks from an ecological point of view. In: D.M. Landers and R.W. Christina (Eds.), *Psychology of motor behavior and sport* (pp. 3-35). Champaign, IL: Human Kinetics. [3]

Flavell, J.H. 1979. Metacognition and cognitive monitoring: A new era of cognitive-developmental inquiry. *American Psychologist* 34: 906-911. [13]

Fleishman, E.A., and M.K. Quaintance. 1984. *Taxonomies of human performance.* New York: Academic Press. [1]

Floor, L., and M. Rosen. 1975. Investigating the phenomenon of helplessness in mentally retarded adults. *American Journal of Mental Deficiency* 79: 565-572. [3]

Fodor, J.A., and Z.W. Pylyshyn. 1981. How direct is visual perception: Some reflections on Gibson's "ecological approach." *Cognition* 9: 139-196. [13]

Fogel, A. 1990. The process of developmental change in infant communicative action: Using dynamic systems theory to study individual ontogenies. In: J. Colombo and J. Fagan (Eds.), *Individual differences in infancy* (pp. 341-358). Hillsdale, NJ: Erlbaum. [12]

Foster, J.B. 2001. Imperialism and "empire." *Monthly Review* 53: 1-9. [3]

Fredericks, H.D.B. 1980. *The teaching research curriculum for moderately and severely handicapped: Gross and fine motor.* Springfield, IL: Charles C Thomas. [10]

French, K., J. Rink, L. Rikard, A. Mays, S. Lynn, and P. Werner. 1991. The effect of practice progressions on learning two volleyball skills. *Journal of Teaching in Physical Education* 10: 261-275. [7]

French, K.E., J.H. Spurgeon, and M.E. Nevett. 1995. Expert-novice differences in cognitive and skill execution components of youth baseball performance. *Research Quarterly for Exercise and Sport* 66: 194-201. [13]

French, K.E., and J.R. Thomas. 1987. The relation of knowledge development to children's basketball performance. *Journal of Sport Psychology* 9: 15-32. [8, 13]

Freysinger, V., and L.A. Bedini. 1994. Teaching for empowerment. *Schole: A Journal of Leisure Studies and Recreational Education* 9: 1-11. [6]

Full, R. 2000. Biomotion: Mystery of motion. Why do animals change gait? http://polypedal.berkeley.edu/ib32/Lectures/gaitfolder/index.htm. [9]

Full, R.J., and D.E. Koditschek. 1999. Templates and anchors: Neuromechanical hypotheses of legged locomotion on land. *Journal of Experimental Biology* 202: 3325-3332. [9]

Gabbard, C. 1998. Considering handedness in studies involving manual control. *Motor Control* 2: 81-93. [5]

Gabel, A., and U.S.L. Nayak. 1984. The effect of age on variability in gait. *Journal of Gerontology* 39: 662-666. [2]

Gallahue, D.L., and F.C. Donnelly. 2003. *Developmental physical education for all children* (4th ed.). Champaign, IL: Human Kinetics. [7]

Gallahue, D.L., and J.C. Ozmun. 2002. *Understanding motor development: Infants, children, adolescents, adults* (5th ed.). Boston: McGraw-Hill. [11]

Gardner, H. 1987. *The mind's new science: A history of the cognitive revolution.* New York: Basic Books. [13]

Gatto, J.T. 1992. *Dumbing us down: The hidden curriculum of compulsory schooling.* Philadelphia: New Society. [3]

Gazzaniga, M.S. 1999. What are brains for? In: R.L. Solso (Ed.), *Mind and brain sciences in the 21st century* (pp. 157-171). Cambridge, MA: MIT Press. [13]

Gelfand, I.M., and M.L. Tsetlin. 1971. Mathematical modeling of mechanisms of the central nervous system. In: I.M. Gelfand, V.S. Gurfinkel, S.V. Fomin, and M.L. Tsetlin (Eds.), *Models of the structural-functional organization of certain biological systems* (pp. 1-27). Cambridge, MA: MIT Press. [2]

Gelinas, J., and G. Reid. 2000. The developmental validity of traditional learn-to-swim progressions for children with physical disabilities. *Adapted Physical Activity Quarterly* 17(3): 269-285. [10]

Gentile, A.M. 2000. Skill acquisition: Action, movement, and neuromotor processes. In: J. Carr and R.B. Shepherd (Eds.), *Movement science: Foundations for physical therapy in rehabilitation* (2nd ed., pp. 111-187). Gaithersburg, MD: Aspen. [11]

Gesell, A. 1933. Maturation and the patterning of behavior. In: C. Murchison (Ed.), *A handbook of child psychology* (2nd ed., pp. 209-235). Worcester, MA: Clark University Press. [11]

Getchell, N., and J. Whitall. 2003. Examining motor coordination in children with learning disabilities: Do children without perceptual motor difficulties show coordination differences? Presented at the Association of University Centers for Disabilities annual meeting and conference, Bethesda, MD, November. [4]

Getchell, N., and J. Whitall. 2004. Transitions to and from asymmetric gait patterns. *Journal of Motor Behavior* 36: 13-27. [4]

Gibson, E.J. 1982. The concept of affordance in development: The renascence of functionalism. In: W.A. Collins (Ed.), *The concept of development: The Minnesota symposia on child psychology* (Vol. 15, pp. 55-81). Hillsdale, NJ: Erlbaum. [4]

Gibson, E.J. 1988. Exploratory behavior in the development of perceiving, acting, and the acquiring of knowledge. *Annual Review of Psychology* 39: 1-41. [12]

Gibson, E.J., and M.S. Schmuckler. 1989. Going somewhere: An ecological and experimental approach to development of mobility. *Ecological Psychology* 1: 3-25. [4]

Gibson, J.J. 1966. *The senses considered as perceptual systems.* Boston: Houghton Mifflin. [2, 4]

Gibson, J.J. 1977. The theory of affordances. In: R.E. Shaw and J. Bransford (Eds.), *Perceiving, acting and knowing: Toward an ecological psychology* (pp. 67-82). Hillsdale, NJ: Erlbaum. [5]

Gibson, J.J. 1979. *An ecological approach to visual perception.* Boston: Houghton Mifflin. [Prologue, 1, 3, 5, 13]

Giddens, A. 1984. *The constitution of society: Outline of the theory of structuration.* Cambridge: Polity Press. [3, 6]

Giddens, A. 1993. *New rules of sociological method* (2nd ed.). Cambridge: Polity Press. [3]

Gilmore, G. 1977. *The ages of American law.* New Haven: Yale University Press. [3]

Ginott, H.G. 1972. *Teacher and child: A book for parents and teachers.* New York: Macmillan. [6].

Glaser, R. 1996. Changing the agency of learning: Acquiring expert performance. In: K.A. Ericsson (Ed.), *The road to excellence: The acquisition of expert performance in the arts and sciences, sports, and games* (pp. 303-312). Mahwah, NJ: Erlbaum. [13]

Glass, D.C., and J.E. Singer. 1972. *Urban stress: Experiments on noise and social stressors.* New York: Academic Press. [3]

Glass, L. 2001. Synchronization and rhythmic processes in physiology. *Nature* 410: 277-284. [2]

Glass, L., and M.C. Mackey. 1988. *From clocks to chaos: The rhythms of life.* Princeton, NJ: Princeton University Press. [2]

Glausier, S.R., J.E. Whorton, and H.V. Knight. 1995. Recreation and leisure likes/dislikes of senior citizens with mental retardation. *Activities, Adaptations, and Aging* 19(3): 43-54. [10]

Gmünder, F. 2003. Swimming technique: Drill to learn wavelike swimming (short axis rotation). Schwimmverein Limmat Zurich. www.svl.ch. [9]

Goodway, J.D., M. Rudisill, and N. Valentini. 2002. The influence of instruction on the development of catching in young children. In: J.E. Clark and J.H. Humphrey (Eds.), *Motor development: Research and reviews* (Vol. 2, pp. 96-119). Reston, VA: NASPE. [7]

Goodwin, D.L. 2001. The meaning of help in PE: Perceptions of students with disabilities. *Adapted Physical Activity Quarterly* 18(3): 289-303. [10]

Gordon, J. 1987. Assumptions underlying physical therapy intervention: Theoretical and historical perspectives. In: J.H. Carr, R.B. Shepherd, J. Gordon et al. (Eds.), *Movement sciences: Foundations for physical therapy in rehabilitation* (pp. 1-30). Rockville, MD: Aspen. [11]

Goswami, A. 2000. *The visionary window: A quantum physicist's guide to enlightenment.* Wheaton, IL: Theosophical Publishing House. [Epilogue]

Gothelf, C.R., D.B. Crimmins, C.A. Mercer, and P.A. Finocchiaro. 1994. Teaching choice-making skills to students who are deaf-blind. *Teaching Exceptional Children* 26: 43-54. [10]

Gove, W.R. 1994. Why we do what we do: Biopsychosocial theory of human motivation. *Social Forces* 73: 363-394. [3]

Grace, M. 1999. When students create curriculum. *Educational Leadership* 57: 49-52. [7]

Graham, G. 2001. *Teaching children physical education: Becoming a master teacher* (2nd ed.). Champaign, IL: Human Kinetics. [7]

Graham, G., S.A. Holt-Hale, and M. Parker. 2001. *Children moving* (5th ed.). Mountain View, CA: Mayfield. [7]

Gravelle, D.C., C.A. Laughton, N.T. Dhruv, K.D. Katdare, J.B. Niemi, L.A. Lipsitz, and J.J. Collins. 2002. Noise-enhanced balance control in older adults. *NeuroReport* 13: 1853-1856. [2]

Greene, P.H. 1972. *Problems of organization of motor systems.* In: R. Rosen and R. Snell (Eds.), *Progress in theoretical biology* (pp. 304-338). New York: Academic Press. [1]

Greenspan, S.I. n.d. Research support for a comprehensive developmental approach to autistic spectrum disorders and other developmental and learning disorders: The Developmental, Individual Difference, Relationship-Based (DIR) Model. [Unpublished paper]. [11]

Greenspan, S.I., and S. Wieder. 1998. *The child with special needs: Encouraging intellectual and emotional growth.* Reading, MA: Perseus Books. [11]

Grehaigne, J.F., and P. Godbout. 1995. Tactical knowledge in team sports from a constructivist and cognitivist perspective. *Quest* 47: 490-505. [8]

Grehaigne, J.-F., P. Godbout, and D. Bouthier. 1997. Performance assessment in team sports. *Journal of Teaching in Physical Education* 16: 500-516. [13]

Gresham, F.M., M.E. Beebe, and D.L. MacMillan. 1999. A selective review of treatments for children with autism: Description and methodological considerations. *School Psychology Review* 28: 559-575. [11]

Gresham, F.M., and D.L. MacMillan. 1998. Early intervention project: Can its claims be substantiated and its effects replicated? *Journal of Autism and Developmental Disorders* 28: 5-13. [11]

Griffin, L.L., S.A. Mitchell, and J.L. Oslin. 1997. *Teaching sport concepts and skills: A tactical games approach.* Champaign, IL: Human Kinetics. [6, 7]

Griffin, L.L., J.J. Oslin, and S.A. Mitchell. 1995. Two instructional approaches to teaching net games. *Research Quarterly for Exercise and Sport* 66 (1): Suppl., 65-66. [8]

Groeneveld, H.J. 1999. Ecological Task Analysis as a model for the development of functional movement and sport skills of children with physical disabilities. Unpublished doctoral dissertation, Stellenbosch, RSA, University of Stellenbosch. [10]

Guckenheimer, J., and P. Holmes. 1983. *Nonlinear oscillations, dynamical systems, and bifurcations of vector fields.* New York: Springer-Verlag. [5]

Guess, D., H.A. Benson, and E. Siegel-Causey. 1985. Concepts and issues related to choice-making and autonomy among persons with severe disabilities. *Journal of the Association for Persons with Severe Handicaps* 10: 79-86. [3, 10]

Guess, D., and W. Sailor. 1993. Chaos theory and the study of human behavior: Implications for special education and developmental disabilities. *Journal of Special Education* 27: 16-34. [12]

Gutmann, A., and D. Thompson. 1999. Democratic disagreement. In: S. Macedo (Ed.), *Deliberative politics: Essays on democracy and disagreement* (pp. 243-279). New York: Oxford University Press. [3]

Haddad, J.M., J.L. Gagnon, C.J. Hasson, R.E. Van Emmerik, and J. Hamill. 2006. Evaluation of time-to-contact measures for assessing postural stability. *Journal of Applied Biomechanics.* 22(2):155-161. [2]

Haken, H. 1977. *Synergetics: An introduction.* Heidelberg: Springer-Verlag. [5]

Haken, H., J.A.S. Kelso, and H. Bunz. 1985. A theoretical model of phase transitions in human hand movements. *Biological Cybernetics* 51: 347-356. [1, 2]

Hamill, J., T.R. Derrick, and K.G. Holt. 1995. Shock attenuation and stride frequency during running. *Human Movement Science* 14: 45-60. [2]

Hamill, J., R.E.A. Van Emmerik, B.C. Heiderscheit, and L. Li. 1999. A dynamical systems approach to lower extremity running injuries. *Clinical Biomechanics* 14: 297-308. [2]

Hanin, Y.L. 1989. Interpersonal and intragroup anxiety: Conceptual and methodological issues. In: D. Hackfort and C.D. Spielberger (Eds.), *Anxiety in sports: An international perspective* (pp. 19-28). Washington, DC: Hemisphere. [11]

Hanson, J. 1993. *The decline of the American empire.* Westport, CT: Praeger. [3]

Harchik, A.E., J.A. Sherman, J.B. Sheldon, and D.J. Bannerman. 1993. Choice and control: New opportunities for people with developmental disabilities. *Annals of Clinical Psychiatry* 5: 151-162. [10]

Harlow, H.R. 1959. Learning set and error factor theory. In: S. Koch (Ed.), *Psychology: A study of a science* (pp. 492-533). New York: McGraw-Hill. [11]

Hausdorff, J.M., S.L. Mitchell, R. Firtion, C.K. Peng, M.E. Cudkowicz, J.Y. Wei, and A.L. Goldberger. 1997. Altered fractal dynamics of gait: Reduced stride-interval correlations with aging and Huntington's disease. *Journal of Applied Physiology: Respiratory, Environmental and Exercise Physiology* 82: 262-269. [2]

Hausdorff, J.M., L. Purdon, C.-K. Peng, Z. Ladin, J.Y. Wei, and A.L. Goldberger. 1996. Fractal dynamics of human gait: Stability of long-range correlations in stride interval fluctuations. *Journal of Applied Physiology* 80: 1448-1457. [2]

Haywood, K.M., and N. Getchell. 2005. *Life span motor development* (4th ed.). Champaign, IL: Human Kinetics. [7]

Heiderscheit, B.C. 2000. Movement variability as a clinical measure for locomotion. *Journal of Applied Biomechanics* 16: 419-427. [2]

Heiderscheit, B.C., J. Hamill, and R.E.A. Van Emmerik. 2002. Variability of stride characteristics and joint coordination among individuals with unilateral patellofemoral pain. *Journal of Applied Biomechanics* 18: 110-121. [2]

Herkowitz, J. 1978a. The design and evaluation of play spaces for children. In: M. Ridenour (Ed.), *Motor development: Issues and applications* (pp. 115-138). Princeton: Princeton Book Co. [7]

Herkowitz, J. 1978b. Developmental task analysis: The design of movement experiences and evaluation of motor development status. In: M. Ridenour (Ed.), *Motor development: Issues and applications* (pp. 139-164). Princeton: Princeton Book Co. [5, 7, 8, 10]

Hesse, S., M. Konrad, and D. Uhlenbrock. 1999. Treadmill walking with partial body weight support versus floor walking in hemiparetic subjects. *Archives of Physical Medicine and Rehabilitation* 80: 421-427. [9]

Hobson, R.P. 1990. On acquiring knowledge about people and the capacity to pretend: Response to Leslie. *Psychological Review* 97: 114-121. [3]

Hobson, R.P. 1993. The emotional origins of social understanding. *Philosophical Psychology* 6: 227-250. [3]

Holt, K.G., S.F. Jeng, R. Ratcliffe, and J. Hamill. 1995. Energy cost and stability during human walking at the preferred frequency. *Journal of Motor Behavior* 27: 164-178. [2]

Holt, K.G., J.P. Obusek, and S.T. Fonseca. 1996. Constraints on disordered locomotion: A dynamical systems perspective on spastic cerebral palsy. *Human Movement Science* 15: 177-202. [11]

Horak, F.B. 1992. Effects of neurological disorders on postural movement strategies in the elderly. In: B. Vellas, M. Toupet, L. Rubenstein, J.L. Albarede, and Y. Christen (Eds.), *Falls, balance and gait disorders in the elderly* (pp. 137-157). Paris: Elsevier. [11]

Horak, F.B., S.M. Henry, and A. Shumway-Cook. 1997. Postural perturbations: New insights for the treatment of balance disorders. *Physical Therapy* 77: 517-533. [2]

Housner, L.D. 1990. Selecting master teachers: Evidence from process-product research. *Journal of Teaching in Physical Education* 9: 201-226. [7]

Howe, M.J.A., J.W. Davidson, and J.A. Sloboda. 1998. Innate talents: Reality or myth? *Behavioral and Brain Sciences* 21: 399-442. [13]

Hresko, W.P., D.K. Reid, and D.D. Hammill. 1988. *Screening children for related early educational needs.* Austin, TX: Pro-Ed. [4]

Hurmuzlu, Y., C. Basdogan, and D. Stoianovici. 1996. Kinematic and dynamic stability of the locomotion of post-polio patients. *Journal of Biomechanical Engineering* 118: 405-411. [2]

Hutchinson, J.R., D. Famini, R. Lair, and R. Kram. 2003. Biomechanics: Are fast-moving elephants really running? *Nature* 422: 493-494. [2]

Hutzler, Y. 2004. *Include me: Examples for including children with disabilities in physical activity.* Ramat Gan: Ilan Sport Center for the Disabled [in Hebrew]. [9]

Hyman, I.A. 1990. *Reading, writing, and the hickory stick: The appalling story of physical and psychological abuse in American schools.* Lexington, MA: Lexington Books. [3]

Ikuenobe, P. 1998. Colonialism in Africa, culturally induced moral ignorance, and the scope of responsibility. *Journal for the Theory of Social Behaviour* 28: 109-128. [3]

Illich, I. 1971. *Deschooling society.* New York: Harper & Row. [3]

Janelle, C.M., D.A. Barba, S.G. Frehlich, L.K. Tennant, and J.H. Cauraugh. 1997. Maximizing performance feedback effectiveness through videotape replay and a self-controlled learning environment. *Research Quarterly for Exercise and Sport* 68: 269-279. [11]

Janelle, C.M., J. Kim, and R.N. Singer. 1995. Subject-controlled performance feedback and learning of a closed motor skill. *Perceptual Motor Skills* 81: 627-634. [11]

Janssen, J. 2002. *Championship team building.* Cary, NC: Winning the Mental Game. [6]

Jeng, S-F., H.G. Holt, L. Fetters, and C. Certo. 1996. Self-optimization of walking in nondisabled children and children with spastic hemiplegic cerebral palsy. *Journal of Motor Behavior* 28: 15-27. [2]

Johnson, C. 2000. *Blowback: The costs and consequences of American empire.* New York: Henry Holt. [3]

Jones, G.S. 1972. The history of US imperialism. In: R. Blackburn (Ed.), *Ideology and social science* (pp. 207-237). London: Fontana. [3]

Juarrero, A. 1999. *Dynamics in action.* Cambridge, MA: MIT Press. [1]

Kamm, K., E. Thelen, and J.L. Jensen. 1990. A dynamical systems approach to motor development. *Physical Therapy* 70: 763-775. [11]

Kantz, H., and T. Schreiber. 1997. *Nonlinear time series analysis.* Cambridge: Cambridge University Press. [2]

Keele, S.W. 1968. Movement control in skilled motor performance. *Psychological Bulletin* 70: 387-403. [1]

Keele, S.W. 1973. *Attention and human performance.* Pacific Palisades, CA: Goodyear. [11]

Kelly, L., J. Dagger, and J. Walkley. 1989. The effects of an assessment-based education program on motor skill development in preschool children. *Education and Treatment of Children* 12(2): 152-164. [7]

Kelso, J.A.S. 1984. Phase transitions and critical behavior human bimanual coordination. *American Journal of Physiology: Regulatory, Integrative and Comparative Physiology* 15: 1000-1004. [11]

Kelso, J.A.S. 1995. *Dynamic patterns: The self-organization of brain and behavior.* Cambridge, MA: MIT Press. [1-3, 11]

Kelso, J.A.S., K.G. Holt, P.N. Kugler, and M.T. Turvey. 1980. On the concept of coordinative structures as dissipative structures: I. Empirical lines of convergence. In: G. Stelmach and J. Requin (Eds.), *Tutorials in motor behavior* (pp. 49-70). Amsterdam: North-Holland. [11]

Kelso, J.A.S., J.P. Scholz, and G. Schöner. 1986. Nonequilibrium phase transitions in coordinated biological motion: Critical fluctuations. *Physics Letters* A134: 8-12. [2]

Kelso, J.A.S., and G.S. Schöner. 1988. Self-organization of coordinative movement patterns. *Human Movement Science* 7: 27-46. [11]

Keogh, J., and D. Sugden. 1985. *Movement skill development.* New York: Macmillan. [Prologue]

Kephart, N.C. 1971. *The slow learner in the classroom* (2nd ed.). Columbus, OH: Merrill. [Intro Part II]

Kern, L., C.M. Vorndran, A. Hilt, J.E. Ringdahl, B.E. Adelman, and G. Dunlap. 1998. Choice as an intervention to improve behavior: A review of the literature. *Journal of Behavioral Education* 8(2): 151-169. [10]

Ketelaar, M., A. Vermeer, H. 't Hart, E. Van Petegem-Van Beek, and P.J.M. Helders. 2001. The effects of a functional therapy program in children with cerebral palsy. *Physical Therapy* 81: 1534-1545. [12]

Kidman, L. 2001. *Developing decision makers: An empowerment approach to coaching.* Christchurch, NZ: Innovative Print Communications. [6]

Kidman, L. 2005. *Athlete-centred coaching: Developing inspired and inspiring people.* Christchurch, NZ: Innovative Print Communications. [6]

Kidman, L., and S.J. Hanrahan. 2004. *The coaching process: A practical guide to improving your effectiveness.* Palmerston North, NZ: Dunmore. [6]

Kishi, G., B. Teelucksingh, N. Zollers, S. Park-Lee, and L. Meyer. 1988. Daily decision-making in community residences: A social comparison of adults with and without mental retardation. *American Journal on Mental Retardation* 92(5): 430-435. [10]

Koehn, D. 1998. *Rethinking feminist ethics: Care, trust and empathy.* London: Routledge. [3]

Kohn, A. 1993. *Punished by rewards.* Boston: Houghton Mifflin. [3, 11]

Konczak, J. 1990. Toward an ecological theory of motor development: The relevance of the Gibsonian approach to vision for motor development research. *Advances in Motor Development Research* 3: 201-224. [4]

Konczak, J., P. Jansen-Osmann, and K.T. Kalveram. 2003. Development of force adaptation during childhood. *Journal of Motor Behavior* 35: 41-52. [4]

Konczak, J., H.J. Meeuwsen, and E.M. Cress. 1992. Changing affordances in stair climbing: How young adult and elderly women perceive maximum climbability. *Journal of Experimental Psychology: Human Perception and Performance* 18: 691-697. [4]

Koot, J.M. 1992. Agresssie en temperamentsstoornissen bij jonge kinderen [Aggression and emotional disorders in young children]. In: F.C. Verhulst and F. Verheij (Eds.), *Kinder-en jeugdpsychiatrie. Onderzoek en diagnostiek* [Child and youth psychiatry. Research and diagnostics] (pp. 551-521). Assen: Van Gorcum. [12]

Kugler, P.N., J.A.S. Kelso, and M.T. Turvey. 1980. On the concept of coordinative structures as dissipative structures: I. Theoretical lines of convergence. In: G.E. Stelmach and J. Requin (Eds.), *Tutorials in motor behavior* (pp. 1-49). New York: North-Holland. [1, 11]

Kugler, P.N., J.A.S. Kelso, and M.T. Turvey. 1982. On the control and coordination of naturally developing systems. In: J.A.S. Kelso and J.E. Clark (Eds.), *The development of movement control and co-ordination* (pp. 5-78). New York: Wiley. [1]

Kugler, P.N., and M.T. Turvey. 1987. *Information, natural law, and the self-assembly of rhythmic movement.* Hillsdale, NJ: Erlbaum. [Prologue, 1-3, 11]

Kuhn, T.S. 1996. *The structure of scientific revolutions* (3rd ed.). Chicago: University of Chicago Press. [1]

Lambeck, J., and F. Coffey Stanat. 2000. The Halliwick concept: Part 1. *Journal of Aquatic Physical Therapy* 8: 6-11. [9]

Lambeck, J., and F. Coffey Stanat. 2001. The Halliwick concept: Part 2. *Journal of Aquatic Physical Therapy* 9: 7-12. [9]

Langer, E.J., and S. Saegert. 1977. Crowding and cognitive control. *Journal of Personality and Social Psychology* 35: 175-182. [3]

Laszlo, E. 2004. *Science and the Akashic field: Integral theory of everything.* Rochester, VT: Inner Traditions. [Epilogue]

Latash, M.L., J.P. Scholz, and G. Schöner. 2002. Motor control strategies revealed in the structure of motor variability. *Exercise and Sport Sciences Reviews* 30: 26-31. [2]

Launder, A.G. 2001. *Play practice: The games approach to teaching and coaching sports.* Champaign, IL: Human Kinetics. [6]

Lazarus, J.C. 1989. Factors underlying inefficient movement in learning disabled children. In: G. Reid (Ed.), *Problems in movement control* (pp. 1-42). Amsterdam: Elsevier Science. [4]

Lee, D.N. 1980. Visuo-motor coordination in space-time. In: G.E. Stelmach and J. Requin (Eds.), *Tutorials in motor behavior* (pp. 281-296). Amsterdam: North-Holland. [1]

Lee, D.N., and P.E. Reddish. 1981. Plummeting gannets: A paradigm for ecological optics. *Nature* 293: 293-294. [2]

Lee, T.D., and R.A. Magill. 1985. Can forgetting facilitate skill acquisition? In: D. Goodman, R.B. Wilberg, and I.M. Franks (Eds.), *Differing perspectives in motor learning, memory, and control* (pp. 3-21). Amsterdam: North-Holland. [11]

Lemke, M.R., T. Wendorff, B. Mieth, K. Buhl, and M. Linnemann. 2000. Spatiotemporal gait patterns during over ground locomotion in major depression compared with healthy controls. *Journal of Psychiatric Research* 34(4-5): 277-283. [9]

Lieberman, L., and C. Houston-Wilson. 2002. *Strategies for inclusion: A handbook for physical educators.* Champaign, IL: Human Kinetics. [9]

Liepert, J., H. Bauder, W.H.R. Miltner, E. Taub, and C. Weiller. 2000. Treatment-induced cortical reorganization after stroke in humans. *Stroke* 31: 1210-1216. [9]

Lipsitz, L.A. 2002. Dynamics of stability: The physiologic basis of functional health and frailty. *Journal of Gerontology A: Biological Sciences and Medical Sciences* 57: B115-125. [2]

Lipsitz, L.A., and A.L. Goldberger. 1992. Loss of "complexity" and aging. *Journal of the American Medical Association* 267: 1806-1809. [1]

Lishman, J.R., and D.N. Lee. 1973. The autonomy of visual kinaesthesis. *Perception* 2: 287-294. [2]

Liu, Y.M. 2001. Discussion on team culture. *Journal of Capital College of Physical Education* 13(1): 28-33, 60. [6]

Locke, J. 1690/1999. Legislative, executive, and federative powers. In: M. Rosen and J. Wolff (Eds.), *Political thought* (pp. 115-117). Oxford: Oxford University Press. [3]

Logan, G.D. 1985. Skill and automaticity: Relations, implications, and future directions. *Canadian Journal of Psychology* 39: 367-386. [13]

Lombardo, B.J. 1987. *The humanistic coach.* Springfield, IL: Charles C Thomas. [6]

Lovaas, O.I. 1987. Behavioral treatment and normal educational and intellectual functioning in young autistic children. *Journal of Consulting and Clinical Psychology* 55: 3-9. [11]

Lovaas, O.I. 1993. The development of a treatment-research project for developmentally disabled and autistic children. *Journal of Applied Behavioral Analysis* 26: 617-630. [11]

Lovelock, J.E. 2000. *Gaia, a new look at life on earth.* Oxford: Oxford University Press. [3]

Lovitt, T.C., and K. Curtis. 1969. Academic response rate as a function of teacher and self-imposed contingencies. *Journal of Applied Behavior Analysis* 2: 49-53. [11]

Lydon, M.C., and J.T.F. Cheffers. 1984. Decision-making in elementary school-age children: Effects upon motor learning and self-concept development. *Research Quarterly for Exercise and Sport* 55: 135-140. [7]

Lyle, J. 2002. *Sport coaching concepts: A framework for coaches' behaviour.* London: Routledge. [6]

Lynch, J. 2001. *Creative coaching: New ways to maximize athlete and team potential in all sports.* Champaign, IL: Human Kinetics. [6]

Magill, R.A. 2001. *Motor learning and control: Concepts and applications* (6th ed.). Boston: McGraw-Hill. [5, 9]

Maki, B.E., P.J. Holliday, and A.K. Topper. 1994. A prospective study of postural balance and risk of falling in an ambulatory and independent elderly population. *Journal of Gerontology* 49: M72-84. [2]

Manning, M.L. 2000. Child-centered middle schools: A position paper of the Association for Childhood Education International. *Childhood Education* 76: 154-159. [7]

Maraj, B.K. 2003. Perceptual judgments for stair climbing as a function of pitch angle. *Research Quarterly for Exercise and Sport* 74: 248-256. [4]

Maraj, B.K., and Domingue, J.A. 1999. Standing distance in climbability of stairs. *Perceptual Motor Skills* 88: 682-684. [4]

Marcus, G. 2004. *The birth of the mind.* New York: Basic Books. [1]

Mark, L.S., 1987. Eye-height scaled information about affordances: A study of sitting and stair climbing. *Journal of Experimental Psychology: Human Perception and Performance* 13: 361-370. [4]

Mark, L.S., and D. Vogele. 1987. A biodynamic basis for perceived categories of action: A study of sitting and stair climbing. *Journal of Motor Behavior* 19: 376-384. [4]

Marteniuk, R.G. 1976. *Information processing in motor skills.* New York: Holt, Rinehart & Winston. [11]

Martinek, T.J., L.D. Zaichkowsky, and J.T.F. Cheffers. 1977. Decision-making in elementary age children: Effects on motor skills and self-concept. *Research Quarterly* 48: 349-357. [7]

McBride, R.E. 1989. Teaching critical thinking in the psycho-motor learning environment: A possibility of a passing phase? *Physical Educator* 46: 170-173. [7]

McBride, R.E. 1999. If you structure it, they will learn: Critical thinking in physical education classes. *Clearing House* 72: 217-220. [7]

McBride, R.E., and R. Bonnette. 1995. Teacher and at-risk students' cognition during open-ended activities: Structuring the learning environment for critical thinking. *Teaching and Teacher Education* 11: 373-388. [7]

McCarthy, D. 1972. *McCarthy scales of children's abilities.* San Antonio, TX: Psychological Corporation. [4]

McCombs, B. 1989. Self-regulated learning and academic achievement: A phenomenological view. In: B.J. Zimmerman and D.H. Schunk (Eds.), *Self-regulated learning and academic achievement: Theory, research, and practice* (pp. 51-82). New York: Springer. [11]

McDermott, W.J., R.E.A. Van Emmerik, and J. Hamill. 2003. Running training and adaptive strategies of locomotor-respiratory coordination. *European Journal of Applied Physiology* 89: 435-444. [2]

McEachin, J.J., T. Smith, and O.I. Lovaas. 1993. Long term outcome for children with autism who received early intensive behavioral treatment. *American Journal of Mental Retardation* 97: 359-372. [11]

McGibbon, C.A., and D.E. Krebs. 2002. Age-related changes in lower trunk coordination and energy transfer during gait. *Journal of Neurophysiology* 85: 1923-1931. [2]

McGinnis, P.M., and K.M. Newell. 1982. Topological dynamics: A framework for describing movement and its constraints. *Human Movement Science* 1: 289-305. [1]

McGraw, M.B. 1943. *The neuromuscular maturation of the human infant.* New York: Columbia University Press. [11]

McNevin, N.H., G. Wulf, and C. Carlson. 2000. Effects of attentional focus, self-control, and dyad training on motor learning: Implications for physical rehabilitation. *Physical Therapy* 80: 373-385. [11]

McPherson, S.L. 1993. Knowledge representation and decision-making in sport. In: J.L. Starkes and F. Allard (Eds.), *Cognitive issues in motor expertise* (pp. 159-188). Amsterdam: Elsevier. [13]

McPherson, S.L., and J.R. Thomas. 1989. Relation of knowledge and performance in boys' tennis. *Journal of Sport and Exercise Psychology* 13: 26-41. [13]

Meeuwsen, H.J. 1991. Variables affecting perceptual boundaries in bipedal stair climbing. *Perceptual Motor Skills* 72: 539-43. [4]

Mentz, G., and S. Mentz. 1982. *Mit Andreas fangt alles an* [It started with Andreas]. Göttingen: Integrationssportverein Göttingen. [12]

Merzenich, M.M., and W.M. Jenkins. 1993. Cortical representation of learned behaviors (pp. 437-454). In P. Anderson (Ed.), *Memory concepts.* New York: Elsevier. [1]

Messier, S.P., and K.J. Cirillo. 1989. Effects of a verbal and visual feedback system on running technique, perceived exertion and running economy in female novice runners. *Journal of Sports Sciences* 7(2): 113-126. [9]

Metzler, M.W. 2000. *Instructional models for physical education.* Boston: Allyn & Bacon. [6, 8]

Meyer, L.H. 1991. Advocacy, research, and typical practices. In: L.H. Meyer, C.A. Peck, and L. Brown (Eds.), *Critical issues in the lives of people with severe disabilities* (pp. 629-649). Baltimore: Brookes. [10]

Michaels, C.F., and C. Carello. 1981. *Direct perception.* Englewood Cliffs, NJ: Prentice-Hall. [1]

Miller, L.J., J.E. Reisman, D.N. McIntosh, and J. Simon. 2001. An ecological model of sensory modulation: Performance of children with fragile X syndrome, autistic disorder, attention-deficit/hyperactivity disorder, and sensory modulation dysfunction. In: S.S. Roley, E.I. Blanche, and R.C. Schaaf (Eds.), *Understanding the nature of sensory integration with diverse populations* (pp. 57-88). San Antonio, TX: Therapy Skill Builders. [11]

Mischel, T. 1969. Scientific and philosophical psychology: A historical introduction. In: T. Mischel (Ed.), *Human action: Conceptual and empirical issues* (pp. 1-40). New York: Academic Press. [1]

Mitchell, S.L., J.J. Collins, C.J. De Luca, A. Burrows, and L.A. Lipsitz. 1995. Open-loop and closed-loop postural control mechanisms in Parkinson's disease: Increased medio-lateral activity during quiet standing. *Neuroscience Letters* 197: 133-136. [2]

Mitchell, S.A., L.L. Griffin, and J.L. Oslin. 1994. Tactical awareness as a developmentally appropriate focus for the teaching of games in elementary and secondary physical education. *Physical Educator* 51 (1): 21-28. [8]

Mitchell, S.A., J.L. Oslin, and L.L. Griffin. 2003. *Sport foundations for elementary physical education: A tactical games approach.* Champaign, IL: Human Kinetics. [8]

Mithaug, D.E. 1996. *Equal opportunity theory.* Thousand Oaks, CA: Sage. [3]

Mittenthal, J.E., and A.B. Baskin (Eds.). 1992. *The principles of organization in organisms.* Reading, MA: Addison-Wesley. [1]

Mobily, K.E. 1985. The ethical dilemma of freedom in therapeutic recreation. *Therapeutic Recreation Journal* 19(4): 22-30. [10]

Montessori, M. 1964. *The Montessori method.* New York: Schocken. [3]

Monty, R.A., E.S. Geller, R.E. Savage, and L.C. Perlmutter. 1979. The freedom to choose is not always so choice. *Journal of Experimental Psychology* 5(2): 170-178. [10]

Monty, R.A., and L.C. Perlmutter. 1987. Choice, control, and motivation in the young and aged. In: M.L. Maehr and D.A. Kleiber (Eds.), *Advances in motivation and achievement* (Vol. 5, pp. 99-122). Greenwich, CT: JAI. [3, 7]

Moos, R.H. 1981. Environmental choice and control in community care settings for older people. *Journal of Applied Social Psychology* 11: 23-43. [3]

Morya, E., R. Ranvaud, and W.M. Pinheiro. 2003. Dynamics of visual feedback in a laboratory simulation of a penalty kick. *Journal of Sports Sciences* 21(2): 87-95. [9]

Mulder, T. 1996. De geboren aanpasser. Ideeën over beweging, beweginsstoornissen en herstel [The born adaptor. Ideas about movement, movement disorders and recovery]. *De Psycholoog* 12: 458-462. [12]

Mulder, T., and J. Hochstenbach. 1997. Motor control and learning: Implications for neurological rehabilitation. In: R.J. Greenwood, M.P. Barnes, T.M. McMillan, and C.D. Ward (Eds.), *Neurological rehabilitation* (pp. 73-81). Hillsdale, NJ: Erlbaum. [12]

Mulder, T., B. Nienhuis, and J. Pauwels. 1996. Prediction of independent mobility following damage to the nervous system. In: B.W. Fries (Hrsg.), *Ambulante und teilstationäre Rehbilitation von Hirnverletzten* [Ambulant and partly institutional rehabilitation of individuals with brain damage] (pp. 52-60). München: W. Zuckschwerdt Verlag. [12]

Munk, D.D., and A.C. Repp. 1994. The relationship between instructional variables and problem behavior: A review. *Exceptional Children* 60(5): 390-401. [10]

Murray, M.P., R.C. Kory, and B.H. Clarkson. 1964. Walking patterns in healthy old men. *Journal of Gerontology* 24: 169-178. [2]

Neisser, U. 1976. *Cognition and reality.* San Francisco: Freeman. [13]

Neisser, U. 1984. Toward an ecologically oriented cognitive science. Emory Cognition Project, unpublished report 1. Atlanta. [13]

Neumayer, R., and M. Bleasdale. 1996. Personal lifestyle preferences of people with an intellectual disability. *Journal of Intellectual and Developmental Disability* 21(2): 91-114. [10]

Nevitt, M., I. Rovegno, and M. Babiarz. 2001. Fourth-grade children's knowledge of cutting, passing and tactics in invasion games after a 12-lesson unit of instruction. *Journal of Teaching in Physical Education* 20: 389-401. [8]

Newell, K.M. 1985. Coordination, control and skill. In: D. Goodman, R.B. Wilberg, and I.M. Franks (Eds.), *Differing perspectives in motor control* (pp. 295-317). Amsterdam: North-Holland. [3, 5]

Newell, K.M. 1986. Constraints on the development of coordination. In: M.G. Wade and H.T.A. Whiting (Eds.), *Motor development in children: Aspects of coordina-*

tion and control (pp. 341-360). Dordrecht: Martinus Nijhoff. [Prologue, Intro Part I, 1, 2, 4, 5, 7, 9, 11]

Newell, K.M. 1989. On task and theory specificity. *Journal of Motor Behavior* 21: 92-96. [1]

Newell, K.M. 1991. Motor skill acquisition. In: M.R. Rosenzweig, and L.W. Porter (Eds.), *Annual review of psychology* (Vol. 42, pp. 213-237). Palo Alto, CA: Annual Reviews. [1]

Newell, K.M. 1996. Change in movement and skill: Learning, retention, and transfer. In: M. Latash and M. Turvey (Eds.), *Dexterity and its development* (pp. 393-429). Hillsdale, NJ: Erlbaum. [1]

Newell, K.M. 2004. Schema theory 1975: Retrospectives and prospectives. *Research Quarterly for Exercise and Sport* 74: 383-388. [1]

Newell, K.M., M.P. Broderick, K.M. Deutsch, and A.B. Slifkin. 2003. Task goals and change in dynamical degrees of freedom with motor learning. *Journal of Experimental Psychology: Human Perception and Performance* 29: 379-387. [1, 2]

Newell, K.M., Y.T. Liu, and G. Mayer-Kress. 2001. Time scales in motor learning and development. *Psychological Review* 108: 57-82. [2]

Newell, K.M., Y.T. Liu, and G. Mayer-Kress. 2003. A dynamical systems interpretation of epigenetic landscapes for infant motor development. *Infant Development and Behavior* 26: 449-472. [1]

Newell, K.M., and P.V. McDonald. 1992. Practice: A search for task solutions. In: American Academy of Physical Education, *Enhancing human performance in sport: New concepts and developments* (pp. 51-59). Champaign, IL: Human Kinetics. [11]

Newell, K.M., P.V. McDonald, and R. Baillargeon. 1993. Body scale and infant grip configurations. *Developmental Psychobiology* 26: 195-205. [4, 11]

Newell, K.M., and P.M. McGinnis. 1985. Kinematic information feedback for skilled performance. *Human Learning* 4: 39-56. [1]

Newell, K.M., D.M. Scully, P.V. McDonald, and R. Baillargeon. 1989a. Task constraints and infant grip configurations. *Developmental Psychobiology* 22: 817-832. [1]

Newell, K.M., D.M. Scully, F. Tenenbaum, and S. Hardiman. 1989b. Body scale and the development of prehension. *Developmental Psychobiology* 22: 1-13. [4]

Newell, K.M., and D. Vaillancourt. 2001. Dimensional change in motor learning. *Human Movement Science* 4-5: 695-716. [1]

Newell, K.M., and J. Valvano. 1998. Therapeutic intervention as a constraint in learning and relearning movement skills. *Scandinavian Journal of Occupational Therapy* 5: 51-57. [1]

Newell, K.M., and R.E.A. Van Emmerik. 1990. Are Gesell's developmental principles general principles for the acquisition of coordination. In: J.E. Clark and J.H. Humphrey (Eds.), *Advances in motor development research* (Vol. 3, pp. 143-164). New York: AMS Press. [1]

Newell, K.M., R.E.A. Van Emmerik, D. Lee, and R.L. Sprague. 1993. On postural stability and variability. *Gait and Posture* 4: 225-230. [2]

Newton, J.S., R.H. Horner, and L. Lund. 1991. Honoring activity preferences in individualized plan development: A descriptive analysis. *Journal of the Association for Persons with Severe Handicaps* 16: 207-212. [3]

Nigg, B.M., and W. Herzog (Eds.). 1994. *Biomechanics of the musculo-skeletal system.* New York: Wiley. [1]

Ning, Z., A. Faro, D. Sue, and N. Hamilton. 1999. Kinesiological analysis of overarm throwing for accuracy with dominant and non-dominant arms. In: R.H. Sanders and B.J. Gibson (Eds.), *XVII International Symposium on Biomechanics in Sports* (pp. 37-41). Perth: Edith Cowan University. [5]

Noddings, N. 1984. *Caring: A feminine approach to ethics & moral education.* Berkeley: University of California Press. [3]

Norman, D.A., and T. Shallice. 1980. *Attention to action: Willed and automatic control of behaviour.* [Technical report]. San Diego: University of California, Center for Human Information Processing. [13]

Ophuls, W. 1997. *Requiem for modern politics: The tragedy of the enlightenment and the challenge of the new millennium.* Boulder, CO: Westview Press. [3]

Oslin, J., and S. Mitchell. 1998. Form follows function. *Journal of Physical Education, Recreation and Dance* 69(6): 46-49. [8]

Overmier, J.B., and M.E.P. Seligman. 1967. Effects of inescapable shock upon subsequent escape and avoidance learning. *Journal of Comparative and Physiological Psychology* 63: 23-33. [3]

Parenti, M. 1995. *Against empire: An expose of the brutal realities of U.S. global domination.* San Francisco: City Lights Books. [3]

Paris, C., and B. Combs. 2000. Teachers' perspectives on what it means to be learner-centered. Paper presented at the annual meeting of the American Educational Research Association, New Orleans. [7]

Parsons, M.B., V.N. Harper, J.M. Jensen, and D.H. Reid. 1997. Assisting older adults with severe disabilities in expressing leisure preferences: A protocol for determining choice-making skills. *Research in Developmental Disabilities* 18(2): 113-126. [10]

Parsons, M.B., J.E. McCarn, and D.H. Reid. 1993. Evaluating and increasing meal-related choices throughout a service setting for people with severe disabilities. *Journal of the Association for Persons with Severe Handicaps* 18: 253-260. [10]

Parsons, M.B., and D.H. Reid. 1990. Assessing food preferences among persons with profound mental retardation: Providing opportunities to make choice. *Journal of Applied Behavior Analysis* 23: 183-195. [10]

Pate, R.R., and R.C. Hohn. 1994. Introduction: A contemporary mission for physical education. In: R.R. Pate and R.C. Hohn (Eds.), *Health and fitness through physical education* (pp. 1-8). Champaign, IL: Human Kinetics. [7]

Paull, G., and D. Glencross. 1997. Expert perception and decision making in baseball. *International Journal of Sport Psychology* 28: 35-56. [13]

Perry, S.B. 1998. Clinical implications of a dynamic systems theory. *Neurology Report* 2: 4-10. [11]

Peters, B.T., J.M. Haddad, B.C. Heiderscheit, R.E.A. Van Emmerik, and J. Hamill. 2003. Limitations in the use and interpretation of continuous relative phase. *Journal of Biomechanics* 36: 271-274. [2]

Peterson, C., S.F. Maier, and M.E.P. Seligman. 1993. *Learned helplessness: A theory for the age of personal control.* New York: Oxford University Press. [3]

Piaget, J. 1952. *The origins of intelligence in children.* Madison, CT: International Universities Press, Inc. [11]

Piaget, J. 1956. *The child's conception of space.* London: Routledge and Kegan Paul. [13]

Piaget, J. 1970. Piaget's theory. In: P. Mussen, (Ed.), *Carmichael's manual of child psychology* (3rd ed., Vol. 1). New York: Wiley. [3]

Piek, J.P. 1998. *Motor behavior and human skill: A multidisciplinary approach.* Champaign, IL: Human Kinetics. [9]

Pigott, B. 1982. A psychological basis for new trends in games teaching. *Bulletin of Physical Education* 18(1): 17-22. [8]

Pihl, R.O., and R. Niauro. 1982. Learning disability: An ability to sustain attention. *Journal of Clinical Psychology* 38: 632-634. [4]

Plomin, R., and J.C. DeFries. 1998, May. The genetics of cognitive abilities and disabilities. *Scientific American* 278: 62-69. [13]

Pohl, M., J. Mehrholz, C. Ritschel, and S. Ruckriem. 2002. Speed-dependent treadmill training in ambulatory hemiparetic stroke patients: A randomized controlled trial. *Stroke* 33(2): 553-558. [9]

Porges, S.W. 1996. Physiological regulation in high risk infants: A model for assessment and potential intervention. *Development and Psychopathology* 8: 43-58. [11]

Potrac, P. 2004. Coaches' power. In: R. Jones, K. Armour, and P. Potrac (Eds.), *Sports coaching cultures: From practice to theory* (pp. 150-162). London: Routledge. [6]

Pozzo, T., A. Berthoz, and L. Lefort. 1990. Head stabilization during various locomotor tasks in humans. I. Normal subjects. *Experimental Brain Research* 82: 97-106. [2]

Prigogine, I., and I. Stengers. 1984. *Order out of chaos.* New York: Bantam Books. [11]

Priplata, A., J. Niemi, M. Salen, J. Harry, L. Lipsitz, and J. Collins. 2002. Noise-enhanced human balance control. *Physical Review Letters* 89 (23): 238101-238104. [2]

Pufall, P.B., and C. Dunbar. 1992. Perceiving whether or not the world affords stepping onto and over. *Ecological Psychology* 4: 17-38. [4]

Raglin, J.S., and Y.L. Hanin. 2000. Competitive anxiety. In: Y.L. Hanin (Ed.), *Emotions in sport* (pp. 93-112). Champaign, IL: Human Kinetics. [11]

Ravizza, K. 1993. Increasing awareness for sport performance. In: J.M. Williams (Ed.), *Applied sport psychology: Personal growth to peak performance* (pp. 148-157). Palo Alto, CA: Mayfield. [6]

Realon, R.E., J.E. Favell, and A. Lowerre. 1990. The effects of making choices on engagement levels with persons who are profoundly multiply handicapped. *Education and Training in Mental Retardation* 25(3): 299-305. [10]

Reed, E.S. 1982. An outline of a theory of action systems. *Journal of Motor Behavior* 14: 98-134. [Prologue, 9]

Reed, E.S. 1988. Applying the theory of action systems to the study of motor skills. In: O.G. Meijer and K. Roth (Eds.), *Complex movement behavior: The motor-action controversy* (pp. 45-86). Amsterdam: Elsevier. [9]

Reed, E.S. 1996. *Encountering the world: Toward an ecological psychology.* New York: Oxford University Press. [3]

Reed, E.S., and R.K. Jones. 1979. James Gibson's ecological revolution in psychology. *Philosophy of Social Science* 9: 189-204. [Epilogue]

Reichle, J., J. Sigafoos, and L. Piche. 1989. Teaching an adolescent with blindness and severe disabilities: A correspondence between requesting and selecting preferred objects. *Journal of the Association for Persons with Severe Handicaps* 14: 75-80. [3]

Reid, D.H., M.B. Parsons, and C.W. Green. 1991. *Providing choice and preferences for persons who have severe handicaps.* Morgantown, WV: Habilitative Management Consultants, Inc. [10]

Reid, G. 2003. Adapted physical activity—what is it? In: R. Steadward, G. Wheeler, and E.J. Watkinson (Eds.), *Adapted physical activity.* Edmonton, AB: University of Alberta Press. [9]

Reid, G., and H. Stanish. 2003. Professional and disciplinary status of adapted physical activity. *Adapted Physical Activity Quarterly* 20: 213-229. [9]

Reiter, S., R. Talmor, and Y. Hutzler. 2004. *Joint sports activities: Research report of a special project.* Jerusalem: National Insurance Institute. [9]

Riccio, G.E. 1993. Information in movement variability. About the qualitative dynamics of posture and orientation. In: K.M. Newell and D.M. Corcos (Eds.), *Variability and motor control* (pp. 317-357). Champaign, IL: Human Kinetics. [2]

Riccio, G.E., and T.A. Stoffregen. 1988. Affordances as constraints on the control of stance. *Human Movement Science* 7: 265-300. [2]

Rink, J. 1998. *Teaching physical education for learning* (3rd ed.). Boston: Brown-McGraw-Hill. [7]

Robb, M.D. 1972. Task analysis: A consideration for teachers of skills. *Research Quarterly* 43(3): 362-373. [10]

Roley, S.S., E.I. Blanche, and R.C. Schaaf. 2001. *Understanding the nature of sensory integration with diverse populations.* San Antonio, TX: Therapy Skill Builders. [11]

Rosenberg, R.M. 1977. *Analytical dynamics of discrete systems.* New York: Plenum Press. [1]

Rosenshine, B., and R. Stevens. 1986. Teaching functions. In: M.C. Wittrock (Ed.), *Handbook of research on teaching* (3rd ed., pp. 376-391). New York: Macmillan. [7]

Rosenstein, M.T., J.J. Collins, and C.J. De Luca. 1993. A practical method for calculating largest Lyapunov exponents from small data sets. *Physica* D 65: 117-134. [2]

Rumelhart, D.E. 1980. Schemata: The building blocks of cognition. In: R. Spiro, B. Bruce, and W. Brewer (Eds.), *Theoretical issues in reading comprehension* (pp. 38-58). Hillsdale, NJ: Erlbaum. [13]

Rush, D.D., M.L. Shelden, and B. Hanft. 2003. Coaching families and colleagues: A process for collaboration in natural settings. *Infants and Young Children* 16: 33-47. [11]

Ryan, R.M., J.P. Connell, and E.L. Deci. 1985. A motivational analysis of self-determination and self-regulation in education. In: C. Ames and R. Ames (Eds.), *Research on motivation in education,* Vol. 2: *The classroom milieu* (pp. 13-51). London: Academic Press. [3]

Ryan, R.M., J. Kuhl, and E.L. Deci. 1997. Nature and autonomy: An organizational view of social and neurobiological aspects of self regulation in behavior and development. *Development and Psychopathology* 9: 701-728. [11]

Saltzman, E.L. 1979. Levels of sensorimotor representation. *Journal of Mathematical Psychology* 20: 91-163. [1]

Saltzman, E.L., and J.A.S. Kelso. 1987. Skilled actions: A task dynamic approach. *Psychological Review* 94: 84-106. [1]

Sanders, S.W. 2002. *Active for life: Developmentally appropriate movement programs for young children.* Washington, DC: National Association for the Education of Young Children. [7]

Saunders, J.B., V.T. Inman, and H.D. Eberhart. 1953. The major determinants in normal and pathological gait. *Journal of Bone and Joint Surgery* 35A: 543-559. [2]

Savelsbergh, G.J.P., W.E. Davis, J. van der Kamp, and M. Singh Badham. 1994. Body scaling and prehension in children with Down syndrome. In: M. Latash, (Ed.), *Motor control in Down syndrome II. Proceedings of the Second International Conference* (pp. 78-83). Chicago: Rush-Presbyterian St. Luke's Medical Center. [4]

Schacter, D.L. 1995. *Searching for memory: The brain, the mind and the past.* New York: Basic Books. [13]

Schafer, R. 1968. *Aspects of internalization.* New York: International Universities Press. [3]

Schempp, P. 1982. Enhancing creativity through children making decisions. In: M. Pieron and J. Cheffers (Eds.), *Studying the teaching in physical education* (pp. 161-166). Leige, Belgium: International Association for Higher Education. [6]

Schempp, P.G., J.T.F. Cheffers, and L.D. Zaichkowsky. 1983. Influence of decision-making on attitudes, creativity, motor skills and self-concept in elementary children. *Research Quarterly for Exercise and Sport* 54: 183-189. [7]

Schindl, M., C. Forstner, H. Kern, and S. Hesse. 2000. Treadmill training with partial body weight support in nonambulatory patients with cerebral palsy. *Archives of Physical Medicine and Rehabilitation* 81: 1-6. [9]

Schloss, P.J., S. Alper, and D. Jayne. 1993. Self-determination for persons with disabilities: Choice, risk, and dignity. *Exceptional Children* 60(3): 215-225. [10]

Schmidt, R.A. 1975. A schema theory of discrete motor skill learning. *Psychological Review* 82: 225-260. [1, 11]

Schmidt, R.A. 1988. *Motor control and learning: A behavioral emphasis* (2nd ed.). Champaign, IL: Human Kinetics. [11]

Schmidt, R.A., and T.D. Lee. 1999. *Motor control and learning* (3rd ed.). Champaign, IL: Human Kinetics. [1, 9]

Scholz, J.P. 1990. Dynamic pattern theory: Some implications for therapeutics. *Physical Therapy* 70: 827-843. [11]

Scholz, J.P., J.A.S. Kelso, and G. Schöner. 1987. Nonequilibrium phase transitions in coordinated biological motion: Critical slowing down and switching time. *Physics Letters* A123: 390-394. [2]

Scholz, J.P., and G. Schöner. 1999. The uncontrolled manifold concept: Identifying control variables for a functional task. *Experimental Brain Research* 126: 289-306. [2]

Schöner, G. 1989. Learning and recall in a dynamic theory of coordination patterns. *Biological Cybernetics* 62: 39-54. [1]

Schöner, G. 1990. A dynamic theory of coordination of discrete movement. *Biological Cybernetics* 63: 257-270. [1]

Schöner, G., W.Y. Jiang, and J.A.S. Kelso. 1990. A synergetic theory of quadrupedal gaits and gait transitions. *Journal of Theoretical Biology* 142: 359-391. [2]

Schöner, G.S., and J.A.S. Kelso. 1988a. Dynamic pattern generation in behavioral and neural systems. *Science* 239: 1513-1520. [2, 11]

Schöner, G.S., and J.A.S. Kelso. 1988b. Dynamic patterns in biological coordination. Theoretical strategy and new results. In: J.A.S. Kelso, A.J. Mandell, and M.F. Schlesinger (Eds.), *Dynamic patterns in complex systems* (pp. 77-102). Singapore: World Scientific. [11]

Schöner, G.S., and J.A.S. Kelso. 1988c. A dynamic theory of behavioral change. *Journal of Theoretical Biology* 135: 501-522. [11]

Schöner, G.S., P.G. Zanone, and J.A.S. Kelso. 1992. Learning coordination patterns as dynamics of dynamics. *Journal of Motor Behavior* 24: 29-48. [11]

Schore, A.N. 1996. The experience dependent maturation of a regulatory system in the orbital prefrontal cortex. *Developmental Psychopathology* 8: 59-97. [11]

Schore, A.N. 1997. Early organization of the nonlinear right brain and development of a predisposition to psychiatric disorders. *Development and Psychopathology* 9: 595-631. [11]

Schrecker, E. 1986. *No ivory tower: McCarthyism and the universities.* New York: Oxford University Press. [3]

Schwartz, B. 1990. The creation and destruction of value. *American Psychologist* 45: 7-15. [3]

Seligman, M. 1975. *Helplessness: On depression, development, and death.* San Francisco: Freeman. [3]

Selman, R.L. 1980. *The growth of interpersonal understanding.* New York: Academic Press. [11]

Semmel, B. 1993. *The liberal ideal and the demons of empire: Theories of imperialism from Adam Smith to Lenin.* Baltimore: Johns Hopkins University Press. [3]

Shea, C.H., D.L. Wright, G. Wulf, and C. Whitacre. 2000. Physical and observational practice afford unique learning opportunities. *Journal of Motor Behavior* 32: 27-36. [11]

Shea, C.H., and G. Wulf. 1999. Enhancing motor learning through external focus instructions and feedback. *Human Movement Science* 18: 553-571. [11]

Shea, C.H., G. Wulf, and C.A. Whitacre. 1999. Enhancing training efficiency and effectiveness through the use of dyad training. *Journal of Motor Behavior* 31: 119-125. [11]

Shebilske, W.L., J.W. Regian, W. Arthur, and J.A. Jordan. 1992. A dyadic protocol for training complex skills. *Journal of Human Factors Society* 34: 369-374. [11]

Sherrill, C. 1995. Adaptation theory: The essence of our profession and discipline. In: I. Morisbak and P.E. Jorgensen (Eds.), *Quality of life through adapted physical activity and sport: A lifespan concept* (pp. 32-34). Proceedings 10th ISAPA, Oslo and Beitostolen, Norway, May 22-26. [9]

Sherrill, C. 2004. *Adapted physical activity, recreation, and sport* (6th ed.). New York: McGraw-Hill. [9]

Shevin, M.M., and N.K. Klein. 1984. The importance of choice-making skills for students with severe disabilities. *Journal of the Association for Persons with Severe Handicaps* 9: 159-166. [3, 10]

Shirley, M.M. 1931. *The first two years: A study of twenty-five babies.* Vol. I. *Locomotor Development.* Minneapolis: University of Minnesota Press. [11]

Shogan, D. 1991. Trusting paternalism? Trust as a condition for paternalistic decisions. *Journal of the Philosophy of Sport* 18: 49-58. [6]

Shogan, D. 1999. *The making of high-performance athletes: Discipline, diversity and ethics.* Toronto: University of Toronto Press. [6]

Shumway-Cook, A., and M. Woollacott. 2001. *Motor control: Theory and practical applications* (2nd ed.). Baltimore: Lippincott Williams & Wilkins. [1, 9, 11]

Siedentop, D. 1994. *Quality PE through positive sport experiences: Sport education.* Champaign, IL: Human Kinetics. [7]

Siedentop, D., and D. Tannehill. 2000. *Developing teaching skills in physical education* (4th ed.). Mountain View, CA: Mayfield. [7]

Silverman, S. 1991. Research on teaching in physical education: Review and commentary. *Research Quarterly for Exercise and Sport* 62: 352-364. [7]

Simpson, C. 1994. *Science of coercion: Communication research and psychological warfare 1945-1960.* New York: Oxford University Press. [3]

Sipma, M. 1996. Orthopedagogische thuisbegeleiding met het Portage Programma Nederland [Special educational home support with the Portage Program Netherlands]. PhD dissertation, Groningen, Stichting Kinderstudies. [12]

Skinner, B.F. 1983. *A matter of consequences.* New York: Knopf. [3]

Skrtic, T.M. 1986. The crisis in special education knowledge: A perspective on perspective. *Focus on Exceptional Children* 18(7): 1-16. [10]

Slobounov, S.M., S.A. Moss, E.S. Slobounova, and K.M. Newell. 1998. Aging and time to instability in posture. *Journal of Gerontology* 53: B71-B78. [2]

Sloman, L., M. Berridge, S. Homatidis, D. Hunter, and T. Duck. 1982. Gait patterns of depressed patients and normal subjects. *American Journal of Psychiatry* 139(1): 94-97. [9]

Smith, J.W. 2002. *Economic democracy: The political struggle of the twenty-first century* (2nd ed.). Armonk, NY: Sharpe. [3]

Smith, L.B., and E. Thelen. 1993. *A dynamic systems approach to development: Applications.* Cambridge, MA: MIT Press. [1]

Smith, M.F.R. 1978. Attribution, achievement motivation, and task difficulty in physical education. Paper presented at the British Columbia conference on the teaching of physical education, Victoria, BC. [13]

Smith, M.D., and C.J. Chamberlin. 1992. Effect of adding cognitively demanding tasks on soccer skill performance. *Perceptual and Motor Skills* 75: 955-961. [13]

Smith, T., A. Groen, and J.W. Wynn. 2000. Randomized trial of intensive early intervention for children with pervasive developmental disorder. *American Journal on Mental Retardation* 104: 269-285. [11]

Southard, D. 1998. Mass and velocity: Control parameters for throwing. *Research Quarterly for Exercise and Sport* 69: 355-367. [5]

Southard, D. 2002. Change in throwing pattern: Critical values for control parameter of velocity. *Research Quarterly for Exercise and Sport* 73: 396-407. [5]

Sparkes, A.C. 2002. *Telling tales in sport and physical activity: A qualitative journey.* Champaign, IL: Human Kinetics. [6]

Sparrow, W.A., E. Donovan, R.E.A. Van Emmerik, and B. Barry. 1987. Using relative motion plots to measure changes in intra-limb and inter-limb coordination. *Journal of Motor Behavior* 19: 115-129. [1]

Sparrow, W.A., and K.M. Newell. 1998. Metabolic energy expenditure and the regulation of movement economy. *Psychonomic Bulletin and Review* 5: 173-196. [2]

Stancliff, R., and M.L. Wehmeyer. 1995. Variability in the availability of choice to adults with mental retardation. *Journal of Vocational Rehabilitation* 5: 319-328. [10]

Stannard, D.E. 1992. *American holocaust: The conquest of the New World.* New York: Oxford University Press. [3]

Sternberg, R.J., G.B. Forsythe, J. Hedlund, J.A. Horvath, R.K. Wagner, W.M. Williams, S.A. Snook, and E.L. Grigrenko. 2000. *Practical intelligence in everyday life.* Cambridge: Cambridge University Press. [13]

Stockmeyer, S. 1967. An interpretation of the approach of Rood to the treatment of neuromuscular dysfunction. *American Journal Physical Medicine* 46: 950-955. [11]

Strogatz, S.H. 1994. *Nonlinear dynamics and chaos: With applications to physics, biology, chemistry, and engineering.* Reading, MA: Addison-Wesley. [2]

Sweeting, T., and J. Rink. 1999. Effects of direct instruction and environmentally designed instruction on the process and product characteristics of a fundamental skill. *Journal of Teaching in Physical Education* 18(2): 216-233. [7]

Szymanski, E.M., and H.T. Trueba. 1994. Castification of people with disabilities: Potential disempowering aspects of classification in disability services. *Journal of Rehabilitation* 60(3): 12-20. [10]

Tam, H. 1996. Introduction. In: H. Tam (Ed.), *Punishment, excuses and moral development* (pp. 1-15). Aldershot, England: Avebury. [3]

Taub, E., and W. Steven. 1997. Constraint induced movement techniques to facilitate upper extremity use in stroke patients. *Topics in Stroke Rehabilitation* 3: 38-61. [9]

Taylor, J. 2001. *Remedial instruction for children with developmental coordination disorder: A manual* (pp. 1-145). Thunder Bay, ON: Lakehead University. [10]

Taylor, J. 2002. Implementing ecological task analysis: Experiences of adolescents with developmental disabilities in a swimming environment. Poster presented at the North American Federation of Adapted Physical Activity Conference, Corvallis, OR. [10]

Thayer, F.C. 1994. God, science, and administrative theory: An unfinished revolution. In: A. Farazmand (Ed.), *Modern organizations* (pp. 229-243). Westport, CT: Praeger. [3]

Thelen, E. 1986. Development of coordinated movement: Implications for early human development. In: M.G. Wade and H.T.A. Whiting (Eds.), *Motor development in children: Aspects of coordination and control* (pp. 107-124). Dordrecht: Martinus Nijhoff. [1]

Thelen, E. 2000. Motor development as foundation and future of developmental psychology. *International Journal of Behavioral Development* 24: 385-397. [11]

Thelen, E., and K. Adolph. 1992. Arnold L. Gesell: The paradox of nature and nurture. *Developmental Psychology* 28: 368-380. [11]

Thelen, E., and L.B. Smith. 1994. *A dynamic systems approach to the development of cognition and action.* Cambridge, MA: MIT Press. [1, 5, 9, 11, 12]

Thelen, E., and L.B. Smith. 1998. Dynamic systems theories. In: W. Damon (Series Ed.) and R.M. Lerner (Eds.), *Handbook of child psychology:* Vol. 1. *Theoretical models of human development* (5th ed., pp. 563-633). New York: Wiley. [11]

Thelen, E., and B.C. Ulrich. 1991. Hidden skills: A dynamic systems analysis of treadmill stepping during the first year. *Monographs of the Society for Research in Child Development* 56: 1-104. [9, 11]

Thompson, J.M.T., and H.B. Stewart. 1986. *Nonlinear dynamics and chaos.* Chichester: Wiley. [1]

Thorpe, R.D. 1990. New directions in games teaching. In: N. Armstrong (Ed.), *New directions in physical education* (pp. 79-100). Champaign, IL: Human Kinetics. [6]

Thorpe, R.D. 2001. Rod Thorpe on teaching games for understanding. In: L. Kidman (Ed.), *Developing decision makers: An empowerment approach to coaching* (pp. 22-36). Christchurch, NZ: Innovative Print Communications. [6]

Titzer, R., J.B. Shea, and J. Romack. 1993. The effect of learner control on the acquisition and retention of a motor task. *Journal of Sport and Exercise Psychology* 15: S84. [11]

Tolman, E.C. 1932. *Purposive behavior in animals and men.* New York: Appleton-Century-Crofts. [1]

Tononi, G., O. Sporns, and G.M. Edelman. 1999. Measures of degeneracy and redundancy in biological networks. *Proceedings of the National Academy of Sciences, USA* 96: 3257-3262. [1]

Townsend, J.S., D.J. Mohr, R.M. Rairigh, and S.M. Bulger. 2003. *NASPE Assessment Series: Assessing student outcomes in sport education: A pedagogical approach.* Reston, VA: AAHPERD. [7]

Treanor, L.J. 1996. Help for the cooperating teacher: How to use high inference techniques. *Strategies* 9(4): 5-8. [7]

Tripp, A., R. French, and C. Sherrill. 1995. Contact theory and attitudes of children in physical education programs toward peers with disabilities. *Adapted Physical Activity Quarterly* 12: 323-332. [10]

Tulving, E. 1972. Episodic and semantic memory. In: E. Tulving and W. Donaldson (Eds.), *Organization and memory.* New York: Academic Press. [13]

Turner, A., and T. Martinek. 1992. A comparative analysis of two models for teaching games (technique approach and game-centered (tactical focus) approach). *International Journal of Physical Education* 29(4): 15-31. [8]

Turvey, M.T. 1990. Coordination. *American Psychologist* 45: 938-953. [1]

Turvey, M.T. 1992. Affordances and prospective control: An outline of the ontology. *Ecological Psychology* 4: 173-187. [3, Epilogue]

Turvey, M.T., and C. Carello. 1996. Dynamics of Bernstein's level of synergies. In: M.L. Latash and M.T. Turvey (Eds.), *Dexterity and its development* (pp. 339-376). Mahwah, NJ: Erlbaum. [2]

Turvey, M.T., K. Holt, M. LaFiandra, and S. Fonseca. 1999. Can the transitions to and from running and the metabolic cost of running be determined from the kinetic energy of running? *Journal of Motor Behavior* 31: 265-278. [4]

Turvey, M.T., R.E. Shaw, and W. Mace. 1978. Issues in the theory of action: Degrees of freedom, coordinative structures and coalitions. In: J. Requin (Ed.), *Attention and performance VII* (pp. 557-598). Hillsdale, NJ: Erlbaum. [1]

Ulrich, B.D., E. Thelen, and D. Niles. 1990. Perceptual determinants of action: Stair climbing choices of infants and toddlers. *Advances in Motor Development Research* 3: 1-15. [4]

Ulrich, B.D., D.A. Ulrich, and D.H. Collier. 1992. Alternating stepping patterns: Hidden abilities of 11-month-old infants with Down syndrome. *Developmental Medicine and Child Neurology* 34: 233-239. [9]

Ulrich, D.A. 1988. Children with special needs: Assessing the quality of movement competence. *Journal of Physical Education, Recreation and Dance* 59(11): 43-47. [7]

Ulrich, D.A. 2000. *Test of gross motor development* (2nd ed.). Austin, TX: Pro-Ed. [9]

Ulrich, D.A., B.D. Ulrich, R.M. Angulo-Kinzler, and J. Yun. 2001. Treadmill training of infants with Down syndrome: Evidence based developmental outcomes. *Paediatrics* 108(5): 1-7. [9, 11]

United States Department of Education, National Center for Education Statistics. 2002. *Digest of Education Statistics 2002,* table 52. [4]

Usher, P. 1997. Empowerment as a powerful coaching tool. *Coaches' Report* 4(2): 10-11. [6]

Vaillancourt, D.E., and K.M. Newell. 2002. Changing complexity in behavior and physiology through aging and disease. *Neurobiology of Aging: Experimental and Clinical Research* 23: 1-11. [1, 2]

Vaillancourt, D.E., and K.M. Newell. 2003. Aging and the time and frequency structure of force output variability. *Journal of Applied Physiology* 94: 903-912. [1]

Van Emmerik, R.E.A., and E.E.H. Van Wegen. 2002. On the functional aspects of variability in postural control. *Exercise and Sport Sciences Reviews* 30: 177-183. [2]

Van Emmerik, R.E.A., and R.C. Wagenaar. 1996a. Dynamics of movement coordination and tremor during gait in Parkinson's disease. *Human Movement Science* 15: 203-235. [12]

Van Emmerik, R.E.A., and R.C. Wagenaar. 1996b. Effects of walking velocity on relative phase dynamics in the trunk in human walking. *Journal of Biomechanics* 29: 1175-1184. [2]

Van Emmerik, R.E.A., R.C. Wagenaar, and E.E.H. Van Wegen. 1998. Interlimb coupling patterns in human locomotion: Are we bipeds or quadrupeds? *Annals of the New York Academy of Sciences* 860: 539-542. [2]

Van Emmerik, R.E.A., R.C. Wagenaar, A. Winogrodzka, and E.Ch. Wolters. 1999. Axial rigidity in Parkinson's disease. *Archives of Physical Medicine and Rehabilitation* 80: 186-191. [2]

Van Gennep, A.Th.G. 1997. *Paradigma verschuiving in de visie op de zorg voor mensen met een verstandelijke handicap* [Paradigm shift in views on the care for persons with intellectual disabilities]. Maastricht: Universiteit Maastricht. [12]

Van Gennep, A.Th.G., A.I. Procee, B.F. Van der Meulen, C.G.G. Janssen, A. Vermeer, and E.A.B. De Graaf. 1997. Effects of early intervention for children with developmental disabilities. *International Journal of Practical Approaches to Disability* 21: 3-7. [12]

Van Manen, M. 1993. The tact of teaching: The meaning of pedagogical thoughtfulness. Ann Arbor, MI: Althouse Press. [10]

Van Wegen, E.E.H., R.E.A. Van Emmerik, and G.E. Riccio. 2002. Postural orientation: Age-related changes in variability and time-to-boundary. *Human Movement Science* 21: 61-84. [2]

Van Wegen, E.E.H., R.E.A. Van Emmerik, R.C. Wagenaar, and T. Ellis. 2001. Stability boundaries and lateral postural control in Parkinson's disease. *Motor Control* 3: 254-269. [2]

Van Wieringen, P.C.W., H.H. Emmen, R.J. Bootsma, M. Hoogesteger, and H.T.A. Whiting. 1989. The effect of video-feedback on the learning of the tennis service by intermediate players. *Journal of Sports Sciences* 7(2): 153-162. [9]

Vars, G.F., and J.A. Beane. 2000. *Integrative curriculum in a standards-based world* (Report No. EDO-PS-00-6). Champaign, IL: ERIC Clearinghouse on Elementary and Early Childhood Education. [7]

Vaughan, C.E. 1993. *The struggle of blind people for self-determination: The dependency-rehabilitation conflict: Empowerment in the blindness community.* Springfield, IL: Charles C Thomas. [3]

Vealey, R.S. 1986. Conceptualization of sport-confidence and competitive orientation: Preliminary investigation and instrument development. *Journal of Sport Psychology* 8: 221-246. [13]

Vealey, R.S., S.W. Hayashi, M. Garner-Holman, and P. Giacobbi. 1998. Sources of sport-confidence: Conceptualization and instrument development. *Journal of Sport and Exercise Psychology* 20: 54-80. [13]

Vereijken, B., R.E.A. Van Emmerik, H.T.A. Whiting, and K.M. Newell. 1992. Free(zing) degrees of freedom in skill acquisition. *Journal of Motor Behavior* 24: 133-142. [2, 3]

Vermeer, A. 2005. Mentale retardatie: Begeleiding van mensen met een verstandelijke beperking [Support of individuals with intellectual disabilities]. In: M.H. van Ijzendoorn and H. de Frankrijker (Eds.), *Pedagogiek in beeld* [The picture of educational sciences] (pp. 267-279). Houten: Bohn Stafleu Van Loghum. [12]

Von Holst, E. 1939/1973. *The behavioral physiology of animals and man.* Coral Gables, FL: University of Miami Press. [2]

Voss, D., M. Ionata, and B. Meyers. 1985. *Proprioceptive neuromuscular facilitation: Patterns and techniques* (3rd ed.). Philadelphia: Harper & Row. [11]

Waddington, C.H. 1957. *The strategy of the genes.* London: Unwin & Unwin. [1]

Wagenaar, R.C., and O.G. Meijer. 1998. Bernstein's revolution in movement medicine: Coordination disorders of and the recovery of walking biodynamics after cerebrovascular injuries. *Motor Control* 2: 181-188. [12]

Wagenaar, R.C., and R.E.A. Van Emmerik. 1994. The dynamics of pathological gait: Stability and adaptability of movement coordination. *Human Movement Science* 13: 441-471. [11]

Wagenaar, R.C., and R.E.A. Van Emmerik. 1996. Dynamics of movement disorders. *Human Movement Science* 15: 161-175. [11]

Wagenaar, R.C., and R.E.A. Van Emmerik. 2000. Resonance frequencies of arms and legs identify different walking patterns. *Journal of Biomechanics* 13: 853-861. [2]

Walker, N. 1991. *Why punish?* Oxford: Oxford University Press. [3]

Wall, A.E. 1986. A knowledge-based approach to motor skill acquisition. In: M.G. Wade and H.T.A. Whiting (Eds.), *Motor development in children: Aspects of coordination and control* (pp. 33-49). Dordrecht: Martinus Nijhoff. [13]

Wall, A.E., J. McClements, M. Bouffard, H. Findlay, and J. Taylor. 1985. A knowledge-based approach to motor development: Implications for the physically awkward. *Adapted Physical Activity Quarterly* 2: 21-42. [13]

Warren, B. 1993. *The right to choose: A curriculum.* New York: State Office of Mental Retardation and Developmental Disabilities. [10]

Warren, W.H. 1984. Perceiving affordances: Visual guidance of stair climbing. *Journal of Experimental Psychology: Human Perception and Performance* 10: 683-703. [4]

Warren, W.H. 1988. Action modes and laws of control for the visual guidance of action. In: O. Meijer and K. Roth (Eds.), *Movement behavior: The motor-action controversy* (pp. 393-379). Amsterdam: North-Holland. [3]

Watkinson, E.J., and A.E. Wall. 1982. *The Prep Play Program: Play skill instruction for mentally handicapped children.* Ottawa: Canadian Association for Health, Physical Education, and Recreation. [10]

Watson, D. 1997. *Against the megamachine: Essays on empire & its enemies.* Brooklyn, NY: Autonomeda. [3]

Watson, J.B. 1930. *Behaviorism.* Chicago: University of Chicago Press. [3]

Wehmeyer, M.L. 1998. Self-determination and individuals with significant disabilities: Examining meanings and misinterpretations. *Journal of the Association for Persons with Severe Handicaps* 23: 5-16. [3]

Wehmeyer, M.L., D.J. Sands, B. Doll, and S. Palmer. 1997. The development of self-determination and implications for educational interventions with students with disabilities. *International Journal of Disability, Development, and Education* 44(4): 305-328. [10]

White, R.W. 1959. Motivation reconsidered: The concept of competence. *Psychological Review* 66: 297-333. [3, 12]

Whiting, W.C., and R.F. Zernicke. 1982. Correlation of movement patterns via pattern recognition. *Journal of Motor Behavior* 14: 135-142. [1]

Whittlesey, S. 2003. An ecological assessment of postural and manual control. Unpublished doctoral dissertation, University of Massachusetts, Amherst. [2]

Williams, M., and K. Davids. 1995. Declarative knowledge in sport: A by-product of experience or a characteristic of expertise? *Journal of Sport and Exercise Psychology* 17: 259-275. [13]

Williams, M.S., and S. Shellenberger. 1996. *"How does your engine run?"* Albuquerque, NM: Therapy Works. [11]

Williams, W.A. 1980. *Empire as a way of life: An essay on the causes and character of America's present predicament, along with a few thoughts about an alternative.* New York: Oxford University Press. [3]

Winfree, A.T. 1980. *The geometry of biological time.* Heidelberg: Springer. [2]

Winfree, A.T. 1987. *The timing of biological clocks.* New York: Scientific American Library. [2]

Winter, D.A. 1995. *A.B.C. (anatomy, biomechanics and control) of balance during standing and walking.* Waterloo, ON: Graphic Services. [2]

Wolk, S., and S. Telleen. 1976. Psychological and social correlates of life satisfaction as a function of residential constraint. *Journal of Gerontology* 31: 89-98. [3]

Wood, E.M. 1995. *Democracy against capitalism.* Cambridge: Cambridge University Press. [3]

Woodard, R.J., and P.R. Surburg. 1999. Midline crossing behavior in children with learning disabilities. *Adapted Physical Activity Quarterly* 16: 155-166. [4]

Woollacott, M., and A. Shumway-Cook. 1990. Changes in postural control across the lifespan, a systems approach. *Physical Therapy* 70: 799-807. [11]

World Health Organization. 2001. *International classification of functioning, disability and health (ICF).* Geneva: Author. [9]

Wraga, M. 1999. The role of eye height in perceiving affordances and object dimensions. *Perceptual Psychophysics* 61: 490-507. [4]

Wulf, G., M. Hoss, and W. Prinz. 1998. Instructions for motor learning: Differential effects of internal vs external focus of attention. *Journal of Motor Behavior* 30: 169-179. [11]

Wulf, G., B. Lauterbach, and T. Toole. 1999. The learning advantages of an external focus of attention in golf. *Research Quarterly for Exercise and Sport* 70: 120-126. [11]

Wulf, G., and T. Toole. 1999. Physical assistance devices in complex motor skill learning: Benefits of a self-controlled practice schedule. *Research Quarterly for Exercise and Sport* 70: 265-272. [11]

Xiaopeng, Z. 1998. An experimental investigation into the influence of the speed and spin by balls of different diameters and weights. In: A. Lees, I. Maynard, M. Hughes, and T. Reilly (Eds.), *Science and racket sports II* (pp. 206-208). London: Spon. [9]

Young, I.M. 1992. Five faces of oppression. In: T.E. Wartenberg (Ed.), *Rethinking power* (pp. 174-195). Albany, NY: State University of New York Press. [3]

Yukelson, D. 1997. Principles of effective team building. *Journal of Applied Sport Psychology* 9(1): 73-96. [6]

Zajonc, R.B. 1980. Feeling and thinking: Preferences need no inferences. *American Psychologist* 35: 151-175. [3]

Zanone, P.G., and J.A.S. Kelso. 1992. Evolution of behavioral attractors with learning: Nonequilibrium phase transitions. *Journal of Experimental Psychology: Human Perception and Performance* 18: 403-421. [11]

Zetlin, A.G., and R. Gillmore. 1983. The development of comprehension strategies through the regulatory function of teacher questions. *Education and Training in Mental Retardation* 18(3): 176-184. [10]

Zijlstra, I. 1997. Evaluatie van het programma "Peuterrevalidatie vanuit opvoedingsperspectief" [Evaluation of the program "Child rehabilitation from an educational perspective"]. PhD dissertation, Groningen, Stichting Kinderstudies. [12]

INDEX

Note: The italicized *f* and *t* following page numbers refer to figures and tables, respectively.

ABOUT THE EDITORS

Walter E. Davis, PhD, is an associate professor in the School of Exercise, Leisure, and Sport at Kent State University in Kent, Ohio. Dr. Davis worked with Allen Burton in originating the Ecological Task Analysis theoretical and applied models, and he implemented the applied model in his teaching lab. He has extended the theoretical model from its focus on biological systems to a focus on social systems, and he has continued to expand on the empowerment aspect of the model in both teaching and writing.

Dr. Davis has edited two books and written nine chapters for edited books. He has published more than 30 journal articles and given nearly 70 national and international presentations. He is currently involved in a grant on democracy and education and further developing an empowerment model for education and society.

Dr. Davis has been active in the International Federation of Adapted Physical Activity, the International Society for Ecological Psychology, the International Society for the Systems Sciences, and the North American Federation of Adapted Physical Activity (NAFAPA). He has received numerous awards and honors, including a Research Achievement Award from the National Consortium of Physical Education Recreation and Dance (now known as the National Consortium for Physical Education and Recreation for Individuals with Disabilities). He also gave a scholar lecture for the Research Consortium at AAHPERD and gave the keynote address at a NAFAPA convention.

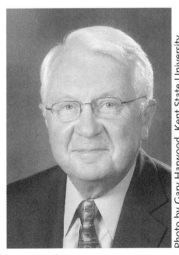

Photo by Gary Harwood, Kent State University

Geoffrey D. Broadhead, PhD, is a professor in the School of Exercise, Leisure, and Sport at Kent State University. Dr. Broadhead has worked in secondary schools in England, a teacher education college in Scotland (now the Institute of Education of Edinburgh University), and in two major universities in the United States. He also has extensive leadership experience, having coordinated university special education and physical education programs and having been a university academic dean.

Dr. Broadhead was a physical education teacher of at-risk children in two schools in England. His research activities over many years have centered on the movement characteristics of individuals with disabilities, the interrelationships of movement and behavioral skills in young children, the efficacy of school physical education programs, and the special education advocacy area of what is now called inclusion. Funds from state, federal, and private sources have supported much of his academic and professional interests.

Dr. Broadhead has coauthored one book and coedited another. He has published more than 80 papers in journals in the United States and Europe and has made almost 90 presentations at national and international conferences. He founded the journal *Adapted Physical Activity Quarterly,* served as its editor for eight years, and is now editor emeritus. He has awards from the English Speaking Union, the Fulbright Commission, the Joseph P. Kennedy Jr. Foundation, and the National Consortium for Physical Education and Recreation for Individuals with Disabilities.